Accelerating Diagnostics in a Time of Crisis

Accelerating Diagnostics in a Time of Crisis

The Response to the COVID-19 Pandemic and a Roadmap for Future Pandemics

Edited by

Steven C. Schachter
Rapid Acceleration of Diagnostics (RADx®) Chief, CIMIT

Wade E. Bolton
RADx–VentureWell

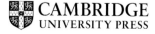
CAMBRIDGE
UNIVERSITY PRESS

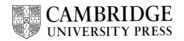

Shaftesbury Road, Cambridge CB2 8EA, United Kingdom

One Liberty Plaza, 20th Floor, New York, NY 10006, USA

477 Williamstown Road, Port Melbourne, VIC 3207, Australia

314–321, 3rd Floor, Plot 3, Splendor Forum, Jasola District Centre,
New Delhi – 110025, India

103 Penang Road, #05–06/07, Visioncrest Commercial, Singapore 238467

Cambridge University Press is part of Cambridge University Press & Assessment,
a department of the University of Cambridge.

We share the University's mission to contribute to society through the pursuit of
education, learning and research at the highest international levels of excellence.

www.cambridge.org
Information on this title: www.cambridge.org/9781009396981

DOI: 10.1017/9781009396998

First published 2024

A catalogue record for this publication is available from the British Library.

Library of Congress Cataloging-in-Publication Data
Names: Schachter, Steven C., editor. | Bolton, Wade E., 1947– editor.
Title: Accelerating diagnostics in a time of crisis : the response to COVID-19 and a roadmap for future pandemics /
edited by Steven C. Schachter, Wade E. Bolton.
Description: Cambridge, United Kingdom ; New York, NY : Cambridge University Press, 2023. | Includes
bibliographical references and index.
Identifiers: LCCN 2023023826 (print) | LCCN 2023023827 (ebook) | ISBN 9781009396981 (paperback) | ISBN
9781009396998 (ebook)
Subjects: MESH: COVID-19 – diagnosis | Pandemics | Emergencies | Rapid Diagnostic Tests | Process Assessment,
Health Care | United States
Classification: LCC RA644.C67 (print) | LCC RA644.C67 (ebook) | NLM WC 506.1 | DDC 616.2/4144–dc23/eng/
20230828
LC record available at https://lccn.loc.gov/2023023826
LC ebook record available at https://lccn.loc.gov/2023023827

ISBN 978-1-009-39698-1 Paperback

....

Dedicated to Lindley Hall for his mentorship, John Parrish for his pioneering work to accelerate health-care solutions and to Wallace and Joe Coulter and their spirit of Science Serving Humanity.

This work was supported by the National Institute of Biomedical Imaging and Bioengineering under Grant 5U54EB015408-06. The views expressed in this manuscript are those of the authors and do not necessarily represent the views of the National Institute of Biomedical Imaging and Bioengineering; the National Heart, Lung, and Blood Institute; the National Institutes of Health; or the US Department of Health and Human Services.

The editors and chapter authors are thankful for the visionary leadership of Francis Collins, Bruce Tromberg, Jill Heemskerk, Tiffani Lash, and Todd Merchak in guiding the development and implementation of the Rapid Acceleration of Diagnostics (RADx®) Tech program and facilitating the close collaboration of crucially essential government agencies and nongovernmental organizations in this effort.

Contents

Contributors

Mara Aspinall
Health Catalysts, Tucson, AZ, USA

Barbara Barnett
Mount Sinai Health System, New York, NY, USA

Leda Bassit
Emory University, Atlanta, GA, USA

Grace Bendinger
Rapid Acceleration of Diagnostics (RADx®)–VentureWell, Hadley, MA, USA Frindle Health, Newnan, GA, USA

Wade E. Bolton
RADx–VentureWell, Hadley, MA, USA Bolton Consulting & Services, Delray Beach, FL, USA

Saralynne Brown
Mount Sinai Health System, New York, NY, USA

Yvette Calderon
Mount Sinai Health System, New York, NY, USA

Cathryn Cambria
Cambria Regulatory Consulting, Atlanta, GA, USA

Devon C. Campbell
Prodct, Boston, MA, USA

Mia Cirrincione
RADx–VentureWell, Hadley, MA, USA

William Clarke
Johns Hopkins University School of Medicine, Baltimore, MD, USA

Marta C. Cohen
Sheffield Children's Hospital, Sheffield, UK

John M. Collins
CIMIT, Boston, MA, USA

Michael K. Dempsey
CIMIT, Boston, MA, USA Massachusetts Institute of Technology, Cambridge, MA, USA

Sam Dolphin
RADx–VentureWell, Hadley, MA, USA

Maren Downing
RADx–VentureWell, Hadley, MA, USA

Erick Eiting
Mount Sinai Health System, New York, NY, USA

Tania Fernandez
DreamCatcher Ventures, San Francisco, CA, USA
RADx-VentureWell, Hadley, MA, USA

Harvey V. Fineburg
Gordon & Betty Moore Foundation, Palo Alto, CA, USA

Adolfo Firpo-Betancourt
Mount Sinai Health System, New York, NY, USA

Jennifer K. Frediani
Emory University, Atlanta, GA, USA

Laura L. Gibson
University of Massachusetts Medical School, Worcester, MA, USA

Morgan Greenleaf
Emory University, Atlanta, GA, USA

Anette E. Hosoi
Massachusetts Institute of Technology,
Boston, MA, USA

Waleed Javaid
Mount Sinai Health System, New York,
NY, USA

Christie Johnson
Prodct, Boston, MA, USA

Emily Kennedy
RADx–VentureWell, Hadley, MA, USA

Manuel Kingsley
Questus Healthcare, Atlanta, GA, USA
RADx–VentureWell, Hadley, MA, USA

Bethany Kranitzky
The Ohio State University Wexner
Medical Center, Columbus,
OH, USA

Wilbur Lam
Emory University, Atlanta, GA, USA

Young Im Lee
Mount Sinai Health System, New York,
NY, USA

Kevin Leite
RADx–VentureWell, Hadley, MA, USA

Jessica Lin
Georgia Institute of Technology, Atlanta,
GA, USA

Yang Lu
Icahn School of Medicine at Mount Sinai,
New York, NY, USA

Yukari C. Manabe
Johns Hopkins University School
of Medicine, Baltimore,
MD, USA

Lina Miyakawa
Mount Sinai Health System, New York,
NY, USA

Sunshine Moore
Sunshine Moore Consulting, Madison, WI,
USA
RADx–VentureWell, Hadley, MA, USA

Emily Muth
RADx–VentureWell, Hadley, MA, USA

Heath Naquin
University City Science Center,
Philadelphia, PA, USA
RADx–VentureWell, Hadley, MA, USA

Anne Piantadosi
Emory University, Atlanta, GA, USA

Enrique M. Rabellino
MedScience Services, Miami, FL, USA

Anuradha Rao
Emory University, Atlanta, GA, USA

Matthew L. Robinson
Johns Hopkins University School of
Medicine, Baltimore, MD, USA

Liz Ruark
covidsafeschools.org, Boston, MA, USA

Adam Samuta
RADx–VentureWell, Hadley, MA, USA

Steven C. Schachter
Harvard Medical School, Boston, MA, USA
CIMIT, Boston, MA, USA

Alexandra Smith
RADx–VentureWell, Hadley, MA, USA
University of South Carolina School of
Medicine Greenville, Greenville,
SC, USA

Julie Sullivan
Emory University, Atlanta,
GA, USA

Paul Tessier
CIMIT, Boston, MA, USA

Erika Tyburski
Atlanta Center for Microsystems
Engineered Point-of-Care
Technologies, Atlanta,
GA, USA

Jose Valdesuso
RADx–VentureWell, Hadley, MA, USA

Eliseo Velasquez
Investors of Color Network, Boston, MA,
USA RADx–VentureWell, Hadley, MA, USA

Brian Walsh
RADx–VentureWell, Hadley, MA, USA

Cassandra Wesselman
ROSALIND Inc., San Diego, CA, USA

Foreword

Harvey V. Fineberg

A deadly pandemic demands a response at multiple levels of government and society and across myriad needs for public health and medical care. As the COVID-19 pandemic took hold in early 2020, the US response faltered. Hospitals lacked sufficient personal protective equipment for staff and, as cases surged, some were overwhelmed by sick patients. Optimal care for extremely ill patients was uncertain. The federal response lacked a clear leadership structure and chain of command. Antivirals were lacking, and an effective vaccine was yet to be developed. Moreover, the Centers for Disease Control and Prevention initially distributed a test kit with a faulty reagent, setting back the national testing strategy for COVID-19.

The nation's premier biomedical research organization, the National Institutes of Health (NIH), focused its COVID-19 efforts on three main goals of research: vaccines, therapeutics, and diagnostics. By April 2020, the NIH had activated a public–private partnership to accelerate the development of COVID-19 therapeutics and vaccines. Through funding and active collaboration, the NIH was instrumental in the development of the Moderna vaccine. With the active engagement of 20 companies and scores of scientists, the NIH screened hundreds of therapeutic candidates, embarked on clinical trials for more than three dozen of the most promising, and obtained six therapeutics approved for clinical use. Fueled by a special congressional appropriation in April 2020, the NIH launched the Rapid Acceleration of Diagnostics (RADx®) initiative. Within six months, the Food and Drug Administration granted emergency use authorization to the first point-of-care – rapid COVID-19 tests funded through RADx – and since then more than four dozen RADx-supported tests (20 point-of-care, 16 laboratory-based, and 13 home-based tests) have received emergency use authorization.

The pandemic demanded unaccustomed speed, intensity, and flexibility in research. All of the institutes of the NIH responded to these pandemic exigencies. However, RADx stands out for its degree of innovativeness and readiness to embrace non-traditional ways of doing business at the NIH.

Led by the National Institute of Biomedical Imaging and Bioengineering, RADx built on years of experience gained through CIMIT and the Point-of-Care Technology Research Network that is coordinated by CIMIT. Rather than consider the aim to be funding brilliant research, RADx adopted an outcomes-oriented approach that embraced every stage, from scientific idea through proof of concept, product development, manufacturing, clinical evaluation, regulatory review, and authorization for use. Rather than traditional peer review, RADx developed a shark-tank approach of presentation, assessment of promise, and investment, followed by an innovation funnel with development milestones and sequential winnowing or intensifying investment. Rather than a hands-off approach after grant approval, RADx adopted venture-capital-like continued support and coaching to overcome any obstacles along the way.

These innovations meant that RADx would seek and foster ideas that had the promise of success and not simply look for reasons that a project might fail. Thus, RADx did not accept an inevitable "valley of death" for biomedical product development; RADx established oases of support that carried easier-to-use, faster, and more reliable diagnostic tests from scientific ideas to clinical laboratories, sites of clinical care, and homes. Because of RADx, as many as 3 billion COVID-19 tests have entered the US market, and rapid home and point-of-care tests have become the norm.

This book describes the concept, organization, implementation, and results of the RADx initiative. It provides many cases to illustrate the varied ways that the RADx model, combining the best of public and private capacities, contributed to the success. It shows how RADx adapted and learned from failures in real time to strengthen its approach. The book positions the quest for more and better diagnostic tests – accurate, easy to use, and widely available – against the backdrop of multiple pandemic demands on clinical care and public health. The RADx experience holds lessons not only for the development of future diagnostics but also for any situation in which multiple scientific scenarios may yield technologies to help meet an urgent health need.

More than three years after the start of COVID-19, the United States and much of the world appear to have weathered the brunt of the pandemic, although the toll on lives and the financial impact continue to mount, and post-acute sequelae of severe acute respiratory syndrome coronavirus 2 (SARS-CoV-2) remain an ongoing clinical dilemma. China, whose zero-tolerance policies held off the full force of COVID-19 for a couple of years, has since found itself in the throes of the pandemic and has lent its weight to the growing, global burden of disease.

With time, we can anticipate many assessments of the pandemic response at the global, national, and subnational levels. Many will proffer lessons, and some will be worth heeding. The RADx story told here meets that high standard, worthy of heeding, in preparing for the next pandemic or for any similarly severe and urgent health threat.

Preface
Wade E. Bolton

In 2019, a unique virus emerged on the world scene that would cause a global affront to our health-care systems. Hundreds of millions of individuals became infected with the virus, resulting in millions of lives lost and catastrophic financial damage. In the United States alone, the pandemic was the most significant medical calamity in the history of our nation, surpassing the lives lost in World War I and World War II combined and even outnumbering the casualties of the 1918 Spanish flu pandemic. As a member of the coronavirus family, which was later named SARS-CoV-2, this raging virus at first appeared to resemble two of its predecessors, SARS and Middle East respiratory syndrome (MERS). The scientific community soon learned, however, that the differences among them were stark.

Through the NIH's RADx initiative, a network of professionals was established to respond to the virus through the development and distribution of diagnostic tests that could accurately diagnose the presence of the virus in patient samples. Our assignment had no boundaries. We reached across international borders, collaborated with the brave men and women in the field, and were welcomed by academic and government institutions willing and able to join in the fight against this common foe. We understood that this was our absolute priority – a national and global mandate with millions of lives at stake.

This book documents how the limits of science and discovery were pushed in a collective effort to contain and manage this pandemic, from the development of diagnostic assays to the surveillance of and response to emerging variants. The authors describe what was done differently to identify, develop, and distribute diagnostic tests in record time and volume. We provide the framework for technical, organizational, practical, and operational action items that are essential to the management of an emergency health crisis. We describe our lessons learned and what we would have done differently to improve the outcomes. And, critically, each chapter includes a roadmap that details the steps necessary to optimally respond to the pandemic. (For a complete roadmap comprising all of the action steps plotted over time, readers will be able to turn to our website, pandemicresponseroadmap .org, once it is live.) We believe this collection of roadmaps is the first comprehensive response plan based on real-life pandemic experiences.

The publication of this book is timely, as the impact of COVID-19 is currently undergoing overall evaluation. We are hopeful that the experiences, roadmaps, approaches, and frameworks herein will serve as scaffolding upon which our colleagues can build when they begin to plan their response to the next health crisis.

The Website

The pandemicresponseroadmap.org website will offer a valuable resource for individuals seeking to enhance their understanding of pandemic response strategies. Through an interactive and customizable pandemic response roadmap, users will be able to gain insights into the complex and evolving nature of pandemics and develop customized strategies to navigate them effectively. Our author biosketches will provide detailed accounts of the training and experiences of each author, enabling readers to trust in and appreciate their unique perspectives and expertise. Additionally, our compiled list of lessons learned during the COVID-19 pandemic will offer insights into successful pandemic response strategies and areas for improvement. By leveraging the collective knowledge and experiences of our authors, our website aims to expand upon the knowledge provided within the book pages to further contribute to a more informed and effective global pandemic response.

Acknowledgments

Project team: Steven Schachter, Wade Bolton, Eric Evans, Tania Fernandez, Enrique Rabellino, D'lynne Plummer, Alexandra Smith, and Mallak Taleb.

RADx® Tech Collaborators

Aaron Black, Aaron Chockla, Abigail Conte, Ace Edwards, Adam Hoffman, Adam Samuta, Adannaya Amadi, Adannaya Pathology, Adriana Quintana, Adrienne Hoey, Agha Mirza, Ahmed Babiker, Ahmed Hassan, Ainat Koren, Albert Lee, Albine Martin, Alec Boudreau, Alema Jackson, Alethea Wieland, Alex Greninger, Alexander Green, Alexis Beatty, Ali Haide, Alicia Loffler, Alison Cernich, Allen Breiner, Allen Graham, Allie Suessmith, Allison Blodgett, Allison Cristman, Allison Eason, Allyson Chabot, Alok Kapoor, Alpdogan Kantarci, Alyssa Owens, Amanda Dion-Schultz, Amanda Foster, Amanda Grindle, Amanda Grindle, Amanda MacLeod, Amanda Riley, Amanda Strudwick, Amanda Sutton, Amber Showers, Amber Thomas, Aminul Joel Islam, Amy Baker, Amy Bucher, Amy Krafft, Amy Miarecki, Andrea Depatie, Andrea Sjostedt, Andrew Adelman, Andrew DiMeo, Andrew Glenn, Andrew Hastings, Andrew Neish, Andrew Perez, Andrew Potter, Andrew Webster, Andrew Weitz, Andy Pekosz, Andy Winffel, Angela Stallworth, Aniket Patel, Anissa Elayadi, Ann Chahroudi, Ann Gawalt, Ann Martin, Anna Horney, Anna Lowe, Anna Wood, Annabelle St. Pierre, Anne Piantadosi, Anne Wyllie, Annette Esper, Annie Miller, Annmarie Walsh, Anthony Curro, Anthony Kirilusha, Anuradha Rao, Anyelo Diaz, Apurv Soni, Arthur Bray-Simon, Arunan Skandarajah, Arynne Wilburn, Asha Storm, Ashley Banks, Ashley Crawley, Asif Rizwan, Atam Dhawan, Austin Tiger Lu, Babar Akhter, Baiba Berzins, Barbara Thompson, Barbara Van Der Pol, Barcey Levy, Benedict Kalibala, Benjamin Helmericks, Bernadette Shaw, Bethanne Giehl, Bethany Trainor, Bethany Watson, Betsy Peters, Beverly Bricker, Beverly Rogers, Bill Heetderks, Bill O'Sick, Bill Riley, Bob Storey, Bonolo Mathekga, Bradley Hanberry, Brandi Limbago, Brandy Mai, Braylon Rumph, Brendan Murphy, Brent Ingraham, Brett Giroir, Brian Mustanski, Brian Walsh, Brittany Goldberg, Brooke Beckman, Brooke Seitter, Brooke Staples, Bruce Barton, Bruce Gay, Bruce Gnade, Bruce Tromberg, Bryan Buchholz, Bryan Du, Cadeidre Washington, Caesar Melendez, Caitlin Pretz, Candace Dufour, Candice Miller, Cangyuan Li, Cara Barnes, Carl Kumpf, Carl Park, Carlos Aparicio, Carlos Moreno, Carlos Perez, Carol Bova, Carol Govern, Carter Usowski, Cassie Bednarek, Cathryn Lapierre, Cathy Cambria, Cecile Davis, Chad Achenbach, Chao Qi, Charles Anamelechi, Charles Daitch, Charles Hart, Charles Hill, Charles Oyesile, Charlette Bronson, Charlotte Gaydos, Cheryl Bastian, Cheryl Maier, Cheryl Shimer, Cheryl Stone, Chiara Ghezzi, Chris Bocus, Chris Bunn, Chris Desrosiers, Chris Elkins, Christian Flanery, Christie Canaria, Christie Johnson, Christina Macauliffe, Christina Rostad, Christine Cooper, Christine Farrell, Christine Hanson, Christine Walter, Christopher Brooke, Christopher Hartshorn, Christopher Porter, Chun Huai Luo, Chung-Jung Chiu, Cindy Pryor, Cindy Teixeira, Clair O'Donovan, Claudia Hawkins, Claudia Morris, Colin Brenan, Colleen Kraft, Colleen Matte, Colleen Sico, Collin Timm, Colton Joseph, Connie Arthur, Connie Rivers, Connor Seabrook, Conrad Tucker, Cornelius Moore, Courtney Lias, Courtney Sabino, Craig Lilly, Crystal Reinhart, Cynthia Hilgren, Cynthia Nicholson, Dale

Gort, Dan Marshak, Dan Wattendorf, Danesh Thirukumaran, Daniel Kalman, Daniel Murphy, Danielle DiMezza, Danielle Howard, Danielle Oliver, Darash Desai, Darci Edmonson, Darwin Salgado, Daveta Brown, David Alter, David D. McManus, David George, David Giarracco, David Goldstein, David Gottfried, David Hoaglin, David Ku, David Mudd, David Sanford, David Smith, Deborah Kelly, Deborah Lee, Denise Ehlen, Denise R. Dunlap, Denise Scholtens, Deniz Peker, Dennis Rose, Devon Campbell, Devon Hartigan, Diana Bianchi, Diane Lawrence, Diane Quinn, Diane Spiliotis, Digvijay Singh, Dilhari Peiris, Dina Simon, Dipanwita Basu, Don Croteau, Donna Matson, Donna McGrath, Doreen Trotta, Dorothy Maxwell, Doug Sheeley, Douglas Bryant, Edith Otabil, Edward Berger, Edward Ehrman, Elaine Kim, Elayn Byron, Elena Koustova, Elias Caro, Eliseo Perez-Stable, Eliseo Velasquez, Elizabeth Bulger, Elizabeth Christian, Elizabeth Heald, Elizabeth Orvek, Elizabeth Walsh, Ellen Clegg, Ellie Brent, Em Beauchamp, Emily Cisney, Emily Muth, Emily Sousa, Emma Wojtowicz, Eri Ortlund, Eric Cecco, Eric Lai, Eric Nehl, Eric Padmore, Eric Stratton, Erica Landis, Ericardo Edwards, Erika Tyburski, Erin Iturriaga, Esmerlda Meyer, Ethan Berke, Etienne Dembele, Eugene Rogers, Eun Mi Lee, Evan Anderson, Evan Bradley, Fajar Nuriddin, Faraz Ilyas, Felicia Qashu, Filipp Viola, Francis Collins, Frank Cable, Franziska Meockel, Frederick Balagadde, Gabriela Varela Heslin, Gail Radclifee, Gallya Gannot, Gary Disbrow, Gary Place, Gary Sudusky, Gaurav Mehta, Gavin Harris, Gene Civillico, Geoff Bonn, Geoffrey Smith, Germán Chiriboga, Glenn Neuman, Gokhan Ozalp, Grace Bendinger, Grace Tran, Graham Threadhil, Greg Gibson, Greg Martin, Gregory Marcus, Gretchen Armington, Gul Nowshad, Guy Benian, Hang Chen, Hans Verkerke, Harold Sullivan, Heath Naquin, Heather Bowers, Heather Tessier, Heba Mostafa, Helene Langevin, Hersh Patel, Hesam Hafizi, Hiba Abbas, Hilary Dupre, Himani Bisht, Holly Alvarez, Holly Sommers, Holly Taylor, Hope Krebell, Howard Golub, Hur Koser, Ian Misner, Ilana Goldberg, J. Christopher Flaherty, Jacob Khouri, Jacqueline Martinez, Jaiprasath Sachithanandhamm, James Anderson, James Patzke, Jane Holl, Janet Figueroa, Janet Hale, Janice Bell, Janice Legace, Jannette Guarner, Jared Kimbrough, Jared O'Neal, Jasmine Chaitram, Jason Ford, Jason Opdyke, Jason Wheeler, Jay Butler, Jean Welsh, Jeanette Daly, Jeanne Keruly, Jeff Evans, Jeff Shuren, Jeff Winner, Jeffrey Brocious, Jeffrey E. Olgin, Jeffrey Holden, Jeffrey Olgin, Jeffrey Williams, Jen Afamefuna, Jenica Patterson, Jennifer Baker, Jennifer Biemer, Jennifer Campbell, Jennifer Fediani, Jennifer Holme, Jennifer Jackson, Jennifer K. Frediani, Jennifer McKenney, Jeremy Boutin, Jeroan Allison, Jesand Sylve, Jessa Waggoner, Jessica Ingersoll, Jessica Meade, Jessica Orozco, Jessica Scott, Jian Lou, Jill Heemskerk, Jill Morgan, Jillian McClain, Jo Hiatt, Joan Davis, Joanna Nathan, Joanne Andreadis, Joanne Lebrun, Joanne Matthew, Joany Jackman, Jocelyn Montgomery, Jodi Black, Jody Ciolino, Joe Davenport, John Barnes, John Blackwood, John Broach, John Click, John Diggs, John Haran, John Healey, John Lear, John Lee, John McQuiston, John Nuckols, John P. Broach, John Parrish, John Roback, Jon McGrath, Jonathan Patton, Jonggyu Baek, Joseph Briggs, Joseph Hutter, Joseph Odorisio, Joseph Valdesuso, Joseph Walsh, Josh Tolkoff, Joshua Jacob, Joshua Levy, Joshua Rumbut, Joshua Wolfe, Jue Chen, Julia Adams, Julia Tisheh, Julia Zakashansky, Julie Flahive, Julie Norton, Julie Stephens, Julie Sullivan, Julie Wilkinson, Jun Guo, Justin Burns, Justin Hardick, Justin McAteer, Justin Tiao, Justin Yang, Kalpana Regarajan, Kamilah Rashid, Kara Palamountain, Kara Penny, Karen Ann Lavallee, Karen Del'Olio, Karen Gilliam, Karen Griffin, Karen Olsen, Karen Wallace, Karl Simin, Kate Klein, Kate Thoma, Katerina Pappas, Katharine Egan, Katherine Immergluck, Katherine Luzuriaga, Katherine Ramirez, Kathryn Lane Musall, Kathryn Marvel, Katie Hambrick, Katie Shapcott, Katrina

Bogan, Kavita Babu, Keivan Zandi, Kelli Malkin, Kelly Army, Kelly Gorman, Kelsey Woods, Ken Beall, Kerry Demarco, Kerry DiBenardo, Kevin Coats, Kevin Leite, Kevin Seiki, Khawar Hamid, Kim Caroline, Kim Noble, Kim Pachura, Kim-Judy You, Kimberlee Cantin, Kimberly Sciarretta, Kira Moresco, Kiran Verma, K. J. Shaikh, Klemens Wengert, Krishna Juluru, Kristen Herzegh, Kristen Weber, Kristi Cooper, Kristian Roth, Kristin Le, Kristina Lowe, Kristopher Bough, Kyle Rose, Kyle Sprow, Kylie Lanman, Kyung Moon, Lacy Wilson, Laia Hussaini, Larry Tabak, Laura Benedit, Laura Ferrara, Laura Gibson, Laura Rose, Laura Sampath, Laurel O'Connor, Lauren Balmert, Lauren Howe, Lea E. Widdice, Leda Bassit, Lee Payne, Leona Wells, Leona Wells, Leonardo Angelone, Leticia Rockenbach, Leyla Kara, Leyla Rose, Li Li, Liesl Warbel, Lifang Hou, Lilliam Martinez Bello, Linda Smith, Lindsey Gieger, Lisa Council, Lisa Hirchhorn, Lisa Ponce, Lisa Portner, Lisa R. Hirschhorn, Lisa Smith, Lisa Waples, Lisa Wei, Liu Xu, Liz DiNenno, Liz McCarty, Liz Ruark, Lori Pbert, Lori Randall, Louis Vuga, Lucie Low, Lucky Jain, Lydia Garcia Jacinto, Lydia McClure, Lynn Furtaw, M. Didem Avcioglu-Ayturk, MacArthur Benoit, Mack Schermer, Madeline Hobbs, Madeline Marx, Madison Conte, Maggie Hassan, Maggie Li, Mahesh Vangala, Mamoudou Maiga, Mandi Blochberger, Mandy O'Reilly, Manuel Kingley, Mara Aspinall, Mara Heng, Marayanaiah Ceedarla, Marc Charette, Maren Downing, Margaret McManus, Margaret Neja, Margaret Ochocinska, Margo Kinney-Petrucha, Maria Cordero, Maria Davilla, Maria Grainger, Marianne Weinell, Marissa Fayer, Mark Bobrow, Mark Bonaficio, Mark Bonifacio, Mark Fisher, Mark Gonzalez, Mark Griffiths, Mark Guitarini, Mark Huffman, Mark Marino, Mark Pletcher, Mark Smith, Mark Snyder, Marshall R. Collins, Mary Ann Picard, Mary Beth Tull, Mary Co, Mary Dubuque, Mary Fadden, Mary Janet McCarthy, MaryAnn Lambert, Marzan Khan, Massiel Mota, Matt Durgin, Matt O'Connell, Matthew Caputo, Matthew Glucksberg, Matthew Hart, Matthew Humbard, Matthew McMahon, Matthew Robinson, Matthew Sanders, Maud Mavigner, Maureen Beanan, Maureen Garner, Maureen Richardson, Megan Schmidt, Megan Shaw, Melanie Peel, Melinda Mathis, Melissa Frangie, Melissa Henson, Melissa Ramos, Melissa Rotella, Melva Steps, Mia Cirrincione, Michael Boyce-Jacino, Michael Brady, Michael Cariseo, Michael Centola, Michael Dempsey, Michael Harsh, Michael Hirsh, Michael Huggins, Michael Iademarco, Michael Kochersperger, Michael Koeris, Michael Lauer, Michael Masterman-Smith, Michael Newcomb, Michael Norton, Michael Palmer, Michael Wolfson, Michele Liston, Michelle Berny-Lang, Michelle McConnell, Michelle Popler, Mike Ryan, Milagros Rosal, Miriam Vos, Monica Lowell, Monica O'Brian, Morgan Greenleaf, Muktha Natrajan, Myla Lai-Goldman, Nadia Hassan, Nancy Elder, Nancy Gagliano, Nancy Mortimer, Nancy Sencabaugh, Naomi Braun, Natalie Bruning, Natalie Lee, Nate Wade, Nathaniel Hafer, Natia Saakadze, Neal Connors, Neal Dickert, Neeta Shenvi, Neil Mucci, Nicholas Gallagher, Nick D'Aimco, Nicole Benevento, Nigistmariam Yasin, Nikki Powell, Nils Schoof, Nimi Fifadara, Nira Pollock, Nisha Fahey, Nitika Gupta, Noah Peyser, Noni Byrnes, Oladapo Olaitan, Olga Brown, Olga Hartman, Oliver Brand, Paige Ezernack, Pamela McGuinness, Pamela Miller, Parang Kim, Paritosh Chandwade, Patricia Helbin, Patricia Wiley, Patti Brennan, Patti O'Neill, Paul Baker, Paul Eder, Paul Tessier, Paul Yoo, Paulina Rebolledo, Peko Hosoi, Penny Ford-Carleton, Peter D'Entremont, Peter Lazar, Peter Rice, Peter Tobin, Petr Sulc, Phil Weilerstein, Punam Mathur, Qiming Shi, Quierra Wells, Rachael Fleurence, Rachel Agoglia, Rachel Factor, Rachel Fink, Rachel Krebs, Rahul Salla, Rana Saber, Randall Morse, Rao Divi, Rashad Wood, Rashida Ferebee, Ray Ebert, Raymond Cariseo, Raymond Felix Schinazi, Raymond MacDougall, Rebecca Cleeton, Rebecca Gore, Rebecca Kirby, Rebekah Neal, Ren Salerno, Renate Myles, Renee Simon, Reshika Mendia, Rhonda Gibson, Ribhi Shawar, Ricardo Ramos, Richard Anderson, Richard Creager, Richard Girards, Richard

Hodes, Richard Rothman, Rick Bright, Rick D'Augustine, Rick Gagliano, Rick Woychik, Rik Madison, Risha Nayee, Rjsekhar Guddneppanavar, Robert Eisinger, Robert Fineberg, Robert Jerris, Robert Kircher, Robert L. Murphy, Robert Mannino, Robert Nobles, Robert Scalese, Rocio Luparello, Rodney Kincaid, Rodney Wallace, Ron Tedesco, Rory Carrillo, Rosemary Humes, Roslyn Seitz, Roxane Burkett, Ruben Salinas, Ruifeng Zhou, Russell Kempker, Ryan Eckmeier, Sadanand Gite, Saja Asakrah, Sal Strods, Sally McFall, Sam Dolphin, Samantha Strickler, Sandeep Patel, Sandra Maher, Sandra Ott, Sara Brenner, Sara Caudillo, Sarah Bank, Sarah Eisenberg, Sarah Farmer, Sarah Fey, Sarah Hernandez, Sarah Huban, Sarah McGee, Sathmurthy Gourisankar, Sauntelle Byfield, Scott Eibel, Scott Tanner, Seegar Swanson, Seila Selimovic, Serena Carroll, Shahid Rashid, Shaminy Manoranjithan, Shanna Bruflodt, Shanna Spencer, Shannon Griffin, Shannon Moore, Sharina Person, Shaukat Soofi, Shawn Mulvaney, Shawn Patel, Sheila Baker, Shirley Coney-Johnson, Shirley Ruiz-Lundgren, Silu Hu, Skyler Ward, Sofia Martinez, Sonia Gales, Sonja Davis, Sonja Dill, Sotirios Geragonis, Sreeram Ramakrishnan, Stacey Carroll, Stacey Spies, Stacy Hellman, Stacy Turner, Stephanie Adams, Stephanie Behar, Stephanie Meisner, Stephenie Lemon, Steve Blanc, Steven Santos, Stewart Ellis, Sumin Koo, Sunita Gopalani, Sunita Park, Sunshine Moore, Susan Gregurick, Susan Moreira, Syed Naeem, Tamara McBrayer, Tamara McKenzie, Tamara Wesley, Tami Hagberg, Tamila Dover, Tammy Beckman, Tammy Falla, Tara Knox, Tara Loomis, Tara Schwetz, Tatia Hodges, Taylor Gilliland, Tempist Evenson, Teresa Zembower, Thanuja Ramachandra, Theodore Zainal, Thomas Grifa, Thomas Johnson, Thomas Pribyl, Thomas Vanderford, Tiffani Lash, Tiffany Wilson, Tim Stenzel, Tim Thurman, Timmy Moore-Simas, Timothy Moulton, Timothy Vanderford, Toby Lowe, Todd Merchak, Todd Sherer, Tony Boiers, Tony Haney, Tony Voiers, Toya Morrison, Traci Leong, Tracy McMahon, Tracy Willoughby, Truc Le, Ugur Celik, Uyen Le, Vi Nguyen, Vicki Anastasi, Victor Sine, Victoria Stittleburg, Vidurshi Gupta, Vijay Dhaka, Vijay Vanguri, Vincent Ahonkhai, Vinton Grant, Viviana Claveria, Vyjayanti Kasinathan, W. O'Neal, Walt Carney, Wayne Wang, Webb Stone, Wendi Kuhnert, Wilbur A. Lam, William Clarke, William Daunch, William Haddad, William Pierce, Wolfgang Krull, Xaivera Martinez-Armenta, Xavier Peralta, Yasmin Haider, Yolanda Zeringue, Yu-Hsiang Hsieh, Yufei Yu, Yukari C. Manabe, Yurima Guilarte-Walker, Zachary Buono, Zachary Ellison, Zachary Favakeh, Zihan Yang, Zina Brown, Ziyue Wang.

Other Acknowledgments

Bill Rodrigues, Marcelle Abell-Rosen, Sergio Carmona, Jim Densmore, Edward Tharp, Bradley Wait, Ben Walker, Justin Valliere, Lisa Butler, Brandi Talkington; Huck Strategies LLC.

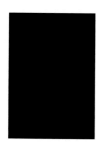

Introduction

Tania Fernandez

The end of 2022 marked three years since the first reports appeared in the news of a potentially novel coronavirus in a seafood market in Wuhan, China. Commencing in December 2019, COVID-19 – caused by the severe acute respiratory disease coronavirus 2 (SARS-CoV-2) – spread rapidly across continents, with the first case of COVID-19 being reported in the United States as early as January 20, 2020. Two months later, with the official announcement being made by the World Health Organization, there was no denying the reality that we were in the midst of a raging pandemic.

At its inception, no one could have predicted the power of the virus. It swept through humanity, infecting more than 700 million people, killing more than 6.9 million people across 215 countries, cutting across caste, creed, and color.

This book is a tribute to the "warriors" who worked in the trenches day and night to combat the virus and wage the deadly war against the pandemic. It is meant to serve as a sobering reminder of the sacrifices made by so many. We dedicate this book to the millions of lives that were lost to COVID-19 and to frontline workers across the globe who sacrificed their lives in the line of duty.

This is our story of how humanity came together during an incredibly challenging time to unite forces and fight a common enemy. It is a story of reflections and lessons learned, a record of what we did right and what we could have done better, but, above all, this is a story that is written in gratitude to the unconquerable spirit of humankind and the relentless pursuit of scientific knowledge to serve humanity.

This book chronicles the power of innovation, the accelerated commercialization of diagnostics, the birth of new business models and creative financing ventures, the perseverance and commitment of entrepreneurs, and the agility and resourcefulness of government institutions as they adapted to meet the imminent needs of the pandemic and serve the community.

Coronaviruses are not new to humankind. Humanity has witnessed three deadly pandemics in the twenty-first century alone, all of which were associated with this group of viruses. In 2002, the world witnessed the first lethal coronavirus-induced disease, which was named severe acute respiratory syndrome coronavirus (SARS-CoV). A decade later, in 2012, a different coronavirus outbreak unraveled in the Middle East, earning the name Middle East respiratory syndrome coronavirus (MERS-CoV). Despite our seeming familiarity with this group of viruses, the global community was unprepared when a novel coronavirus reared its ugly head and swept through humankind with a ferocity last witnessed only during the Spanish influenza pandemic of 1917 caused by the H1N1 virus and often referred to as the greatest medical holocaust in history.

Despite previous appearances, this coronavirus was labeled as novel because a comparison of the viral genome revealed that it had only 79.5% homology with SARS-CoV and 40% homology with MERS-CoV. Thus, it was battle time again. We had no armamentarium to fight the virus or any specialized knowledge of what we were dealing with. Our understanding of the evolution of SARS CoV-2 and how it spread was particularly unclear during the early stages of the COVID-19 pandemic. Misconceptions and myths about its origin and its mode of transmission raged like wildfires across continents, fueling panic and chaos.

The pandemic had made its way into the life of the masses, and the scientific community was forced to meet the demands of questioning and angry communities demanding answers. Whatever side of the fence one was on with regard to the quality of scientific rigor on social media, it cannot be denied that the media served to disseminate knowledge and information at an unprecedented speed.

In the world that we live in today, where COVID-19, social distancing, lockdowns, contact tracing, super spreader events, antigen tests, and polymerase chain reaction (PCR) tests have all become common household parlance, let us not forget that, in December 2019, the world was a different place. Awareness of pandemics was at an all-time low, despite the occasional visionary messages of caution that were voiced by a select few but largely neglected.

The depth and breadth of scientific knowledge that we have amassed since that fatal day that SARS-CoV-2 interrupted humanity serves as a tribute to all the scientists, clinicians, and health-care workers who worked tirelessly at an unprecedented pace to advance coronavirus research. During its early spread in January, thousands of viral genomes were rapidly sequenced by research laboratories around the world and shared in open-access databases such as the EpiCoV database from the Global Initiative on Sharing All Influenza Data (GISAID) and the Our World in Data COVID-19 dataset. Within a month of the release of the SARS CoV-2 genome, the CDC had developed the first SARS-CoV-2 diagnostic test kit which got FDA EUA approval on February 4, 2020.

A glimmer of hope arose that widespread testing and early detection might serve to intervene in disease progression and thus counteract the increasing mortality that humanity was witnessing. Accordingly, many countries rushed to implement population-based testing to monitor spread and implement quarantining to reduce viral transmission. This created enormous pressure for high-quality, reliable tests to be developed and commercialized at record-breaking pace. The planet morphed into the largest global testing ground for humanity. Governments across the world rose to the occasion, as they have traditionally done, to fund research and innovation. From sequencing the SARS-CoV-2 genome and sharing it with the world to characterizing methods of viral entry and spread, as well as ongoing surveillance of an assault of viral variants and dealing with the confusion and utter despair of those who were asymptomatically spreading the virus, the scientific community worked tirelessly to push the boundaries of understanding the biology of the virus.

The chapters in this book are written by a wide range of authors with varying experiences and expertise, who have worked across the spectrum from research and development to commercialization of COVID-19 diagnostics. Given the multidisciplinary nature of this initiative, each chapter has been written by authors with relevant expertise and provides an in-depth narrative from their own unique perspectives. The chapters have been compiled to take the reader on a journey with us as we chronicle the early stages of the pandemic, the historical events, and the effectiveness of the decision-making processes during crucial phases of the pandemic. We delve briefly into the immunology of the virus and its rapid evolution through mutagenesis and touch upon the controversial topic of immunity to the virus.

In the United States, SARS-CoV-2 spread rapidly, and with it grew the inability to keep pace with the increasing demands for COVID-19 diagnostic testing. In April 2020, as mortality continued to soar and the need for testing within the United States became imminent, the National Institutes of Health (NIH) received a $1.5 billion appropriation from Congress to expand testing capacity in the USA. Thus, it was that, while the world continued to operate in a chaotic frenzy, a new innovative program was born within five days after the legislation was signed into law.

The NIH launched the Rapid Acceleration of Diagnostics (RADx®) program. The RADx Tech initiative was created to support the development, validation, production, and commercialization of accurate, point-of-care, and home tests, as well as to improve existing clinical tests that could detect SARS-CoV-2. This brainchild initiative pushed diagnostics, a much-neglected sector, to the forefront through a focus on the compression of a diagnostic prototype-to-product launch from over five years to under a year. Many of the chapters in this book are written by authors who were part of the RADx initiative and worked in the trenches. These chapters go into intricate detail on each aspect of the journey, from development to deployment, and what it took to accelerate diagnostic capacity in a time of crisis.

Overall, the RADx Tech initiative was an unprecedented program that invested a huge amount of capital into COVID-19 diagnostics across the spectrum, from tests performed in reference laboratories to point-of-care diagnostics and over-the-counter home tests. The program used a rigorous "deep dive" diligence process and a "shark tank" model run by leading industry experts to select companies and projects with innovative technologies that had the potential to scale up and address the testing needs in different segments of society. Beyond the capital investments, RADx Tech proved to be a fertile ground for the evolution of a public–private partnership model such as the industry had not witnessed before. Combining the best of both worlds, it set out on its mission not just to finance innovation in companies and de-risk technology, but to provide companies with an ecosystem built to maximize success in commercialization. Its focus on external verification and validation through key institutions, data-driven go/no-go decisions, stringent timelines, and outcomes was responsible for the success of the program.

Another unique aspect of the initiative was the leverage of the Point-of-Care Technology Research Network (POCTRN), run by the National Institute of Biomedical Imaging and Engineering (NIBIB), which through three cycles of prior NIH funding had previously identified a critical gap in diagnostic device development around the clinical use case. Thus, as companies developed their technologies for COVID-19 tests, they were guided by experts in the areas of infectious disease and emergency medicine; ambulatory, pediatric, and adult clinicians; medical directors of certified laboratories; diagnostic developers; and marketing experts with real-world experience. At the time of writing this book, hundreds of millions of COVID-19 tests have been developed and marketed.

It was initially thought that, with SARS-CoV-2 being well adapted to humans, there was minimal need for concern about mutations among circulating viruses (because of the historically slow mutation rate of coronaviruses and their inherent self-editing mechanism). This changed during the later months of 2020, when the first reports appeared of emergent SARS-CoV-2 variants that were associated with increased transmissibility and disease severity.

Diagnostic tests, which were based on the original Wuhan sequence of SARS-CoV-2, were found to be affected by these mutations. The repeated emergence of new SARS-CoV-2 variants presented challenges to the development of high-performing diagnostics. The RADx Variant Task Force – an interdisciplinary group composed of representatives of federal agencies, diagnostic device manufacturers, private and public bioinformatics companies and organizations, large laboratory organizations, and academic institutions – was thus created as a program within the larger RADx initiative that focused on assessing RADx technologies against variants.

The clinical management chapter (Chapter 3) focuses on patient care during a time of absolute crisis and the significant shift in clinical practice from using evidence-based medicine to being forced to use experimental methods of treatment. It highlights the innovation in health-care delivery models as hospital leaders sought to incorporate telemedicine to widen patient reach while not compromising on quality.

A quote from George Santayana (*The Life of Reason*, 1905) comes to mind: "Those who do not remember the past are condemned to repeat it." So, let us not forget. Let us never cease to remember the sacrifice of doctors, health-care workers, and frontline responders across the globe. Humanity will always be grateful to them for their sacrifice during these unprecedented times. This book captures case studies of how strong and selfless leaders made it their mission to focus on the care of patients in a time when there were no rules on how to combat this enemy.

Can we prevent the next pandemic? As we continue to reflect on that question, we look back not just at the mistakes that were made during the pandemic but also at what we did right and the key contributions that were made in this period. A few of the noteworthy successes include but are not limited to controlling supply-chain bottlenecks, the rapid commercialization of diagnostics in a time of crisis, the unprecedented rollout of COVID-19 testing, vaccine development, accelerated regulatory approvals, and ensuring that affordable tests were made available as much as possible. A key differentiator of this book is the fact that, in each chapter, readers will find meticulously detailed roadmaps that are specific to the chapter. We hope that these will serve as useful tools for the next generation of health-care leaders to create, implement, and execute operational strategies in the face of chaos and uncertainty during successive disease outbreaks.

We are cognizant of the fact that, in this book, we have analyzed the pandemic through what could be considered a very US-centric lens. While part of this was choice, a large part of it was necessity. To be able to communicate with our readers with the experience and expertise that is required to tell this story, we had to write it from the battlefield we operated from, which was the United States. In no way do we mean to diminish the heroic efforts of other nations that fought this battle, and they should be applauded. Where possible, we have referenced global efforts and drawn attention to them in select chapters.

A pandemic affects various aspects of society. The closure of essential and nonessential businesses, restrictions on travel, requiring individuals to isolate to combat rising rates of mortality and morbidity all took their toll, and society faced existential threats as economies began to shut down. Varied national responses to the threat of the virus, as well as economic and racial differences across nations, led to societal disparities and vastly different pandemic impacts across the globe. This has not been ignored and is also a focus of this book.

There is no doubt in anyone's mind that the effect of the pandemic have been severe, and we are still witnessing and will continue to witness its long-term damage to society worldwide. The power of sharing scientific data, the strength of partnerships, the creativity of collaborations, and the refusal to admit defeat in the presence of a common enemy should never be forgotten. These memories will serve us well for building a better and more resilient world.

Through this book, we hope to address the main components of the pandemic as it evolved and to provide strategies and guidelines for the management of outbreaks beyond COVID-19, thus serving as a legacy for many future generations.

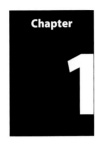

Early Detection, Response, and Surveillance of the COVID-19 Pandemic Crisis

Enrique M. Rabellino, Alexandra Smith,
and Marta C. Cohen

Introduction

This chapter provides foundational knowledge of the occurrences, events, and disease manifestations during the early stages of the COVID-19 pandemic, including the responses and
measures that were undertaken to contain the transmission of severe acute respiratory
syndrome coronavirus 2 (SARS-CoV-2), the virus that causes COVID-19. The importance
of early intervention is discussed throughout this chapter to illustrate the impact that timely
action – or, in many cases, inaction – had on the development of the pandemic. This chapter
explores the data collection and analysis mechanisms utilized to monitor disease spread in
different geographies. The necessity of information that is derived from early disease vigilance
and subsequent surveillance programs is stressed. This chronological account is intended to
create a roadmap for health and governmental authorities to follow for future undertakings,
programs, and decision-making processes at the earliest phases of future pandemics.

Disease Outbreak

The spread of infectious diseases affects both individuals and entire communities. Early
detection of a new outbreak is crucial so that containment measures can be implemented
quickly enough to minimize the need for large-scale quarantine, especially when resources
are limited. When primary care, public health, laboratories, and involved communities
collaborate effectively, early identification and mitigation initiatives are achievable. This
section outlines the initial detection of the COVID-19 outbreak and the responses of
governments, public health officials, and communities. Figure 1.2 is designed to help
visualize the significant occurrences during the earliest phases of the COVID-19 pandemic.

First Cases

On December 19, 2019, a case of pneumonia of unknown origin was detected in Wuhan,
China, a city of 11 million people and the capital of Hubei province in central China. By
December 29, 2019, four more cases had been reported to the Chinese Center for Disease
Control and Prevention (CCDC).[1] All initially reported cases were related to the Wuhan
South China Seafood Market (Huanan Seafood Wholesale Market). These cases had been
identified through a surveillance mechanism for "pneumonia of unknown etiology,"
a concept designed to allow timely identification of novel infectious organisms introduced
following the 2003 SARS-CoV outbreak.[2] Due to varying disease severity and clinical
manifestations, these cases attracted the attention of local physicians. While little was
known about the cause of these infections, there were indications of a possible new
emerging virus that diverged from the classical influenza virus.

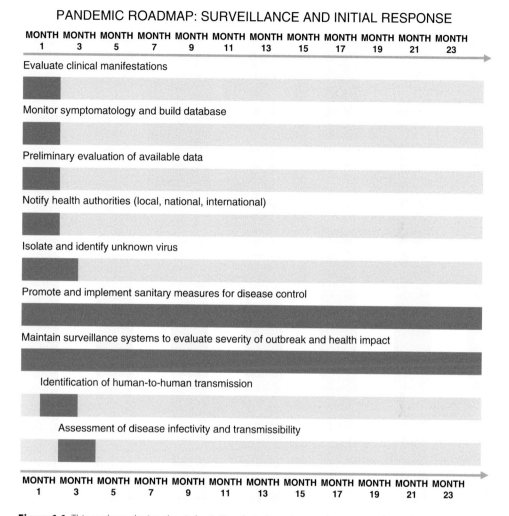

Figure 1.1 This roadmap depicts the vital activities, their chronology, and an estimated time frame in months. In the case of the SARS-CoV-2 pandemic, month 1 was December 2019, the month in which the virus was isolated, sequenced, identified, and published.

Roughly 10 days later, the medical administration of the Wuhan Municipal Health Commission (http://wjw.wuhan.gov.cn/) issued and distributed a document announcing the outbreak, reporting 27 new cases of pneumonia, mostly in stallholders at the Wuhan South China Seafood Market. Seven of these patients were in critical condition. Various hospitals in Wuhan held emergency symposia, where they defined a suspected case as a patient who met all four of the following criteria: fever, with or without recorded temperature; radiographic evidence of bilateral pneumonia; low or normal white blood cell count or low lymphocyte count; and no improvement in symptoms after three days of antimicrobial treatment, as per standard clinical guidelines. A patient who met the first three criteria and had an epidemiological link to the Wuhan South China Seafood Market could also be considered a suspected case.[3]

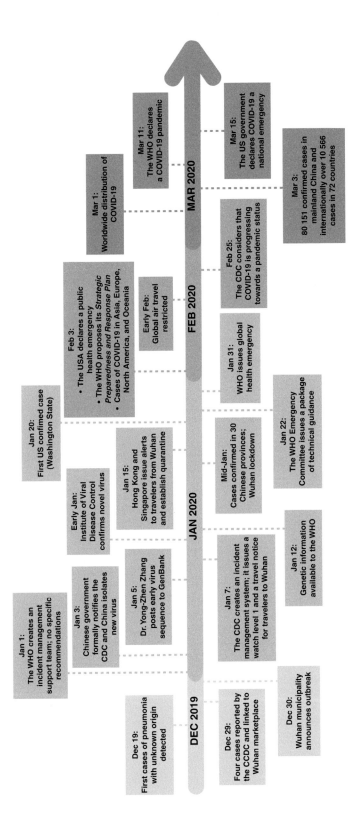

Figure 1.2 Pandemic evolution: from early detection to the declaration of the COVID-19 pandemic.

CCDC, Chinese Center for Disease Control and Prevention; CDC, US Centers for Disease Control and Prevention; WHO, World Health Organization.

Local authorities responded by initiating virus-typing studies, implementing population isolation, and closing the market. While most patients were linked to the Wuhan market, it soon became evident that human-to-human transmission had been occurring since mid-December and that the number of cases was doubling every 7.4 days.

Early reports referred to the outbreak as "viral pneumonia," suggesting that bacterial agents had been ruled out. Although the exact virus that caused the outbreak was unknown, the similarity in symptomatology to the previous SARS-CoV and Middle East respiratory syndrome coronavirus (MERS-CoV) outbreaks led health officials to hypothesize that it was another SARS-CoV outbreak.

Initially, Chinese health officials were free to share information about the newly emerging infectious disease; however, China's federal authorities quickly began inhibiting global medical and scientific communication. The Chinese government began to censure doctors who, in December 2019, raised the alarm about this pneumonia of unknown origin. For example, at the Central Hospital of Wuhan, a young ophthalmologist expressed his concerns to coworkers about a virus that he felt resembled SARS-CoV, a disease that originated in China and spread to four countries in 2003. The police summoned and admonished him, together with seven other doctors, on January 3, 2020. He was instructed to "stop making false comments" and investigated for "spreading rumors."[3] Tragically, he contracted COVID-19 and, on February 7, 2020, he passed away at the age of 33.[4]

By January 1, 2020, according to the World Health Organization (WHO) Newsroom, "the causal agent had not yet been identified or confirmed."[5] Further requests were made to the Chinese authorities for information that would enable assessment of the risk posed by the virus. On the same day, the Wuhan South China Seafood Market was closed, and the Chinese National Health Commission set daily meetings to monitor potential pneumonia epidemics. While it was clear that humans were infected with pneumonia of unknown etiology, the initial theories seemed to suggest a link to a wholesale fish and live animal market, indicating possible exposure to animals. Up to this point, information about the situation was only reaching local and international communities informally or through news released by the press, and they had received limited information to determine and monitor the potential risks.[3,5] The WHO assembled an incident management support team, which recommended continued public health measures and surveillance of influenza and severe acute respiratory infections. These recommendations did not include any specific measures for travelers.

On January 3, 2020, the Chinese government formally notified the director of the US Centers for Disease Control and Prevention (CDC) of the outbreak, revealing that 44 patients with pneumonia of unknown etiology had been reported, 11 of whom were critically ill, with the remaining 33 in stable condition.[3,6] In January 2020, Chinese scientists at the National Institute for Viral Disease Control and Prevention announced the discovery of a new coronavirus.[7] This novel coronavirus was the pathogenic cause of the viral pneumonia of unknown etiology, designating the disease as a novel coronavirus-infected pneumonia.

Responding to a surge in pneumonia cases with unknown etiology, on January 7, 2020, the CDC established an "incident management system" and issued watch level 1 travel precautions for Wuhan, China. The CDC recommended that visitors to Wuhan avoid contact with sick people; avoid animals (alive or dead), animal markets, and products that originated from animals (such as undercooked meat); and wash their hands often with soap and water. Additionally, the CDC advised anyone who had traveled to Wuhan and felt sick to isolate at home, except when seeking medical attention. At this stage, the WHO was uncertain of the cause of the 59 pneumonia-like cases, but it began to suspect that a novel coronavirus was to blame. Further research was required to correctly diagnose the individuals infected with the emerging virus.

Viral Pathogen Sequencing

Genomic sequencing is a laboratory technique used to decipher the full genetic composition of an organism (a virus in this case) or cell type. This approach may also be used to detect changes in specific regions of the genome. Viral sequencing was a quickly emerging technology that was critical in the diagnosis of COVID-19 and for understanding the transmission and management of the novel coronavirus.

On January 5, 2020, researchers at Fudan University, Shanghai, at the Shanghai Public Health Clinical Center and at the Fudan University School of Public Health published the sequence of SARS-CoV-2, the virus that causes COVID-19.[8, 9] The sequence was published to GenBank and the Global Initiative on Sharing All Influenza Data, both of which are online databases that are open and accessible to the public.

The genetic information became available to the WHO on January 12, 2020, opening the gateway for laboratories in different countries to produce specific, diagnostic polymerase chain reaction (PCR) tests that could detect the novel infection. The isolation and sequencing of the new virus confirmed it was a coronavirus.[10] While the Chinese researchers provided an essential tool for developing diagnostic tests, the Chinese authorities reacted negatively once again, closing the sequencing laboratory and ordering the "rectification" of disclosed statements on the virus, as well as the censorship of "misleading information" on social media.[3]

Assessment of Infectivity

In early January 2020, the Wuhan Municipal Health Commission stated that there was "no clear evidence of person-to-person transmission and while the possibility of limited person-to-person transmission cannot be ruled out, the risk of sustained person-to-person transmission was low."[11] A retrospective analysis of initial data shows that this was not true, the data highlights the necessity for early assessments of disease infectivity. Assessments of disease infectivity provide vital insight into how easily a disease is transmitted from human to human, which better informs officials on the best mitigation practices. Finally on January 20, 2020, China confirmed person-to-person transmission of the novel coronavirus and infections among medical workers.[3]

A universal measurement of disease transmission is the reproduction index (R_0). The R_0 index is defined as the number of susceptible people that one person with the disease can infect. It is a function of the following variables: the period of infectivity after infection, the chance of infection transmission per contact between a susceptible and an infectious individual, and the contact rate.[12]

Studies found that the initial Wuhan SARS-CoV-2 strain exhibited an estimated R_0 value between 1.4 and 2.5. For context, this value is displayed in Table 1.1 in comparison with other coronaviruses and known respiratory viral diseases with potential epidemic spread.[13] It is important to note that the infectivity of SARS-CoV-2 changed with the introduction of new variants.[14-16] Each variant presented structural changes to the viral spiral proteins that control binding to epithelial angiotensin converting enzyme 2 (ACE2) receptors and thus affect the infectivity of the virus. For more information on the impact of variant infectivity, see Chapter 9.

Table 1.1 Viral infectivity: basic reproductive number (R_0) of various known respiratory viral diseases[12–16]

Virus	Disease	R_0	Transmission
SARS-CoV-2: original Wuhan strain	COVID-19	2.4–2.6	Respiratory droplets/aerosol
SARS-CoV-2 alpha (B.1.1.7)	COVID-19	4–5	Respiratory droplets/aerosol
SARS-CoV-2 delta (B.1.617.2)	COVID-19	5–8	Respiratory droplets/aerosol
SARS-CoV-2 omicron (B.1.1.529)	COVID-19	8.2	Respiratory droplets/aerosol
SARS-CoV	Severe acute respiratory syndrome	2.2–3.6	Respiratory droplets
MERS-CoV	Middle Eastern respiratory syndrome	1.7–3.1	Direct contact or large virus-laden droplets
Influenza A	Influenza	0.9–3.1	Respiratory droplets
Respiratory syncytial virus	Bronchiolitis	1.2–3.0	Respiratory droplets/fomites
Rhinovirus	Cold-like illness	2.0–3.0	Respiratory droplets
Measles virus	Measles	12.0–18.0	Small particles/aerosol
Mumps virus	Mumps	10.0–12.0	Respiratory droplets
Ebola virus	Ebola virus disease	1.5–2.5	Body fluids
Adenovirus	Human adenoviruses systemic infection	2.3	Respiratory, fecal–oral

Disease Progression

While the Wuhan Municipal Health Commission was reporting no new infections or deaths, stating that the cumulative number of cases in the city had remained steady at 41, cases were being detected internationally. The first COVID-19 case inside the United States was detected on January 21, 2020, in a passenger returning from Wuhan. The CDC quickly set up a team to investigate the case and began tracing the patient's contacts. Similarly, cases were identified in the Republic of South Korea, Japan, Thailand, Singapore, France, Germany, Italy, the United Kingdom, and Spain.[17]

On January 22 and 23, 2020, the WHO Director-General convened an emergency committee under the 2005 International Health Regulations (IHR), issuing a comprehensive package of technical guidance on how to detect, test for, and manage potential cases.

On January 23, 2020, the Chinese government placed Wuhan in lockdown. By this time, the virus had spread to other provinces, and nearly 5 million people had left Wuhan to celebrate the Lunar New Year. Approximately one-third of those individuals traveled to locations outside Hubei province. The measures introduced by the Chinese government included strict social distancing, isolation requirements, the use of masks in public places, and the extension of the Lunar New Year holiday until March 10 for Hubei province and February 9 for many other provinces.[18, 19]

By the end of January, new epidemiological information revealed increases in the number of confirmed cases, suspected cases, and affected provinces, and in the proportion of deaths among the cases that had been reported to date (~3%; 17 of 557). Fourth-generation cases in Wuhan and second-generation cases outside Wuhan were reported, as well as some clusters outside Hubei province. Figure 1.3 shows the first reported analysis of the COVID-19 epidemic undertaken using the information system of the CCDC. The analysis showed that, over 30 days, the disease had spread from Hubei province to the rest of mainland China. It provided information on patient characteristics, calculations of case fatality and mortality rates, a geo-temporal analysis of viral spread, and an epidemiological curve construction based on location, contacts, disease severity, comorbidity, and geography.

The identification of the events that led to the infection of patient zero is crucial in investigating any epidemic outbreak. For SARS-CoV-2, these events were never clearly identified; thus, the possibility that SARS-CoV-2 was already circulating in Wuhan at the time of the outbreak has led to the proposition that the seafood market was a consequence, rather than the source, of the SARS-CoV-2 virus.[19] A study published in 2021 applied a technique known as the "mutational order approach" – which was initially developed to identify the evolutionary history of malignant tumor clones – to reconstruct the ancestral sequence and mutational history of SARS-CoV-2 genomes.[21] The results demonstrated the worldwide presence of SARS-CoV-2 well before the pandemic began, which makes it nearly impossible to identify patient zero.

Unfortunately, when the pandemic began, there was no surveillance system in place that could efficiently reflect the severity of the outbreak, its impact, or the required mitigation measures. Such a surveillance system would have facilitated and improved international coordination, including research efforts for developing medical countermeasures. Additionally, a lack of transparency from the Chinese government negatively affected the investigation of the initial outbreak in Wuhan. While general measures for controlling the crisis were eventually advised in specific countries and geographies, there were no conclusive or specific recommendations of measures to be implemented internationally, including for international travel.

Declaration of Health Emergency

On January 30, 2020, the WHO COVID-19 IHR Emergency Committee reconvened and, on January 31, 2020, the WHO issued recommendations for a global health emergency to be declared. Three days later, the United States declared a public health emergency. Despite this and the progressive spreading of virus infections and indications of intercontinental distributions of the disease, several members of the WHO committee considered it still too early to declare a public health emergency of international concern (PHEIC). With cases continuing to increase and in the face of an evolving epidemiological situation, the WHO's resistance to declaring a PHEIC was questionable. Issuing an intermediate-level alert could have reflected the severity of the outbreak. In the absence of conclusive recommendations, international travel continued and cases spread globally in alarming numbers.

Research and Development Prioritization

On February 4, 2020, the WHO published the *2019 Novel Coronavirus (2019-nCoV): Strategic Preparedness and Response Plan*, which included accelerating research and development (R&D) processes as one of three major strategies. On February 11 and 12, 2020, the

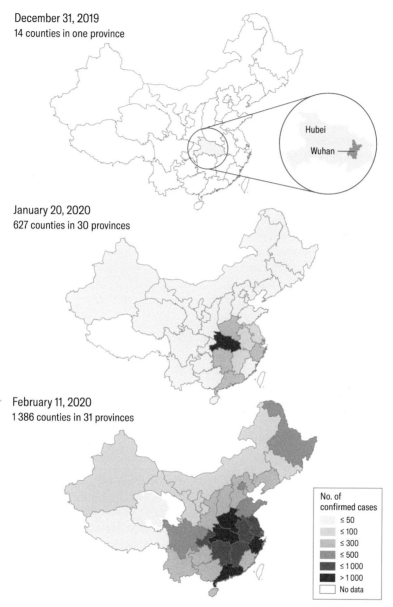

December 31, 2019
14 counties in one province

Hubei
Wuhan

January 20, 2020
627 counties in 30 provinces

February 11, 2020
1 386 counties in 31 provinces

No. of
confirmed cases
≤ 50
≤ 100
≤ 300
≤ 500
≤ 1 000
> 1 000
No data

Figure 1.3 Series of graphs illustrating the spread of SARS-CoV-2 within China's provinces before the declaration of the COVID-19 pandemic.[20]

WHO held the "Global Research and Innovation Forum: Towards a Research Roadmap for COVID-19." The fact that a COVID-19 R&D forum was the first meeting convened after the PHEIC declaration testifies to the importance of R&D in response to emerging infectious diseases.[22]

The prioritization of research allowed for rapid identification of the pathogen behind the SARS-CoV-2 outbreak and successful sequencing of the genome by February 7, 2020. In parallel, international research resulted in the prompt understanding of the physiopathology of viral infection and the disease progression, with the initiation of vaccine research by early March 2020.

Very judiciously, in February 2020, The Jenner Institute of the University of Oxford started developing the Oxford–AstraZeneca vaccine. By April 2020, 115 vaccines were in development, 73 of which were in the exploratory phase; however, only a handful of the vaccine projects succeeded. These R&D achievements were crucial and led to the development of vaccines in just 9 to 10 months, with these vaccines being granted temporary and conditional authorization. In December 2020, a 90-year-old female patient became the first person to receive a SARS-CoV-2 vaccine. Nevertheless, the R&D infrastructure was poorly coordinated overall and was still an inadequate response to a pandemic of this size.

A report prepared by the Independent Panel for Pandemic Preparedness and Response (IPPPR) highlighted the benefit that science and researchers provided during the COVID-19 pandemic.[23] The panel stated that the expertise and technology from decades of work – specifically on HIV, Ebola, and cancer vaccine research and immunology – were available and ready to apply to the new virus.

Global Response

One of the first coordinated efforts to curtail transmission occurred on a cruise ship that originated in Japan on January 20, 2020, with stops in Hong Kong, Vietnam, and Taiwan before returning to Japan on February 3, 2020. A passenger on board presented with symptomatology and subsequently tested positive for the novel virus. The ship was thus placed in quarantine. From the information collected, it was clear then that substantial transmission of COVID-19 had been occurring before the implementation of quarantine, that the quarantine intervention was effective in reducing transmission among passengers, and that, among contacts, there were asymptomatic cases requiring at least 14 days of isolation to reduce transmission.[24]

Data analysis on patient characteristics is critical for calculations of case fatality, mortality rates, a geo-temporal analysis of viral spread, and an epidemiological curve construction based on location, contacts, disease severity, comorbidity, and geography.[20, 25]

By February 2020, Korea had demonstrated remarkable research capacity by conducting high-throughput COVID-19 testing and utilizing innovative drive-through sampling. These measures for early detection and the screening of cases should have been followed by full global efforts to produce research-based evidence by thoroughly analyzing epidemiological, clinical, and immunologic data, which would facilitate the development of vaccines and therapeutics for COVID-19. However, there was no globally directed, concerted effort in place to facilitate the coordination. Korea was a key global partner in COVID-19 research and actively participated in the development of immediate and mid-/long-term priorities, which was jointly led by WHO partners.

Figure 1.4 illustrates the emergence of SARS-CoV-2 in Europe and the United States, mapping the path followed by infected travelers from China.[17] This identification of the various transmission networks was essential for the later demonstration of the effectiveness of countermeasures for the spread of the disease, including testing, isolation, quarantine, and air traffic control.

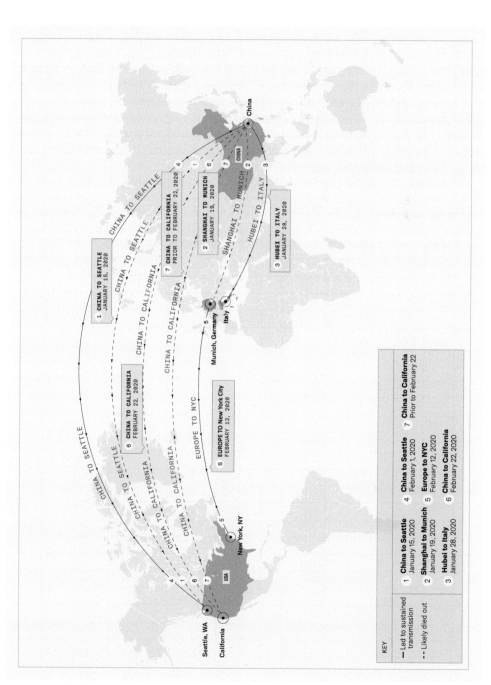

Figure 1.4 SARS-CoV-2 introductions to the United States and Europe. Credit: Modified from Worobey (2020).[17]

Several clusters of cases were initially identified in 37 European countries, with variability in the incidence rate (IR) and mortality rate (MR) related to the population age and diverse national approaches to the crisis.[16, 26] From February 28 to May 21, 2020, the most severely impacted countries in terms of the IR and MR were Spain, Belgium, Ireland, Sweden, the United Kingdom, Italy, France, and the Netherlands, which had IRs and MRs higher than the European average. While the IR and MR are determined by multiple factors, the lack of initial unity in the various countries' responses to the COVID-19 crisis may have led to some diversity in the numbers of cases and deaths. In Europe, the largest and most serious clusters of COVID-19 cases were in the Lombardy region of Italy in early March. The disease in this region was considered particularly severe owing to the unprecedented number of patients, including healthcare workers, and the very high case-fatality rate among elderly people, despite aggressive containment efforts.

The pandemic unfolded in the United States following the recognition of the first cases on the west coast (Santa Clara, CA, and Seattle, WA), and clusters of infection began developing from people traveling back from the Far East who were infected and showing clinical symptoms. This made it very clear that we were dealing with a pandemic of massive proportions. The exponential growth of reported cases in the United States is indicated in Figure 1.5. The cases reported at that time may have represented only a fraction of the total number of actual cases, as testing and contact tracing were not fully implemented at that time.

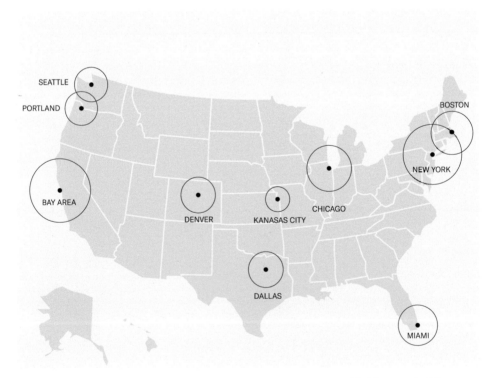

Figure 1.5 Relative infections in the United States as of March 1, 2020. Credit: Modified from *New York Times*, www.nytimes.com/interactive/2020/us/coronavirus-spread.html.

On March 11, 2020, the WHO declared COVID-19 to be a pandemic, with the Director-General declaring "the alarming levels of spread and severity of the outbreak followed by alarming levels of inaction."[26, 27] Soon after, on March 15, 2020, the President of the United States declared COVID-19 to be a national emergency, offering billions of dollars in federal funding to combat the disease.

Pandemic Development and Consolidation

From March 2020 onwards, the pandemic spread globally, affecting different continents, countries, and cultures and impacting society at virtually all levels and types of activities. The spread of COVID-19 skyrocketed in the United States, with the fatality rate reaching 100 000, 300 000, and 1 million deaths by, respectively, May 23, 2020, December 12, 2020, and May 14, 2022.

Public health policies needed to be implemented for isolation, quarantine, and the control of human travel. The enacting of a social lockdown (March 21, 2021, in the United States) that restricted circulation, banned large gatherings, and promoted the closing of schools and business activities resulted in an unprecedented situation in which the entire global community underwent a shutdown that lasted for variable amounts of time, up to several months in some countries. Mechanisms to recognize COVID-19 transmission among presymptomatic and asymptomatic cases were of particular significance. Prompt contact tracing, including close and non-close contact from 2 days before clinical symptoms started, was demonstrated as effective in stopping further transmission.

Early experiments showed that SARS-CoV-2 aerosol and fomite transmission was extremely probable, and that social distancing (of 1 meter or more), the use of face masks (preferably N95) as personal protective equipment (PPE), and the use of eye protection were associated with less infection and could be efficient deterrents of virus spread.[28] Surprisingly, it took over 6 months for the WHO to announce new guidance for the use of face masks (June 7, 2020).

One of the most basic measures for containing a pandemic is identifying infected people and putting measures in place for contact tracing, finding their contacts, and preventing them from infecting others. A major challenge for the United States was to remedy testing gaps by developing and providing nationwide the rapid diagnostic tests that were needed for an accurate diagnosis. The United States quickly rose to the challenge, with the CDC, Food and Drug Administration (FDA), and National Institutes of Health (NIH) working expeditiously to create and finance the bio-network needed to develop appropriate assay diagnostic systems.

The CDC developed protocols to utilize reverse transcriptase PCR as a highly specific diagnostic test. The NIH, working collaboratively with multiple partners across government, academia, and the private sector, created the Rapid Acceleration of Diagnostics (RADx®) initiative (April 29, 2020). The mission of RADx was to accelerate the development, validation, and commercialization of innovative point-of-care and home-based tests. Chapter 7 describes in detail the entire strategy and process to develop appropriate molecular tests for prompt and specific disease diagnosis. The FDA authorized the CDC's test via an Emergency Use Authorization at the end of February 2020 under growing pressure to expand testing capacity. During 2020, 2021, and 2022 and potentially into 2023, many individual Emergency Use Authorizations for antigen and molecular diagnostic tests for SARS-CoV-2 were or are expected to be authorized, as described in Chapter 4. More details on the regulatory steps involved in granting Emergency Use Authorizations can be found in Chapter 10.

To analyze the actions taken by individuals, institutions, communities, local and national governments, and international bodies to suppress or stop the spread of disease, the WHO provides longitudinal public health and social measures (PHSM). The composite PHSM Severity Index expresses the average of six indicators, including wearing face masks; closing schools, offices, businesses, institutions, and operations; and restrictions on gatherings. The PHSM Severity Index has been useful to endorse the implementation of effective measures in areas where there was reluctance toward such measures.

Pandemic Preparedness

It became very evident as the pandemic progressed that no country was fully prepared for an epidemic or pandemic, and there was no consensual, comprehensive, global operational preparedness plan in place to respond to COVID-19, despite multiple efforts by many states and leading governmental organizations.[29] As a result, countermeasures for controlling and preventing disease spread failed or achieved only partial results. Therefore, the Pandemic Response Accountability Committee was created for overseeing and guiding both national and international organizations and stakeholders on operating and synchronizing activities. Many organizations started working on the advancement of national preparedness at the federal, state, private, and academic levels.

One example is the Public Health Emergency Medical Countermeasures Enterprise, which coordinates and collaborates with partners to ensure that medical countermeasures and associated capabilities are available where needed. Another example is the Global Health Security (GHS) Index, which is intended to assess and improve national and international capabilities to address infectious disease outbreaks. Recent GHS Index reports reveal that, while many countries can develop the capabilities to confront a crisis, the majority remain unprepared to face future epidemics and pandemics. Gaps were detected in the level of financial investment, the fitness of the health systems, and the lack of mechanisms to detect outbreaks. In the United States, only 34% of states showed indicators of readiness for state emergency preparedness. Funding being revoked at the state level is in part responsible for some states' poor performance.

There are several federal documents addressing various aspects of the governmental and administrative management of the crisis. For instance, the Pandemic Response Accountability Committee provides information on and strategies for how federal government funding for pandemic programs can be allocated, resources/monies can be appropriated, and spending can be tracked. The committee was established to promote transparency and coordinate oversight of the pandemic response.

The White House released the *National Strategy for the COVID-19 Response and Pandemic Preparedness*, a document produced by the federal government to coordinate the pandemic response across all federal departments and agencies and improve the effectiveness of our fight against COVID-19. This is a comprehensive document covering many aspects of the COVID-19 crisis and defining government participation, but with less emphasis on operational protocols.[29]

Crisis in the Health-Care System

The abrupt eruption of cases with severe disease placed tremendous pressure on health and hospital systems, as first seen in Italy.[30, 31] The medical community had to adapt to the crisis and develop capabilities to assist thousands, if not millions, of patients requiring special management, starting with isolation, transmission containment, monitoring disease severity, and critical care in intensive care units. Chapter 3 meticulously describes the impact of the numbers of patients with COVID-19 on emergency medicine and health-care organization in general in the United States.

The medical supply chain, which provides essential tools, medical supplies, medication, and PPE, was under tremendous strain to comply with increasing demands. The challenge for the network was to quickly develop efficient new production lines of products and services while lacking guidelines on allocation and distribution amidst changing regulations and pricing. Medical and surgical attention for all non-COVID-19 illnesses were limited, which resulted in delays in diagnostic and therapeutic interventions, including cancelations. Waiting lists for non-COVID-19 conditions soon reached millions of patients worldwide, and it is estimated that the waiting list will only be cleared by the end of 2023.

Disease Origin: Zoonotic Transference

With millions of people dead and even more hospitalized due to SARS-CoV-2, the burning question is: Where did this disease come from? All data at the time of writing this book suggest that SARS-CoV-2 originated from a zoonotic source. The WHO defines zoonosis as any disease or infection that is naturally transmissible from vertebrate animals to humans.[32] The disease or infection can be passed from an animal to a human through direct contact (saliva, urine, blood, etc.), indirect contact (contact with the animal's home [e.g. aquarium water or chicken coop]), or vector-borne (e.g. an insect bite), waterborne, or foodborne sources.

Zoonotic transference poses a large public health threat, as there is a close relationship between humans and animals in agriculture, in zoological settings, as domestic pets, and in nature. Scientists have estimated that three out of every four emerging infectious diseases have come from a zoonotic source. To strengthen this theory, and in trying to understand the source of the new virus, a researcher at the Fred Hutchinson Cancer Center investigated the virus's evolution and identified a dataset containing SARS-CoV-2 sequences from early in the Wuhan epidemic. He was then able to reconstruct partial sequences of early viruses and concluded that they likely contained three mutations relative to the market viruses that made these sequences more similar to the bat coronavirus relatives of SARS-CoV-2.[33]

More recently, studies on the distribution within the Wuhan market of animals susceptible to being infected with SARS-CoV-2 and humans infected with SARS-CoV-2 revealed that there was a spatial relative risk, even though it was not possible to establish a direct correlation. Because of the prevalence of cases and the disease distribution among the Wuhan population, it is understood that the Wuhan South China Seafood Market was the early epicenter of the COVID-19 pandemic.[19, 34–36] However, as mentioned earlier, some studies have shown that SARS-CoV-2 was already circulating before December 2019, and so it has also been proposed that the seafood market was a consequence, rather than the source, of the SARS-CoV-2 virus.[21, 36]

Recent human coronaviruses, SARS-CoV and MERS-CoV, have been caused by zoonotic transmission. In 2003, SARS-CoV emerged through zoonotic spillover at a live animal market in China's Guangdong province. Antibodies against SARS-CoV were detected in animals being sold at the market: masked palm civets and raccoon dogs. Further research discovered that the masked palm civets and raccoon dogs were most likely intermediate hosts, with the disease originating from horseshoe bats (*Rhinolophus affinis*), a species demonstrating a 99.8% nucleotide match with the human isolates. MERS-CoV is another human coronavirus likely originating from bats, as the disease has been detected in 14 distinct bat species. Anti-MERS-CoV antibodies have been isolated in camels in the Middle East, Africa, and Asia. Thus, the likely intermediate host between bats and humans for MERS-CoV has been identified as camels.

SARS-CoV-2 has been detected in several species, but no animal reservoir has been documented. It has been suggested that the most likely source of SARS-CoV-2 is the horseshoe bat species. Studies have found that there is about a 96% nucleotide identity match between the coronaviruses of humans and horseshoe bats (RaTG13 GenBank: MN996532.1). Additionally, phylogenetic analyses of a large subgenomic dataset of bat coronaviruses from China further support the claim that SARS-CoV and SARS-CoV-2 both likely originated in horseshoe bats. As humans do not commonly come into close contact with bats, the transmission to humans likely occurred through an intermediate host. This intermediate host would need to be one more commonly handled by humans, such as a domestic animal, livestock, or a domesticated wild animal. At the time of writing, no intermediate host for SARS-CoV-2 has been identified.

Reverse Zoonosis and Secondary Zoonosis

While the search for the zoonotic host continues, it is important to conduct research in parallel into which other animal species are susceptible to SARS-CoV-2 infection. This research will help epidemiologists better prevent secondary zoonotic events (transmission of the infection from animals back to humans) and possible reverse zoonosis (also referred to as zooanthroponosis: the transmission of the infection from humans to animals).[37, 38]

There have been several cases of dogs, cats, and zoo animals testing positive for SARS-CoV-2 in countries such as Belgium, France, Spain, Germany, the United States, and Hong Kong.[39, 40] Clinical manifestations in animals have ranged from asymptomatic to severe respiratory illness. When symptoms are present, they can include coughing, sneezing, respiratory distress, nasal discharge, ocular discharge, vomiting, diarrhea, fever, and lethargy. Although there is no definitive evidence that dogs, cats, or zoo animals can transmit SARS-CoV-2 to humans, it is important to be cautious of how the virus may behave in other animal species. For this reason, increased continuous monitoring and planned targeted surveillance of high-risk animals and their caretakers should be implemented at local and national levels.

There is not enough SARS-CoV-2 testing currently being done for companion and zoo animals. It is important to note that IDEXX Laboratories in the United States has released a diagnostic test, "SARS-CoV-2 (COVID-19) Real PCR Test," for screening companion animals. Serological assays and nucleic acid-based tests for the diagnosis of SARS-CoV-2 in domestic and zoo animals are also being developed and used by several other private and government veterinary laboratories.

Zoonotic Monitoring

As explained previously, controlling and monitoring zoonosis is critical for responding quickly and effectively to emerging infectious diseases. Several organizations controlling and monitoring zoonosis include the:

- CDC National Center for Emerging and Zoonotic Infectious Diseases
- CDC Division of High-Consequence Pathogens and Pathology
- National Animal Health Laboratory Network
- WHO Scientific Advisory Group for the Origins of Novel Pathogens
- World Organisation for Animal Health

These organizations collectively constitute a network through which new infectious agents are communicated and possible zoonosis reservoirs are monitored that represent a risk of epidemics and pandemics to humans. Furthermore, the Global Virome Project is an international initiative to map zoonotic viruses around the world through the creation of a database of animal viruses. In many ways, this project parallels the Human Genome Project, which has revolutionized our understanding of human diseases.

Therefore, the next question to ask ourselves is: What should we do in anticipation or even for the prevention of an upcoming pandemic? As the major source of novel infectious agents is zoonosis, comprehensive monitoring of animals for detecting zoonosis at the preemergence stage would be ideal, that is, at the stage when the disease is still in its natural reservoir before being transmitted to humans. However, given the high number of animal species and novel agents continuously emerging, this strategy would be extremely difficult, costly, and practically impossible to carry out to its full extent. Nevertheless, pandemic threat programs are emerging that aim to prevent pandemics at the source before they infect humans. These programs are based on the building of health-care capacity, surveillance and diagnostic programs, and the implementation of predictive disease modeling. Another important tool in zoonotic monitoring is viral molecular sequencing, which can provide useful information about virus dynamics, such as the viral mutation rate and the detection of selective sequences compatible with human receptors that can facilitate infection of human tissues. While these recent advancements are useful for monitoring and controlling the spread of infectious diseases, additional research and resources are needed to fully assess the dangers of zoonotic transmission.

A mathematical model developed to simulate potential hotspots of future viral sharing under climate change and land-use scenarios for 2070 predicted that species will aggregate in new combinations at high elevations, in biodiversity hotspots, and in areas of high human population density in Asia and Africa, driving the novel cross-species transmission of their viruses an estimated 4 000 times.[41, 42] The model identified bats as the most likely mammal to share viruses along evolutionary pathways that will facilitate future emergence in humans.

Surveillance

From February 2020 to the present, an extraordinary surge of information has pervaded communications across the medical, scientific, epidemiological, statistical, social, and financial fields. Information provided in different formats – from recognized professional journals to media news – has helped enormously in the understanding, management, and control of the pandemic crisis.[42] Nevertheless, the analytical processing, interpretation, archiving, and overall evaluation of the current pandemic, as well as of future pandemics, is still under scrutiny and will require profound analysis before being incorporated as pre-scribed pandemic preparedness protocols.[43]

The epidemiological and clinical characteristics of COVID-19 were further clarified by a landmark communication in *The Lancet* in 2020, with the clinical description of 99 patients with COVID-19, 49 of whom had a history of exposure to the Wuhan South China Seafood Market.[25] This revealed the importance of rapid communication and the publication of all types of information related to pandemic evolution.[42, 43] Around this time, the major publishers and university presses opened their archives with regard to articles related to COVID-19, a fortunate decision that helped tremendously in understanding the 2019 outbreak and in the decision-making process to develop appropriate diagnostic tools and countermeasures.

The implementation and management of effective surveillance systems are essential for early detection and effective responses to emerging infectious diseases.[39] Surveillance systems provide officials with an understanding of when, where, and in which demographics an infectious disease is being transmitted. The data from surveillance systems are then used to inform decisions surrounding countermeasures, controls, prevention, and patient man-agement. Inaccurate or incomplete data can drastically impact decision-making and poten-tially place people at higher risk of severe disease.

Surveillance has been a pillar of public health systems since the first recorded epidemic in Egypt in 3180 BC.[43] Since then, surveillance has evolved with each epidemic and pandemic, including the first public health action as a result of surveillance during the 1348 bubonic plague epidemic, commonly coined the "Black Death," when public health officials imposed the first quarantine by refusing the entrance of ships with infected passengers. More recently, we have seen both the strong and the weak points of our current surveillance systems through the COVID-19 pandemic.

One of the most vital data points tracked through the surveillance system is the number of cases. This information can be used to determine incidence (the number of new cases in a specific period), prevalence (the number of cases at one specific point in time), hospital-ization (the number of cases resulting in the hospitalization of the patient), and deaths (the number of cases resulting in death). Based on WHO guidance, the minimum testing rate should be maintained as 1 person tested per 1 000 population per week to ensure sufficient data collection.

Additionally, the WHO suggests that strong surveillance systems include:

- immediate notification of changes in epidemiological patterns
- tracking of morbidity and mortality statistics
- calculation and monitoring of disease impact on health-care capacity, including hospitalizations, intensive care unit admissions, the financial health-care burden, and the number of health-care workers
- monitoring of variants through strategic and geographic genomic surveillance
- effective monitoring of potential animal reservoirs
- special studies (on the impact on high-risk groups, the characterization of new variants, and long COVID)
- monitoring of vaccination doses when available; this should include both primary series and boosters

The delay between data collecting and analysis and the absence of data reporting from at-home testing are two significant challenges facing our current surveillance systems. For the most effective disease predictions and decisions, data must be analyzed in real time. One potential solution is to develop and deploy an electronic case-reporting system that would supply data seamlessly from a health-care provider's electronic health record to a public health agency. These systems should be implemented both nationally and globally before the next pandemic.

A unique characteristic of the COVID-19 pandemic was the unprecedented number of at-home diagnostic tests being performed. This was a major accomplishment in slowing the spread of COVID-19, but it did impose difficulties in tracking the tests performed and the confirmed cases, as individuals were not required to report their results. Many individuals who tested positive on an at-home test had a confirmatory test done at a health-care facility, and these confirmatory tests were required to be reported. However, those who tested negative at home were not required to report and thus there was the possibility of overinflation of the positivity rate. Most at-home tests do have a reporting component for individuals to report their results, whether it be a mobile application or a website, but this is not often used. Further changes need to be made to address issues surrounding the lack of at-home reporting and the potential subsequent positivity rate inflation.

Scientists in California developed a nanobeads technique that allowed the identification of coronavirus strains circulating in a community up to 14 days earlier. This technique applied PCR to sewage and could become an early warning system to be used in surveillance.[44, 45] According to the study published in *Nature*, the use of the nanobeads technique increases the amount of viral ribonucleic acid (RNA) that can be sequenced from a wastewater sample from 40% to nearly 95%.[44] In addition, the California team also developed a method that allows the identification of the variants present in each wastewater sample and a determination of their concentrations.

The use of machine learning as a tool to extract concealed information patterns, mine huge raw datasets, and establish high-quality clinical predictive models has proven to be very helpful. Similarly, digital medicine and artificial intelligence programs supporting data analysis and decision processes of clinical, genomics, and even sociocultural information have been successfully introduced through the COVID-19 pandemic.

Surveillance took several different formats across multiple media during the COVID-19 pandemic. This was largely due to many professional and nonprofessional media and government agencies advocating for the collection of critical information. The CDC is a leading surveillance institution in the United States. The CDC plays a key role in issues related to emerging infections by developing and implementing infectious disease surveillance and laboratory activities and providing an initial rapid response capability. A short example of the different survey programs conducted by different organizations/groups and potential benefits to disease control are listed in Table 1.2.

Progressing from Response to Pandemic Control

The main strategies to manage the pandemic have evolved since the initial phases of the crisis. Currently, the approach is based on the combination of control measures directed at creating global immunity, primarily through effective vaccination, monitoring the emergence of new variants, and assessing pandemic progression through the appearance of new outbreaks, breakthrough infections, and the impact of long COVID.

Table 1.2 Epidemiological parameters helpful for characterizing emerging pandemics

Epidemiological parameter	Organization/tool that measures the parameter	Purpose/benefits
Emergence of new zoonotic and vector-borne diseases	• CDC National Center for Emerging and Zoonotic Infectious Diseases (NCEZID) • WHO COVID-19 IHR Emergency Committee • Coronaviridae Study Group (CSG) of the International Committee on Taxonomy of Viruses (ICTV)	Early identification of possible zoonotic emergence and the exact mechanism responsible for its initial transmission
Case information	• National Notifiable Diseases Surveillance System (NNDSS) • CDC COVID Data Tracker • District Health Information Software (DHIS2) • Surveillance, Outbreak Response Management and Analysis System (SORMAS®) • Go.Data • Epi Info™	Detection of subclinical and asymptomatic infections Monitoring for typical symptoms, atypical symptoms, and complications
Laboratory diagnostic tools (monitoring test results)	• RADx program • Diagnostic industry • Laboratory design tests	Improvement of the accuracy of diagnostics and the introduction of new technologies and diagnostic systems
Tracking and monitoring disease	• CDC, WHO, and national, state, and county health departments • COVID-19 dashboard of the Johns Hopkins University • Community and social organizations	Statistic information on basic epidemiological parameters such as prevalence, hospitalization, death rate, and demographic information
Novel disease contact tracing	• Detect study by Scripps Research Digital Trials Center and The Rockefeller University • Use of artificial intelligence and expert systems	Early detection of clinical manifestations, such as fever
Social and cultural response, such as willingness to accept a COVID-19 vaccine	• Multiple official and nongovernmental organizations and community organizations	Essential for pandemic control, disease management, and transmission reduction

Table 1.2 (cont.)

Epidemiological parameter	Organization/tool that measures the parameter	Purpose/benefits
Immune protection at public and individual levels	• Health departments, international organizations, and university hospital diagnostic centers	Antibody levels induced by vaccination and/or natural immunity following viral infection
	• Serology surveillance (or antibody) testing	Establishing seroprevalence in a population and uncovering missed infections
Vaccination monitoring	• CDC COVID-19 vaccine reporting systems	Vaccination distribution
	• WHO	Monitoring vaccine safety and effectiveness
	• American Medical Association	Vaccine concerns, government control
	• Various national and international organizations	

Challenges for the global control of COVID-19 remain at the forefront of anti-COVID-19 activities and countermeasures. Testing still plays a major role in pandemic control. However, despite the hundreds of brands of tests available, difficulties with testing remain in many areas, particularly in low- and middle-income countries, due to a lack of infrastructure for countermeasure implementation and global competitive pricing for access to diagnostic kits and supplies.

Studies on the effectiveness of testing have expanded to areas such as diagnostics in clinical practice, screening of populations at an increased risk of acquisition and transmission, and public health in terms of testing travelers, testing in schools, and testing large communities. The impact of home tests and over-the-counter kits has been quite significant in terms of increasing the numbers of asymptomatic individuals taking tests and confirmed cases. Furthermore, comprehensive contact-tracing programs with testing and effective isolation or quarantine have been crucial for successful outbreak control.[46]

WHO COVID-19 Dashboard

One example of a publicly available surveillance system is the WHO COVID-19 dashboard, which has provided official daily counts of COVID-19 cases, deaths, and vaccine utilization reported by countries, territories, and areas since early 2020. Data interpretation, especially at the early stage of a pandemic, needs to be taken as a partial overview of the developing pandemic, because the data provided by some countries may be incomplete or of variable integrity. While steps are taken to ensure accuracy and reliability, all data are subject to continuous verification and change. Despite some deficits, the WHO dashboard has been very useful for clinical management, monitoring pandemic evolution, and measuring the effectiveness of vaccination programs. At the time of writing of this book, there are **769 774 646** confirmed cases of COVID-19, including **6 955 141** deaths (as of August 25, 2023). A total of **13 498 570 620** vaccine doses have been administered (as of August 25, 2023). Updated global data are available at covid19.who.int.

Surveillance of pandemic parameters conducted at various phases helped to assess the COVID-19 pandemic evolution, decode processes of transmission, and control spreading. Modifications and adaptations of surveillance programs were necessary to respond to evolving needs through the various pandemic phases (i.e. from antibody and PCR testing to adverse events following immunization and the acceptance of vaccination). Surveys of the multiple social, medical/scientific, epidemiological, and environmental components require significant participation of public health systems and cooperation with government and political organizations. While the information gained in the initial phases was very useful, at the same time, informal or poorly structured and conducted surveys provided information of lesser quality. Overall, the major constraints were associated with data collection, analysis, interpretation, and, more importantly, data integration and distribution. The latter remains a major challenge and certainly needs to be strongly considered during future pandemic and epidemic conditions.

What Went Wrong?

Reflections on the events of the COVID-19 pandemic – the largest medical-social global crisis of modern times – provides great insights into the areas that were successful and those that failed. A prime example of such reflection on a global scale can be seen in the IPPPR's May 2021 report.[47] The IPPPR is an independent panel that was established in May 2020 by the WHO Director-General to construct an evidence-based course for the future based on lessons learned from the past and present to ensure that nations and international organizations, specifically the WHO, successfully address health risks.

The IPPPR's May 2021 report outlined key errors within the COVID-19 pandemic response:

- Warning signs from previous pandemics were ignored. These included the SARS-CoV epidemic (2003), the H1N1 influenza pandemic (2009), the Ebola outbreak in West Africa (2014–2016), and the Zika virus and MERS-CoV outbreaks. The SARS-CoV outbreak led to an update of the IHR in 2005. Several recommendations added to the 2005 IHR were never implemented.
- Pandemic preparedness was underfunded. A great opportunity exists to improve the capacities and capabilities of underserved populations.
- No appropriate system of zoonotic disease surveillance was implemented. The necessity of such a system is heightened, as most new pathogens are zoonotic in origin due to increasing deforestation for land use and food production.

The message from the WHO when declaring the PHEIC fell short of communicating the severity of the COVID-19 threat. As a consequence, the international response was divided: proactive countries were successful and those that denied and delayed were unsuccessful. The declaration of a PHEIC did not lead to an urgent, coordinated, worldwide response. The IPPPR concluded that February 2020 was a lost month of opportunity to contain the outbreak. There was a worldwide shortage of equipment, supplies, diagnostic tests, funds, and workforce, which led to health-care systems and health-care workers not being properly prepared to face a prolonged crisis. The bureaucracy of many governments was too slow, with governments taking actions only when the WHO declared a pandemic. The panel stressed that measures could and should have been taken to eradicate the epidemic and prevent the pandemic.

Successful vaccine development with initial shortages introduced vaccine nationalism, leading to high-income countries purchasing doses to cover 200% of their population, while the program COVAX – launched by the WHO and partners to equitably deliver vaccines – failed to achieve its goal.

Among other recommendations, the IPPPR report highlighted the need for an improved system for surveillance and alerts that works at a speed that can combat viruses such as SARS-CoV-2. The report also recommended that authority be given to the WHO to publish information and dispatch expert missions immediately.[47]

At the national level, the United States was lacking a national strategic pandemic plan that was subscribed to by major stakeholders, including multiple government agencies; health-care, public health, and professional organizations; industry; and socially relevant entities. Such a national plan should clearly define the capabilities, capacities, and responsibilities of operating groups and the coordination of the various components.

As the COVID-19 pandemic progressed, many new challenges arose. Thus, in addition to an initial national pandemic plan, a committee needs to be established to monitor and synchronize pandemic-related policies.

A lack of strong leadership was revealed at multiple levels, both internationally and at the domestic level, by the delayed response and implementation of countermeasures. The mismanagement of human circulation with poor control of air traffic and trade activities failed to stop the virus from spreading soon after the outbreak. Additionally, leadership was varied in terms of public health communications, with messaging often conflicting.

Finally, pandemic education was lacking in many populations. Pandemic education should provide correct and accurate information on disease countermeasures. This information can be delivered through social media and diverse instruction campaigns at work sites, schools, churches, and community centers. Strong education programs on vaccine benefits are particularly needed to counterbalance negative opinions on vaccinology that have been so detrimental to society. Can COVID-19 vaccination perception change and become a social norm in the same way that society has adopted wearing seatbelts, stopping at red lights, wearing bike helmets, and living in smoke-free environments? In the same way that these behaviors have become social norms, we need society to view COVID-19 vaccination as another such social norm before full global vaccination can be reached. It should also be remembered that smallpox and poliomyelitis were globally controlled and are in the process of eradication thanks to vaccination.

Lessons Learned

Recognizing the failures presented in the previous section, we must now look toward implementing the following lessons learned to prevent these failures in the future:

- aim for early recognition of infectious ailments with unique clinical manifestations different from known diseases
- monitor symptomatology and gather all clinical information to develop databases
- report all suspicious or confirmed infectious diseases immediately to health authorities and international health forums
- attempt to identify and isolate the agent microorganism(s)
- identify the origin of clusters of cases
- assess disease infectivity and human-to-human transmission

- promote and implement sanitary measures and recommendations, starting from universal countermeasures
- establish surveillance systems of the severity of the outbreak and its impact on health at individual and social levels
- provide clear control indications based on the emergent conditions of the disease
- upon declaration of a pandemic, consider the spread of disease and transmission to different geographies and continents
- develop surveillance programs in different areas related to patient care, disease spread, control countermeasures, diagnostics, therapies, and vaccination programs, and secure appropriate data analysis, integration, interpretation, and broad distribution as required
- set up pandemic/endemic oversight committees at the national and international levels to manage information, announcements, and countermeasures for disease control
- promote information notification and diffusion among different countries and communities
- maintain the fitness of health systems to meet the health needs associated with the crisis
- develop robust programs of pandemic control in coordination with national and international health organizations (the WHO, CDC, CCDC, the UK health system, and country health ministries)
- demonstrate robust leadership by prominent representatives of the various crisis constituents and elected and nonelected governmental officials through strong commitment and conviction
- develop strong policies to tackle inequalities – the COVID-19 pandemic demonstrated how rich countries put their interests ahead of those of low- and middle-income countries, putting "their relationship with the big pharma ahead of ending this pandemic."[48]

References

1. Q. Li, X. Guan, P. Wu, et al., Early transmission dynamics in Wuhan, China, of novel coronavirus-infected pneumonia. *N Engl J Med*, **382**, 13 (2020), 1199–1207.

2. N. Xiang, F. Havers, T. Chen, et al., Use of national pneumonia surveillance to describe influenza A(H7N9) virus epidemiology, China, 2004–2013. *Emerg Infect Dis*, **19** (2013), 1784–1790.

3. Congressional Research Service, COVID-19 and China: A Chronology of Events (December 2019–January 2020). Updated May 13, 2020 (2020). https://crsreports.congress.gov/product/pdf/r/r46354 (accessed November 20, 2022).

4. Wikipedia, Li Wenliang (2023). https://en.wikipedia.org/wiki/Li_Wenliang (accessed June 23, 2022).

5. K. Huang, World Health Organisation in touch with Beijing after mystery viral pneumonia outbreak, *South China Morning Post* (January 1, 2020). https://tinyurl.com/yup3a8rs (accessed June 14, 2023).

6. World Health Organization, Pneumonia cases in China's Wuhan could be due to a new type of virus, WHO news article (January 9, 2020). https://tinyurl.com/4942ejhd (accessed February 7, 2020).

7. N. Khan, New virus discovered by Chinese scientists investigating pneumonia outbreak, *The Wall Street Journal* (January 8, 2020). https://tinyurl.com/5dve5nh4 (accessed February 8, 2020).

8. Y. Z. Zhang, Novel 2019 coronavirus genome, *Virological* (2020). https:/

virological.org/t/novel-2019-coronavirus-genome-/319 (accessed June 23, 2022).

9. National Library of Medicine, Severe acute respiratory syndrome coronavirus 2 isolate Wuhan-Hu-1, complete genome, National Library of Medicine (2022). www.ncbi.nlm.nih.gov/nuccore/1798174254 (accessed June 23, 2022).

10. F. Wu, S. Zhao, B. Yu, et al., A new coronavirus associated with human respiratory disease in China. *Nature*, **579**, 7798 (2020), 265–269.

11. Wuhan Municipal Health Commission, Bulletin on the situation regarding viral pneumonia of unknown cause (January 5, 2020). http://wjw.wuhan.gov.cn/front/web/showDetail/2020010509020 (no longer available).

12. H. J. Chang, Estimation of basic reproduction number of the Middle East respiratory syndrome coronavirus (MERS-CoV) during the outbreak in South Korea, 2015. *Biomed Eng Online*, **16**, 1 (2017), 79.

13. J. C. Lindstrøma, S. Engebretsen, A. B. Kristoffersen, et al., Increased transmissibility of the alpha SARS-CoV-2 variant: evidence from contact tracing data in Oslo, January to February 2021. *Infect Dis (Lond)*, **54**, 1 (2022), 72–77.

14. Y. Liu and J. Rocklöv, The reproductive number of the Delta variant of SARS-CoV-2 is far higher compared to the ancestral SARS-CoV-2 virus. *J Travel Med*, **28**, 7 (2021), table 1.

15. M. Gjorgjievska, S. Mehandziska, A. Stajkovska, et al., Case report: Omicron BA.2 subvariant of SARS-CoV-2 outcompetes BA.1 in two co-infection cases. *Front Genet*, **13** (2022), 892682.

16. Y. Fan, X. Li, L. Zhang, et al., SARS-CoV-2 Omicron variant: recent progress and future perspectives. *Sig Transduct Target Ther*, 7, 1 (2022), 141.

17. M. Worobey, J. Pekar, B. B. Larsen, et al., The emergence of SARS-CoV-2 in Europe and North America. *Science*, **3070**, 6516 (2020), 564–570.

18. S. Chen, J. Yang, W. Yang, W. Wang, and T. Barnighausen, COVID-19 control in China during mass population movements at New Year. *Lancet (Lond)*, **395**, 10226 (2020), 764–766.

19. J. Cohen, Wuhan seafood market may not be source of novel virus spreading globally, *Science Insider* (January 26, 2020). https://tinyurl.com/mrxu6wd5 (accessed January 20, 2023).

20. The Novel Coronavirus Pneumonia Emergency Response Epidemiology Team, Vital surveillances: the epidemiological characteristics of an outbreak of 2019 novel coronavirus diseases (COVID-19) – China, 2020. China CDC Weekly, 2, 8 (2020), 113–122. https://doi.org/10.46234/ccdcw2020.032.

21. S. Kumar, O. Tao, S. Weaver, et al., An evolutionary portrait of the progenitor SARS-CoV-2 and its dominant offshoots in COVID-19 pandemic. *Mol Biol Evol*, **38**, 8 (2021), 3046–3059.

22. Y. Jee, WHO international health regulations emergency committee for the COVID-19 outbreak. *Epidemiol Health*, **42** (2020), e2020013.

23. Independent Panel for Pandemic Preparedness and Response, Main report and documents, The Independent Panel (2023). https://theindependentpanel.org/documents/ (accessed January 20, 2023).

24. National Institute of Infectious Diseases, Field briefing: Diamond Princess COVID-19 cases (2020). www.niid.go.jp/niid/en/2019-ncov-e/9407-covid-dp-fe-01.html (accessed January 20, 2023).

25. N. Chen, M. Zhou, X. Dong, et al., Epidemiological and clinical characteristics of 99 cases of 2019 novel coronavirus pneumonia in Wuhan, China: a descriptive study. *Lancet*, **395**, 10223 (2020), 507–513.

26. H. Zach, M. Hanová, and M. Letkovičová, Distribution of COVID-19 cases and deaths in Europe during the first 12 peak weeks of the outbreak. *Cent Eur J Public Health*, **29**, 1 (2021), 9–13.

27. D. K. Chu, E. A. Akl, S. Duda, et al., Physical distancing, face masks, and eye protection to prevent person-to-person transmission of SARS-CoV-2 and COVID-19: a systematic review and meta-analysis. *Lancet*, **395**, 10242 (2020), 1973–1987.

28. World Health Organization, Coronavirus Disease 2019 (COVID-19) Situation Report – 53 (2020). https://tinyurl.com/25 64hs7j (accessed January 20, 2023).

29. The White House, National Strategy for the COVID-19 Response and Pandemic Preparedness (2021). https://tinyurl.com/y peyuaju (accessed January 20, 2023).

30. A. Remuzzi and G. Remuzzi, COVID-19 and Italy: what next? *Lancet*, **395**, 10231 (2020), 1225–1228.

31. G. Onder, G. Rezza, and S. Brusaferro, Case-fatality rate and characteristics of patients dying in relation to COVID-19 in Italy. *JAMA*, **323**, 18 (2020), 1775–1776.

32. World Health Organization, Zoonoses (July 29, 2020). www.who.int/news-room/ fact-sheets/detail/zoonoses (accessed January 20, 2023).

33. J. D. Bloom, Recovery of deleted deep sequencing data sheds more light on the early Wuhan SARS-CoV-2 epidemic. *Mol Biol Evol*, **38**, 12 (2021), 5211–5224.

34. K. G. Andersen, A. Rambaut, W. I. Lipkin, E. C. Homes, and R. F. Garry The proximal origin of SARS-CoV-2. *Nat Med* 2020, **26** (4): 450–452.

35. C. Huang, U. Wang, X. Li, et al., Clinical features of patients infected with 2019 novel coronavirus in Wuhan, China. *Lancet*, **395**, 10223 (2020), 497–506.

36. M. Worobey, J. I. Levy, L. M. Serrano, et al., The Huanan Seafood Wholesale Market in Wuhan was the early epicenter of the COVID-19 pandemic. *Science*, **377**, 6609 (2022), 951–959.

37. I. V. Goraichuk, V. Arefiev, B. T. Stegniy, A. P. Gerilovych, Zoonotic and reverse zoonotic transmissibility of SARS-CoV-2. *Virus Res*, **302** (2021), 198473.

38. K. Munir, S. Ashraf, I. Munir, et al., Zoonotic and reverse zoonotic events of SARS-CoV-2 and their impact on global health. *Emerg Microbes Infect*, **9**, 1 (2020), 2222–2235.

39. World Health Organization, Public health surveillance for Covid-19: interim guidance (July 22, 2022). https://tinyurl .com/2pakdfus (accessed January 20, 2023).

40. C. J. Carlson, G. F. Albery, C. Merow, et al., Climate change increases cross-species viral transmission risk. *Nature*, **607**, 7919 (2022), 555–562.

41. J. D. Sachs, S. S. Abdool Karim, L. Aknin, et al., The Lancet Commission on lessons for the future from the COVID-19 pandemic. *Lancet*, **400**, 10359 (2022), 1224–1280.

42. B. Kufferschmidt, "A completely new culture of doing research." Coronavirus outbreak changes how scientists communicate (February 26, 2020). https:// tinyurl.com/54zk68nu (accessed January 20, 2023).

43. B. C. Choi and A. W. Pak, Lessons for surveillance in the 21st century: a historical perspective from the past five millennia. *Soz Präventivmed*, **46**, 6 (2001), 361–368.

44. S. Karthikeyan, J. I. Levy, P. De Hoff, et al., Wastewater sequencing reveals early cryptic SARS-CoV-2 variant transmission. *Nature*, **609**, 7925 (2022), 101–108.

45. G. Bonanno Ferraro, C. Veneri, P. Mancini, et al., A state-of-the-art scoping review on SARS-CoV-2 in sewage focusing on the potential of wastewater surveillance for the monitoring of the COVID-19 pandemic. *Food Environ Virol*, **14**, 4 (2022), 315–354.

46. R. W. Peeling, D. L. Heymann, Y. Y. Teo, and P. J. Garcia, Diagnostics for COVID-19: moving from pandemic response to control. *Lancet*, **399**, 10326 (2022), 757–768.

47. The Independent Panel for Pandemic Preparedness and Response, An evidence-based quest to protect human health (2023). https://theindependentpanel.org/ (accessed December 29, 2022).

48. E. Mahase, Covid-19: rich countries are putting "relationships with big pharma" ahead of ending pandemic, says Oxfam. *BMJ*, **373** (2021), n1342.

Immunology of COVID-19 and Ineffective Immunity

Adolfo Firpo-Betancourt and Enrique M. Rabellino

Introduction

Immunology is the study of immunity, namely the condition of being protected from infection by a pathogenic microorganism, including a virus. The study of immunity enables us to improve our understanding of how our bodies resist infectious diseases and lends an effective and broad perspective to medical research, biology, chemistry, and population health.

As described in this chapter, the immune response to severe acute respiratory syndrome coronavirus 2 (SARS-CoV-2) is known to involve several immune system components for viral elimination and recovery from the infection. As we seek to better understand the pathophysiological responses of the human body to this virus, we can better identify those at risk of infection and those for whom the disease will be more severe and possibly lethal. Additionally, a better understanding of immunity (or lack of it) could shed light on the risk of recurrent infections and the long-term complications of infection.

Ultimately, we aim to anticipate the natural progression of the virus among different patient subgroups and explore ways to enhance the immune system to induce effective immunity. By further understanding COVID-19 immunopathogenesis, we can continue to design more effective diagnostic, therapeutic, and prophylactic strategies.

SARS-CoV-2 Immune Response

In this chapter, we focus on a selected few key components in the immune responses to SARS-CoV-2. We follow the viral infection of susceptible cells in the respiratory tract, the spread of viral infection, and the possible ways infection may progress to clinical disease expression. We also touch upon immune responses elicited by vaccination to induce host adaptive immunity specific against the agent and to control the infection's spread. We will frequently refer to various components of SARS-CoV-2, as shown in Figure 2.2.

SARS-CoV-2 Entry into a Cell

SARS-CoV-2 infections occur when contact occurs between a susceptible cell and the SARS-CoV-2 virus. This can happen only under several specific conditions, all of which are influenced by the amount of virus exposure and its duration.

For SARS-CoV-2, the conditions are as follows:

1. Infective viral particles must contact an exposed cell surface that expresses an angiotensin-converting enzyme 2 (ACE2) receptor molecule

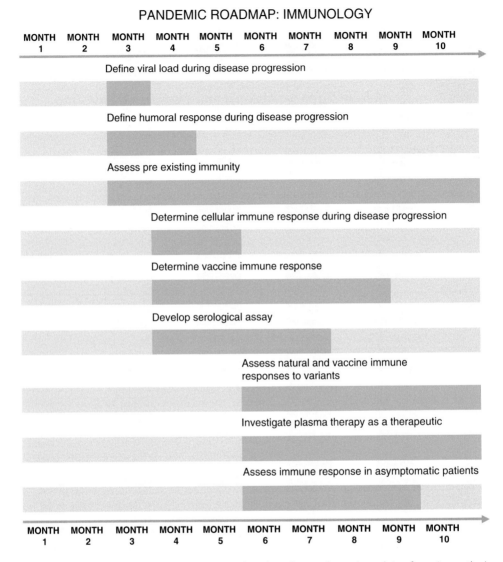

Figure 2.1 This roadmap depicts the vital activities, their chronology, and an estimated time frame in months. In the case of the SARS-CoV-2 pandemic, month 1 was December 2019, the month in which the virus was isolated, sequenced, identified, and published.

2. The viral particle must orient so that its receptor-binding domain (RBD) region is close enough to a specific region on the ACE2 receptor for the two molecules to bind. The binding occurs through multiple weak van der Waals forces, which collectively produce a strong bond of high affinity between the two molecules at the points of highest complementarity

3. These forces bring the molecules together so that other neighboring molecules on the cell membrane can split the SARS-CoV-2 spike (S) protein. This allows the external

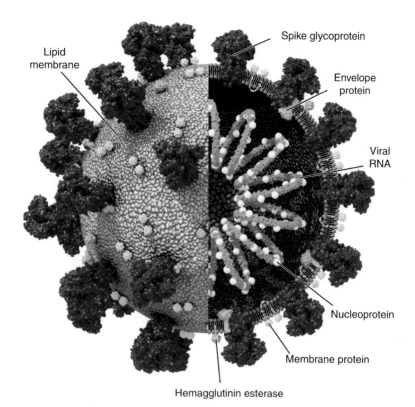

Figure 2.2 SARS-CoV-2 structure.

RNA, ribonucleic acid.

surface of the virus to fuse with the cell membrane so that the viral ribonucleic acid (RNA) enters the cytoplasm of the cell

4. The SARS-CoV-2 genetic material, a single strand of RNA, takes over the metabolic machinery of the infected cell to produce viral proteins and all of the other components necessary to replicate the virus

This sequence constitutes a successful viral infection of the host by SARS-CoV-2. However, more must happen for COVID-19, the clinical expression of SARS-CoV-2 infection, to occur or be prevented from manifesting.

The interactions between the RBD of the viral particle and ACE2 receptor molecules on the cell surface have been studied closely since early 2003 following the severe acute respiratory syndrome coronavirus (SARS-CoV) epidemic in China.

Research on how coronaviruses invade cells intensified in 2012 after the occurrence of a second coronavirus epidemic known as the Middle East respiratory syndrome coronavirus (MERS-CoV). The goal of the research was to discover possible ways to prevent cellular coronavirus infections spreading to others and discover effective and efficient ways for virus elimination from infected hosts and eventually from affected communities.[1]

The unobstructed process and mechanism of SARS-CoV-2 pathogenicity, from attachment to a susceptible cell to intracellular viral replication, is described in Figure 2.3.[2, 3] When

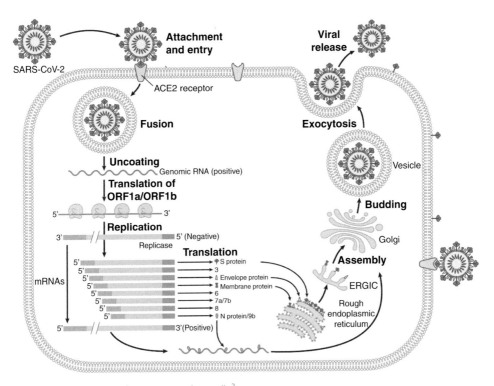

Figure 2.3 The life cycle of SARS-CoV-2 in host cells.[2]
ERGIC, endoplasmic reticulum–Golgi intermediate compartment.

an unvaccinated person or someone previously unexposed to the virus comes into contact with the virus, there is no interferon (IFN) being produced and therefore the infection proceeds unopposed. Viral growth in infected cells eventually triggers the recognition of the virus' distinct molecular patterns, stimulating innate cellular immunity. This produces a cascade of other reactions, resulting in a variable inflammatory response at the site of infection. During the early inflammatory response, chemical mediators of inflammation called cytokines mobilize various cellular elements to fight infection by different means, including the destruction of virally infected cells and the removal of their remains. This process also involves the production and release of regulatory molecules that keep the intensity of the response in check.

Collectively, these events represent an expression of innate immunity, and the effectiveness of these responses influence the host's defense against SARS-CoV-2 during the early stages of infection – they influence how the local spread of SARS-CoV-2 evolves, going on to infect neighboring and distant cells and resulting in increasingly worse outcomes of infection. In addition, in some patients, the production of some cytokines becomes uncontrolled, with cytokines reaching very high levels (known as a cytokine storm), and this has been related to more severe COVID-19 and higher risk of mortality. Together, all of these factors are thought to account for the observed differences in clinical outcomes among different populations.[4]

Overview of the Immune System

The immune system mounts the first defensive response of the body following the colonization or infection by a microorganism or foreign agents. Upon detection of the foreign agents, the immune system activates multiple responses to attack and destroy the invading organism – innate, humoral adaptive, and cell-mediated adaptive responses. These systemic responses often coordinate their approach via signaling pathways, as shown in Figure 2.4.

Innate Immune Response to a SARS-CoV-2 Infection

As the SARS-CoV-2 viral RNA is reproduced in an infected cell, transient double-stranded viral RNA molecules appear and are recognized as foreign by existing intracellular molecules.[5] These molecules, called pattern recognition receptors, trigger the earliest innate immune response against the virus, inducing the production and release of a variety of small proteins called cytokines.[6] These cytokines function as alarms that indicate the presence of a foreign entity (viral RNA undergoing reproduction) in the affected living tissue.

At this early stage of infection, IFNs are the most important cytokines and result from the innate immune response. Because they interfere with viral reproduction to stop the spread of the infection, IFNs are critical.[7] The primary benefit of the first wave of IFNs is that they bind noninfected cells in the surrounding environment. This binding triggers a complex physiological process resulting in a refractory state of the cells, making them resistant to SARS-CoV-2 infection.

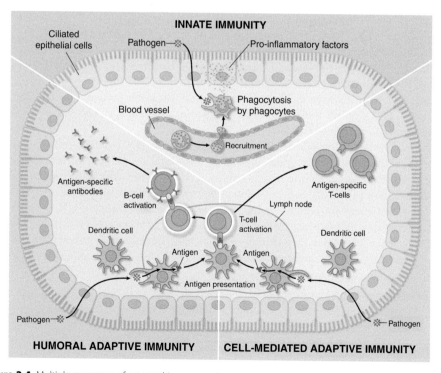

Figure 2.4 Multiple responses of a normal immune system.

However, viral RNA already inside the cell can escape the effects of IFNs. The viral RNA can activate other immune system components causing a broad defense response. These mechanisms are driven by the overarching processes of discrimination (between self and nonself), inactivation, and elimination of the threatening virus (or other foreign agent or substance) and are mediated by a variety of different effector molecules produced in response to cell death and tissue injury caused by the virus. In viral infections, the effectors recruit mononuclear cells to the site of infection and interactions among these cells induce the production of cytokines in a highly regulated fashion. However, at the very start of the viral infection of susceptible healthy cells, the dominant metabolic response of innate immunity is the production of type I interferon (IFN-I).

Signaling by IFN-I leads to protective responses in both infected and uninfected cells. The level of IFN-I signaling varies drastically between host cells. Some cells will not produce IFN-Is, even while being infected and/or being activated by other infected cells through paracrine signaling.

Initially, IFN-I responses were recognized for their role in antiviral immunity, but IFN-I's many immunomodulatory functions are now widely recognized, including its role in antimicrobial defenses, autoimmune manifestations, and antitumor responses.[8]

The cellular heterogeneity found in the mammalian IFN-I system results from multiple random events over three distinct, but intertwined, stochastic layers: viral, host, and spatiotemporal, see figure 2.5.

Each layer originates chronologically over the course of a viral infection, starting with the elements introduced by the virus or other stimuli. In this viral layer, the random distribution of viral particles and genetic variability leads to differences in infectiousness, replication inside the host, and so on.

The second layer (host) involves all elements introduced by the host cell state at the time of infection, comprising both deterministic and stochastic cellular processes. This layer is statistically probable but difficult to predict, resulting in differences in susceptibility to the virus, IFN-I production, viral replication, etc.

The third layer involves different spatiotemporal diffusion gradients of viral progeny and IFN-I. This exposes individual cells to different gradients, a process that is further enhanced by complex tissue structures.

The multilayered probabilistic effect in the mammalian IFN-I system creates a massive degree of cellular heterogeneity, drastically increasing over the course of a viral infection. As the heterogeneity increases, it leads to multiple different cellular states, which then lead to different cellular decisions. During the early infection phase, cellular heterogeneity is still relatively low, with minor variations introduced by the virus. However, when infected cells start to elicit antiviral responses, their heterogeneity increases, see figure 2.6. Given that individual host cells are in different cellular states, they are exposed to different quantities of viral particles. All these cells undergo drastic all-or-nothing decisions, which result in one of two different outcomes:

1. Cells become major sources of viral replication
2. Cells undergo drastic reprogramming, leading to massive IFN-I production, the inhibition of viral replication, and then programmed cell death (apoptosis)

Innate Cellular Immunity: A Double-Edged Sword

The innate immune system recognizes invading pathogens by sensing their pathogen-associated molecular patterns (PAMPs) using various pattern recognition receptors. Viral

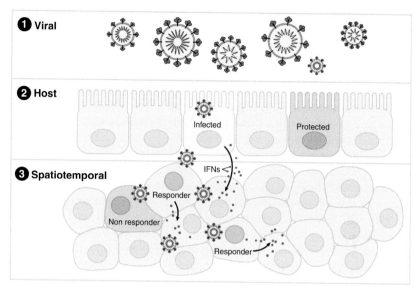

Figure 2.5 Stochasticity layers of the mammalian IFN-I system.[8]

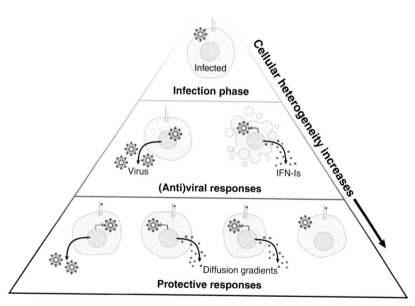

Figure 2.6 Different cellular states due to varying levels of cellular heterogeneity.[8]

PAMPs are often distinct molecular signatures not found in host cells, such as unique nucleic acid structures of the viral genome or viral replication intermediates.[9] Within endosomes, Toll-like receptors (TLRs) recognize viral RNA. In the cytosolic compartment, retinoic acid-inducible gene I (RIG-I)-like receptors (RLRs) perform this function. Most host cells have cytosolic RLRs. Endosomal TLRs are mostly expressed by innate immune cells. White blood cells are key players in innate immunity and different populations predominate depending on the infective agent; for example, bacterial infections typically lead to the accumulation of neutrophils at sites of infection.[10]

Natural killer (NK) cells are the most important effector lymphocytes in viral infections. They are critically important against SARS-CoV-2 infection.[11] NK cells contain large cytoplasmic granules and are cytotoxic without the need to specifically recognize the infecting virus. They induce programmed cell death (apoptosis) of virally infected cells. This process also occurs during normal embryological development and tissue differentiation.[12] Apoptosis prevents the spilling of intracellular components into the interstitial space and thereby avoids triggering an additional inflammatory response. The fragmented remains of apoptotic cells are ingested by tissue macrophages that were recruited to the site by specific cytokines. The uptake of apoptotic cell debris by macrophages is part of the clean-up function of these cells at sites of tissue injury or infection. The cellular debris also contains viral proteins that are further degraded during metabolism. During this process, some fragments or peptides of viral proteins are incorporated into the human leukocyte antigen type II (HLA-II) cell membrane molecules to be expressed on the external surface of the macrophage. These self molecules, when occupied by peptide derived from foreign proteins such as a virus, are detected as foreign by T lymphocytes (T-cells), which become activated by various pathways. These events represent the cellular phase of the adaptive immune response to the viral infection to be described in detail in the next section.

Returning to the innate cellular immune response, we add that, besides apoptosis, other cell death mechanisms, such as necrosis from tissue damage as a result of injury or bacterial infection, produce additional signals that mobilize other inflammatory cells such as neutrophils in the affected location. Necrosis results in acute inflammation with the production of pus and abscess formation, which are not features of viral infections or diseases and are thus not a major primary feature of COVID-19.

The NK cells play a key role in viral infections, including SARS-CoV-2. These innate immune effector cells belong to the rapidly expanding family of known innate lymphoid cells and represent 5–20% of all circulating lymphocytes in humans. Innate lymphoid cells also play important roles in innate defense responses against SARS-CoV-2 and are different from the traditional T-cell responses of acquired immunity activated by viral peptides detected in the context of HLA-I and -II molecules. The mechanisms by which SARS-CoV-2 evades an otherwise effective and normal innate immune response to cause COVID-19 have been reviewed in detail and are beyond the scope of this discussion.[13] The role of NK cells and details of the innate immune response evoked by vaccination based on messenger RNA (mRNA) preparations has also been examined formally in normal and immunocompromised individuals.[14]

As with many infectious diseases, the immune response to coronavirus infection may act as a double-edged sword. Although necessary for promoting antiviral host defense, it may also incite life-threatening immunopathology. These responses may help explain the underlying pathophysiology of the most severe cases of COVID-19, at least over some phase of the viral infection.[15]

Adaptive Immune Response to a SARS-CoV-2 Infection

An essential function of the innate immune system is to trigger the adaptive immune response. This response primarily involves three major cell types, each with its distinct function:

1. B lymphocytes (B-cells) possess membrane receptors for soluble antigens. When the B-cell antigen receptor is occupied by a specific antigen, the cell becomes activated and migrates to secondary lymphoid organs where it interacts with CD4+ T-cells with a receptor to the same or a very similar antigen, resulting in enhanced activation, proliferation, and differentiation into plasma cells that produce a high volume of specific antibodies and memory cells for a faster response upon reexposure to the antigen

2. CD4+ T-cells that recognize a specific cell-bound antigen become activated, proliferate and expand. In this process, they acquire a variety of help/effector functions, including enhancing the production of specific antibodies by B-cells and their differentiation into plasma cells

3. CD8+ T-cells are cytotoxic and kill virus-infected cells that are recognized by specific receptors in their cell membrane when the antigens are detected within HLA-I molecules on the surface of infected cells. This is different from the effector function of NK cells, which do not require recognition of the antigen as part of the cell-killing process

Adaptive immune response to a viral infection generally occurs 6–10 days after the initial infection because of the small number of randomly produced virus-specific effector cells among the large pools of naive B- and T-cells. Detection and activation of a few effector T-cells (CD4+ and CD8+) and B-cells triggers proliferation of cells with the same antigen specificity, causing an expansion in the number of cells specific for the same antigen. This process is called clonal expansion and it is a cornerstone of our understanding of acquired immunity. The effective acquired immune response to the virus involves the close interaction of these diverse cells, and different immune response regulatory signals are produced at different stages of the infection as the disease runs its natural course in any given patient.

While T-cell responses are detected after almost all SARS-CoV-2 infections, the CD4+ T-cell response is associated with the control of the primary SARS-CoV-2 infection, as CD4+ T-cells are crucial for enhancing and amplifying the response of B-cells and the production of progressively more specific antibodies to the virus.[16] These cells are detected as early as two to four days after the onset of symptoms.[16–18] The rapid induction of this subset of cells is associated with a reduction in COVID-19 disease severity owing to their key role in enhancing the specificity of the antibodies produced by B-cells, while the absence of these cells is often associated with severe COVID-19, probably because of the less than optimal antibody responses of different possible types.[17–19] T-cells make up approximately 60% of all lymphocytes in normal blood. CD8+ T-cells can develop rapidly after infection and are associated with better outcomes.[16, 20] However, they have been less consistently observed than CD4+ T-cells.[21]

The primary role of the mature humoral immune response is the production of high-affinity neutralizing antibodies for controlling the spread and progression of the infection, for protecting against reinfection or ameliorating the severity of the reinfection by a variant of concern, and for the induction of long-term immunity. Neutralization is one of the most important protective functions of antibodies capable of generating sterilizing immunity in infected patients. Serum from most patients who have been infected with SARS-CoV-2 exhibit neutralizing activity.[22]

The most immunogenic structural proteins encoded by the genome of SARS-CoV-2 are the S protein that contains the RBD and the nucleocapsid protein (NCP).

Of particular interest are neutralizing antibodies directed against epitopes of the S protein, namely anti-RBD antibodies that block the virus from binding to the specific ACE2 receptors on human cells. The anti-NCP is not a neutralizing antibody but instead interferes with the virus replication and the packing of the viral RNA into new virions. Anti-NCP antibodies have been intensively investigated in relation to the disease severity and patient outcome. Anti-NCP immunoglobulin (Ig) M and IgG began to be observed on days 7 and 10 and peaked on days 28 and 49, respectively. These antibodies appear earlier in the disease and antibody titers are higher in patients with severe clinical manifestations than in non-severe patients. S-specific IgG development also occurs early, and higher IgG titers are detected in survivors of severe disease compared to non-survivors, indicating that rapid and potent IgG class switching is related to survival.

Secretory IgA is the prevalent antibody isotype in mucosal surfaces with potent neutralizing activity. Recent studies on SARS-CoV-2-specific IgA antibodies in the serum, saliva, and bronchoalveolar fluid show that IgA antibodies are predominant in the early phase of SARS-CoV-2 infection.

Using mutant virus neutralization assays at each time point of testing longitudinal samples supports the idea that immune responses to some variants tested may be weaker[23] but formal comparative studies of differences in avidity of antibodies specific to different epitope configurations of SARS-CoV-2 variants compared to the original strain have not been performed using clinically calibrated serological assays for a definitive conclusion.

The endurance (persistence) of the immune memory response is critical for long-term protection from pathogen reinfection. There are several studies showing that antibodies remain stable for several months after infection. Other studies claim a rapid decline in antibody levels within three or four months.[24] The reasons for this discrepancy need to be further studied. Of note is the fact that the number of RBD-specific memory B-cells did not change up to six months after infection. Also of interest is the fact that the waning of anti-SARS-CoV-2 IgA antibodies seems to be affected less than IgM and IgG antibodies.

In summary:

- Antibody titers specific for SARS-CoV-2 do not directly correlate with disease severity. However, the kinetics of seroconversion, antibody isotype, and antigen specificity of antibodies appear to regulate the effect of the response on disease severity
- The neutralizing activity of antibodies against SARS-CoV-2 can offer preventive protection for COVID-19 infection, and the identification of such antibodies provides the basis for the development of vaccines
- Human monoclonal antibodies capable of neutralizing SARS-CoV-2 are strong candidates for effective COVID-19 therapeutics and prophylaxis tools

These results reinforce the need to continue monitoring the levels of neutralizing antibodies in patients infected with emergent variants.

Herd Immunity

Another aspect resulting from adaptive immunity in a population is "herd immunity." Herd immunity is a strategy to help thwart the spread of the virus. In its simplest terms it can be best described as population or community-based immunity that occurs when a virus cannot spread anymore because it keeps encountering people who are protected against an infection. In fact, some epidemiologists prefer the term "herd protection" as opposed to herd immunity. With that caveat we will, however, continue to use the term herd immunity throughout this chapter, given that it evokes greater familiarity in any given audience.

Herd immunity works by achieving a threshold immunity within the population that theoretically should be able to cut the spread of an infectious disease agent. This could be through either natural infection or vaccination. Once this level of herd immunity is reached, people who are not immunized are supposed to be protected by those who are, and this is referred to as the "herd immunity threshold." It is important to remember, though, that even when herd immunity is achieved, it is still possible to have outbreaks for several reasons, including low vaccination rates or the existence of a susceptible population.

Given that SARS-CoV-2 was a novel pathogen, many features of its transmission were not understood and, to date, it continues to be studied extensively. The herd immunity threshold required to stop the spread of SARS-CoV-2 remains extremely difficult to determine because of a host of complicating factors. One of the uniquely challenging aspects is the presence of asymptomatic carriers of the virus. Clinical manifestations do not suffice as an indicator of transmissibility, as asymptomatic hosts can be highly infectious and contribute to the spread of the disease.

There are two potential approaches to establishing herd immunity to SARS-CoV-2: (1) massive vaccination campaigns and (2) natural immunization of the entire population with the virus through infection.

In November 2020, when herd immunity was being considered as a strategy by some, the nation's epidemiologists warned against an approach of surrendering to the virus to achieve immunity because it would lead to catastrophic loss of human life. Despite these warnings, the use of herd immunity in this way to combat the spread of the virus was continuously debated among policymakers in several countries including Sweden, Brazil, the United Kingdom, and the United States.

Clinical Manifestations of a SARS-CoV-2 Infection

Although SARS-CoV-2 mostly affects the respiratory tract, it can also infect other tissues and organs. This is because ACE2 receptor molecules are present in many different types of cells all over the body, including endothelial cells, cardiomyocytes, enterocytes, parietal cells, Leydig cells, spermatogonia, and Sertoli cells.[25, 26] For example, infected cells or free infective virions can enter the gastrointestinal system and take hold of ACE2 receptor-expressing cells. Local inflammation can occur in these organs when immune cells detect the foreign agent and respond with a physiological attack. As the infection progresses, the virus can enter the blood circulation to spread throughout the body and, in some patients, it may cause systemic infection and affect multiple organs; it may even lead to death in some, more vulnerable, patients.[27]

The various levels of intensity of the responses elicited in these tissues by the viral infection cause different degrees of alterations in the tissues. This may interfere with normal physiological function, such as the absorption of oxygen by the respiratory system resulting

Table 2.1 Clinical characteristics of the earliest cases of SARS-CoV-2 pneumonia (the first 99 patients)

Symptom	No. of cases	Percent of cases
Fever	82	83
Cough	81	82
Shortness of breath	31	31
Muscle ache	11	11
Confusion	9	9
Headache	8	8
Sore throat	5	5
Rhinorrhea	4	4
Chest pain	2	2
Diarrhea	2	2
Nausea and vomiting	1	1

in abnormally low blood oxygen levels and shortness of breath. In susceptible patients, this may get progressively worse, requiring medical attention and management with assisted mechanical ventilation.

We have seen these varying levels of response in a wide range of symptoms and clinical outcomes. The first detailed account of the clinical features of COVID-19 was based on 99 patients with confirmed infection with the novel coronavirus (2019-nCov), as detected by real-time reverse transcription polymerase chain reaction (RT-PCR) between January 1 and 20, 2020. The report describes epidemiological, demographic, clinical, and radiological features, as well as laboratory data.[28] The key clinical findings are summarized in Table 2.1. Overall, fever was the dominant sign of systemic infection, and cough was the most frequent symptom suggestive of respiratory illness. Other signs and symptoms were variable among the cases, including several that suggested the involvement of the cardio-vascular, gastrointestinal, and neuromuscular systems.[28]

In all cases, the same coronavirus was recovered from throat swab samples and, of all 99 patients, 74 (75%) had bilateral pneumonia on chest X-ray, 14 (14%) showed multiple mottling and ground glass opacity, and one (1%) showed a pneumothorax. Seventeen patients (17%) exhibited acute respiratory syndrome. Despite the pulmonary imaging abnormalities in most patients (74%), the degree of clinical pulmonary distress was not consistent. Only 17 patients (17%) developed clinical SARS and, of these, 11 (11%) worsened over a short period of time and died of complications of multiple organ failure.[28]

Based on the demographic and personal characteristics of this cohort of confirmed cases, the investigators concluded that "2019-nCoV infection was of clustering onset, more likely to affect older males with comorbidities, and can result in severe and even fatal respiratory diseases such as acute respiratory distress syndrome."[28]

As the pandemic evolved, some populations succumbed to SARS-CoV-2 infection in large numbers, while others presented milder or no symptoms, validating the outcomes in the report of the initial 99 clinical cases.[28] A subsequent report of 2 199 hospitalized patients with COVID-19 in New York City, the epicenter of the epidemic in the United States at that time, focused on in-hospital mortality at a major quaternary urban hospital system. This report compared patients who died in the hospital with those who were discharged alive.[29] The investigators concluded that mortality was high in their cohort of hospitalized patients and that their patients often required intensive care. Confirming previous clinical reports, the patients who died had more preexisting conditions and greater perturbations in inflammatory markers than those who survived.

These and further observations continued to suggest that varying immune responses to the virus could explain intrinsic differences among hosts and be the underlying reason for the variability in severity of SARS-CoV-2 infections.[30]

Serological Assays

The World Health Organization (WHO) issued updated interim guidance on May 27, 2020,[31] which included information for laboratory testing for COVID-19 in suspected human cases and expanded the clinical guidance to areas not covered in the earlier laboratory testing strategy recommendations of March 21.[32] The WHO guidance anticipated that "serological assays will play an important role in research and surveillance." However, despite this explicit recognition of the value of serological testing, the WHO did not recommend its use for acute case detection, which was the primary concern at that time.

Serological assays are important tools for detecting and measuring a major component of the immune response to a viral infection in symptomatic and asymptomatic infected hosts. These assays can provide unique information for tracking the spread and progression of infection in a group or community. However, the WHO's caution in recommending the use of serological assays at that time is understandable, as the inappropriate use of serological tests for the diagnosis of SARS-CoV-2 would present major risks to epidemiological studies. First, antibodies to SARS-CoV-2 can be detected in the blood of patients or persons exposed only 14–21 days after infection, on average. This well-known delay in the appearance of antibodies led to a concern that antibody tests for diagnosis using samples taken too soon after infection would give false-negative results. False-negative diagnoses would allow infected persons to continue spreading the infection to other susceptible people. In addition, detected antibodies may not be specific for the epidemic virus, resulting in false-positive results and overestimation of the magnitude of the epidemic. Until more was learned about the reliability of the clinical serological tests, the WHO recommended that the diagnosis of SARS-CoV-2 rely exclusively on the presence of specific viral RNA in samples obtained from the respiratory tract of exposed or symptomatic persons suspected of viral infection or COVID-19.

Therefore, the WHO guidance emphasized screening for the virus with nucleic acid amplification tests such as RT-PCR in suspected cases, as informed by the expanding clinical descriptions of COVID-19 cases and suggestions for the appropriate management of suspected and confirmed cases.[31]

Vaccination Immunity

From the beginning of the SARS-CoV-2 pandemic, it was clear that, in addition to the physical preventive countermeasures (i.e. quarantine, isolation, and the use of face mask), specific anti-SARS-CoV-2 vaccines would be required to effectively control the viral spread and ultimately defeat the pandemic. In December 2019, there was no vaccine against the novel coronavirus and prior coronavirus infections were not providing sufficient immune protection. The scientific community, several governments, and academic and private organizations recognized the urgent need to quickly develop vaccines by setting up groups of biologists, virologists, immunologists, and epidemiologists to work on different vaccine development strategies.

In April 2020, the National Institutes of Health (NIH) set up a public–private partnership to speed up the COVID-19 vaccine and treatment options. This partnership brought together leading pharmaceutical companies to accelerate the pandemic response.[33] The NIH and the Foundation for the NIH initially assembled the following organizations to develop an international strategy for a coordinated research response to the COVID-19 pandemic:

- 15 biopharmaceutical companies
- the US Department of Health and Human Services Office of the Assistant Secretary for Preparedness and Response
- the Centers for Disease Control and Prevention
- the US Food and Drug Administration
- the European Medicines Agency

The Accelerating COVID-19 Therapeutic Interventions and Vaccines (ACTIV) partnership[34] created a framework for collaboration and for prioritizing vaccine and drug candidates, facilitating clinical trials, coordinating regulatory processes, and reinforcing assets among all partners to promote a rapid response to COVID-19. ACTIV provided the infrastructure, subject matter expertise, and funding to identify, prioritize and facilitate the entry of some of the most promising vaccine and drug candidates into clinical trials. ACTIV was led by a highly motivated working group of senior scientists representing government, industry, and academia.

The first initiative to develop an anti-SARS-CoV-2 vaccine was announced in February 2020 by the Jenner Institute of the University of Oxford to develop the Oxford–AstraZeneca vaccine. By April 2020, 115 vaccines were already under development and 73 had reached the exploratory phase. Of these, only a handful of the vaccine projects succeeded. These research and development efforts were crucial for the development of vaccines and were exceptional in that they gained temporary and conditional authorization in a record time of 9–10 months. The first person to receive the SARS-CoV-2 vaccine, in December 2020, was a 90-year-old female patient in the United Kingdom. Nevertheless, the research and development infrastructure at that time was still unable to respond to a pandemic of this size.

Several vaccine platforms were available at the time to develop anti-SARS-CoV-2 vaccines. Historically, vaccine development has been achieved only after many years of intense research and clinical validation. The COVID-19 crisis required prompt action to expedite development within a few months.[35] To support this effort, the WHO classified COVID-19 vaccines into the following categories: inactivated, live attenuated, vector, RNA, DNA, protein subunit, and virus-like particle vaccines, as set out in Table 2.2.

In the Western world, the most administered vaccines were constructed with viral vectors and mRNA. Both existing mRNA vaccines (Pfizer BioNTech and Moderna) elicited good immune responses and have proven to decrease the spread of disease and reduce the severity of the disease based on symptomatology, rate of hospitalization, and mortality rate.[36] Some viral vector or mRNA vaccines resulted in adverse events including pain at the injection site and fever. In some cases, complications such as

Table 2.2 The features of various COVID-19 vaccine platforms[35]

Vaccine platforms	Vaccine components	Mechanism of induction antibody	WHO approved vaccines
Inactivated vaccine	Entire viruses cultured in vitro; inactivated by chemical reagents[35]	Entire virus as an immunogen induces a wide range of antibodies against different epitopes	BBIBP-CorV (Sinopharm) CoronaVac (Sinovac Biotech) COVAXIN (Bharat Biotech International)
Live attenuated vaccine	The virus is obtained by reverse genetics or adaptation	(1) The retained viral amino acid sequences induce extensive responses, including innate, humoral, and cellular immunity (2) Induces mucosal immunity through nasal inhalation to protect the upper respiratory tract	N/A
Viral vector vaccine	Engineered viruses with replication attenuated, carrying genetic material of viral proteins or polypeptides	Viral vector vaccines can induce Th1 cell responses, thus inducing strong protective effects	AZD1222 (AstraZeneca and University of Oxford) Ad26.COV2.S (Johnson & Johnson) COVISHIELD (Serum Institute of India)
Protein subunit vaccine	Cell-expressing systems express viral proteins or peptides systemically	Induces Th1 cell responses	NVX-CoV2373 (Novavax) COVOVAX (Serum Institute of India)
DNA vaccine	Viral antigens encoded by a recombinant plasmid	Induces neutralizing antibodies	N/A
mRNA vaccine	mRNA encapsulated by vectors, viral proteins, or polypeptides	Induces strong Th1 cell responses and germinal center B-cell responses and simultaneously produces long-lived plasma cells and memory cells to elicit neutralizing antibodies	BNT162b2 (Pfizer BioNTech) mRNA-1273 (Moderna)
Virus-like particle vaccine	Noninfectious particles consisting of viral structural proteins and viral polypeptides	Antigens loading on the protein particles induce neutralizing antibodies against immune epitope	N/A

thrombocytopenia, myocarditis, immune diseases, and neurological and lymphatic system diseases have been reported, raising concerns about the safety of these COVID-19 vaccines. Complications have been described mostly in patients with comorbidities such as immunodeficiency, cancer, transplants, and immunosuppressed AIDS. The rate of complication is extremely low given the millions of vaccine doses administered.[37] Adverse events related to vaccination are continuously monitored and analyzed. Currently, several strategies are under evaluation to reduce the impact of adverse events and improve sustained postvaccination immunity, including mix-and-match vaccination, developing new vaccines such as nanoparticle vaccines, and optimizing immune adjuvants to improve vaccine safety and efficacy. The health status of the elderly and patients with underlying diseases are carefully assessed prior to immunization. In addition, new vaccine reformulation will be under consideration if new variants of concern, such as the omicron variant, continue emerging. Variants with distinct infectivity of the upper respiratory tract may require changing the vaccine administration route, optimizing vaccine formulation, and generating a new family of vaccines inducing stronger IgA immunity to protect the nasal-pharyngeal mucosa.

Finally, vaccine-induced immunity remains a pivotal tool for pandemic control. The WHO, governments, and other relevant agencies continue to recommend the acceleration of vaccine immunization programs.

Conclusion

It is critical that we understand and map the immune response to any new virus in a comprehensive and coordinated fashion. In the "Lessons Learned and Next Steps" section, we make a broad attempt to list some of the basic tenets of immune response that are important for monitoring a patient's status, designing approaches to amplify the response, assessing therapeutic efficacy, assessing the response to variants, stratifying patients for therapy and care, and using vaccines to induce a comprehensive response.

For SARS-CoV-2, multiple international institutions investigated "pieces" of the immune response profile. However, there were no established standards for collecting, transporting, and storing patient samples or for performing and evaluating immune response and functional response assays. This lack of standards resulted in conflicting and often confusing outcomes. In the initial six to nine months of the pandemic, a few of our associates attempted to piece together a comprehensive "immune map" based on scientific communications, but the outcome was sketchy (data not shown). There needs to be an established protocol for this assessment that can be coordinated among several institutions, such that the data generated can yield solid and successful immune response maps.

When we better understand the pathophysiological responses to this virus, we can better identify those at risk of infection and those for whom the disease will be more severe and possibly lethal. Additionally, our understanding of immunity could shed light on the risk of recurrent infections and the long-term complications of infection. Ultimately, we aim to anticipate the natural progression of the virus among different patient subgroups and explore ways to enhance the immune system to induce effective immunity. By further understanding COVID-19 immunopathogenesis, we can continue to design more effective diagnostic, therapeutic, and prophylactic strategies.

Lessons Learned and Next Steps

- Establish a permanent procedure or standard protocol for monitoring the status of natural immunity to a virus posing a potential risk of becoming an epidemic or pandemic
- Promote and plan key studies to develop vaccines for selective agents and virus groups that could potentially infect humans, such as the coronavirus family
- Continue to explore immunologic and molecular research to develop molecular strategies to better understand infection transmission to humans, as well as technologies to develop innovative vaccine systems, including innovative approaches to serological studies aiming to better characterize the key functional features of antibody-mediated immunity, such as quantitative assays of high sensitivity and specificity, and that correlate with binding affinity to the various antigenic determinants of the agents
- Develop and improve the sensitivity and specificity of diagnostic and screening tests to assess and control pandemic evolution and implement serological testing for antibodies to monitor the immune response to vaccines to identify weak antibody responses to vaccination or nonresponders, which interfere with effective herd immunity
- Foster basic studies on the control and possible therapeutic use of a cytokine storm as a means to abate the severe impact of massive mediator release
- Recognize the value of immune therapy, including plasma therapies and manufactured monoclonal antibodies targeting the selective phase of virus transmission and infectivity

References

1. J. Shang, G. Ye, K. Shi, et al., Structural basis of receptor recognition by SARS-CoV-2. *Nature*, **581**, 7807 (2020), 221–224.

2. M.A. Shereen, S. Khan, A. Kazmi, N. Bashir, and R. Siddique, COVID-19 infection: origin, transmission, and characteristics of human coronaviruses. *J Adv Res*, **24** (2020), 91–98.

3. J. Shang, Y. Wan, C. Luo, et al., Cell entry mechanisms of SARS-CoV-2. *Proc Natl Acad Sci USA*, **117**, 21 (2020), 11727–11734.

4. S. Amor, L. Fernandez Blanco, and D. Baker, Innate immunity during SARS-CoV-2: evasion strategies and activation trigger hypoxia and vascular damage. *Clin Exp Immunol*, **202**, 2 (2020), 193–209.

5. K. Onomoto, K. Onoguchi, and M. Yoneyama, Regulation of RIG-I-like receptor-mediated signaling: interaction between host and viral factors. *Cell Mol Immunol*, **18**, 3 (2021), 539–555.

6. M. Stravalaci, I. Pagani, and E. M. Paraboschi, et al., Recognition and inhibition of SARS-CoV-2 by humoral innate immunity pattern recognition molecules. *Nat Immunol*, **23**, 2 (2022), 275–286.

7. I. Busnadiego, S. Fernbach, M. O. Pohl, et al., Antiviral activity of type I, II, and III interferon counterbalances ACE2 inducibility restricts SARS-CoV-2. *mBio*, **11**, 5 (2020), e01928–20.

8. L. C. Eyndhoven, A. Singh, and J. Tel, Decoding the dynamics of multilayered stochastic antiviral IFN-I responses. *Trends Immunol*, **42**, 9 (2021), 824–839.

9. A. Iwasaki, A virological view of innate immune recognition. *Annu Rev Microbiol*, **66**, 1 (2012), 177–196.

10. Y. Ma, Y. Zhang, and L. Zhu, Role of neutrophils in acute viral infection. *Immun Inflamm Dis*, **9**, 4 (2021), 1186–1196.

11. N. K. Bjorkstrom, B. Strunz, and H. G. Ljunggren, Natural killer cells in

antiviral immunity. *Nat Rev Immunol*, **22**, 2 (2022), 112–123.

12. Y. Fuchs and H. Steller, Programmed cell death in animal development and disease. *Cell*, **147**, 4 (2011), 742–758.

13. W. Gu, H. Gan, Y. Ma, et al., The molecular mechanism of SARS-CoV-2 evading host antiviral innate immunity. *Virol J*, **19**, 1 (2022), 49.

14. A. Cuapio, C. Boulouis, I. Filipovic, et al., NK cell frequencies, function and correlates to vaccine outcome in BNT162b2 mRNA anti-SARS-CoV-2 vaccinated healthy and immunocompromised individuals. *Mol Med*, **28**, 1 (2022), 20.

15. S. Majumdar and P. M. Murphy, Chemokine regulation during epidemic coronavirus infection. *Front Pharmacol*, **11** (2020), 600369.

16. G. J. Gorse, G. B. Patel, J. N. Vitale, and T. Z. O'Connor, Prevalence of antibodies to four human coronaviruses is lower in nasal secretions than in serum. *Clin Vaccine Immunol*, **17** (2010), 1875–1880.

17. A. W. D. Edridge, Seasonal coronavirus protective immunity is short-lasting. *Nat Med*, **26** (2020), 1691–1693.

18. G. Saletti, Older adults lack SARS CoV-2 cross-reactive T lymphocytes directed to human coronaviruses OC43 and NL63. *Sci Rep*, **10**, (2020), 21447.

19. F. Tang, Lack of peripheral memory B cell responses in recovered patients with severe acute respiratory syndrome: a six-year follow-up study. *J Immunol*, **186** (2011), 7264–7268.

20. L. P. Wu, Duration of antibody responses after severe acute respiratory syndrome. *Emerg Infect Dis*, **13** (2021), 1562–1564.

21. N. Le Bert, A. T. Tan, K. Kunasegaran, et al., SARS-CoV-2-specific T cell immunity in cases of COVID-19 and SARS, and uninfected controls. *Nature*, **584** (2020), 457–462.

22. K. Röltgen and S. D. Boyd, Antibody and B cell responses to SARS-CoV-2 infection and vaccination. *Cell Host Microbe*, **29** (2021), 1063–1075.

23. SARS-CoV-2-specific antibody and T-cell responses 1 year after infection in people recovered from COVID-19: a longitudinal cohort study Li Guo, Geng Wang, Yeming Wang, Qiao Zhang, et al. Lancet Microbe. 2022 May;3(5):e348-e356.

24. D. H. Jo, D. Minn, J. Lim, et al., Rapidly declining SARS-CoV-2 antibody titers within 4 months after BNT162b2 vaccination. *Vaccines (Basel)*, **9**, 10 (2021), 1145.

25. S. Verma, S. Saksena, and H. Sadri-Ardekani, ACE2 receptor expression in testes: implications in coronavirus disease 2019 pathogenesis. *Biol Reprod*, **103**, 3 (2020), 449–451.

26. A. M. Poma, D. Bonuccelli, R. Giannini, et al., COVID-19 autopsy cases: detection of virus in endocrine tissues. *J Endocrinol Invest*, **45**, 1 (2022), 209–214.

27. C. Bryce, Z. Grimes, E. Pujadas, et al., Pathophysiology of SARS-CoV-2: the Mount Sinai COVID-19 autopsy experience. *Mod Pathol*, **34**, 8 (2021), 1456–1467.

28. N. Chen, M. Zhou, X. Dong, et al., Epidemiological and clinical characteristics of 99 cases of 2019 novel coronavirus pneumonia in Wuhan, China: a descriptive study. *Lancet*, **395**, 10223 (2020), 507–513.

29. I. Paranjpe, A. J. Russak, J. K. Freitas, et al., Retrospective cohort study of clinical characteristics of 2199 hospitalised patients with COVID-19 in New York City. *BMJ Open*, **10**, 11 (2020), 040736.

30. R. Z. Raza and S.W. Abbasi, An evolutionary insight into the heterogeneous severity pattern of the SARS-CoV-2 infection. *Front Genet*, **13** (2022), 859508.

31. World Health Organization, Clinical Management of COVID-19: Interim Guidance, May 27, 2020 (2020).

32. World Health Organization, Laboratory Testing for Coronavirus Disease (COVID-19) in Suspected Human Cases: Interim Guidance, March 19, 2020 (2020), https://apps.who.int/iris/handle/10665/331501.

33. NIH, NIH to launch public-private partnership to speed COVID-19 vaccine and treatment options (April 17, 2020), https://tinyurl.com/dpve3adr.

34. FNIH, Accelerating COVID-19 Therapeutic Interventions & Vaccines (ACTIV), https://tinyurl.com/2uz7amzc.

35. M. Li, H. Wang, L. Tian, et al., COVID-19 vaccine development: milestones, lessons and prospects. *Signal Transduct Target Ther*, 7, 1 (2022), 146.

36. R. Link-Gelles, A. A. Ciesla, K. E. Fleming-Dutra, et al., Effectiveness of bivalent mRNA vaccines in preventing symptomatic SARS-CoV-2 infection – increasing community access to testing program, United States, September–November 2022. *MMWR Morb Mortal Wkly Rep*, 71, 48 (2022), 1526–1530.

37. National Center for Immunization and Respiratory Diseases (NCIRD), Division of Viral Diseases. Selected Adverse Events Reported after COVID-19 Vaccination (2023), https://tinyurl.com/aucame4v.

Clinical Management: A Roadmap Based on One New York City Hospital's Response to the COVID-19 Pandemic

Barbara Barnett, Yvette Calderon, Bethany Kranitzky, Young Im Lee, Erick Eiting, Lina Miyakawa, Waleed Javaid, and Saralynne Brown

Introduction

This chapter outlines the events that took place during the COVID-19 pandemic at Mount Sinai Beth Israel (MSBI) medical center, an academic teaching tertiary care facility in the East Village of Manhattan that is part of the Mount Sinai Health System. We also include the clinical case study of two patients, Harold[1] and Danny[1], a father and son who were admitted to our hospital during the pandemic. We quickly discovered that traditional approaches to managing severe acute respiratory syndrome coronavirus 2 (SARS-CoV-2), the virus that causes COVID-19, were ineffective, and new strategies were needed to manage the psychosocial needs of our patients.

Our purpose is to outline a roadmap of how our leadership and clinical teams navigated caring for patients and staff during a time of absolute crisis. Our goals are to recount the feelings of uncertainty, confusion, and chaos that permeated our city as the record-breaking pandemic unfolded and discuss how the pandemic permanently changed our operations. We strive to share the lessons learned during this journey and provide a framework for future health-care leaders to successfully manage and efficiently operationalize strategies for the next pandemic.

Pre-Pandemic Operations

As January 2020 dawned at MSBI, our workforce was energized for a new year. Our focus was on "No Wait for Perfect Care," an institution-wide initiative to train leaders and employees in the Kata approach to problem-solving to optimize throughput, quality, and patient safety. Key stakeholders had signed off on plans for a new state-of-the-art hospital that would leverage technology and operationalize throughput, and construction was set to begin. We then began to hear about the novel coronavirus in Wuhan, China, and there was a sense of increased urgency as cases began to be detected in New York City.

On March 1, 2020, the Mount Sinai Health System saw its first confirmed patient with COVID-19. On March 11, 2020, the World Health Organization (WHO) declared the COVID-19 outbreak a pandemic. The number of patients with COVID-19 continued to grow exponentially by the day, and it became clear that New York City was the epicenter of

---

[1] Names have been changed for privacy. Note, this chapter describes the unique personal experiences of health-care providers and patients at one hospital and does not attempt to reflect the varied experiences of health-care professionals or patients in other hospital systems/parts of the country. However, many of these lessons learned are applicable to a wide variety of health-care systems.

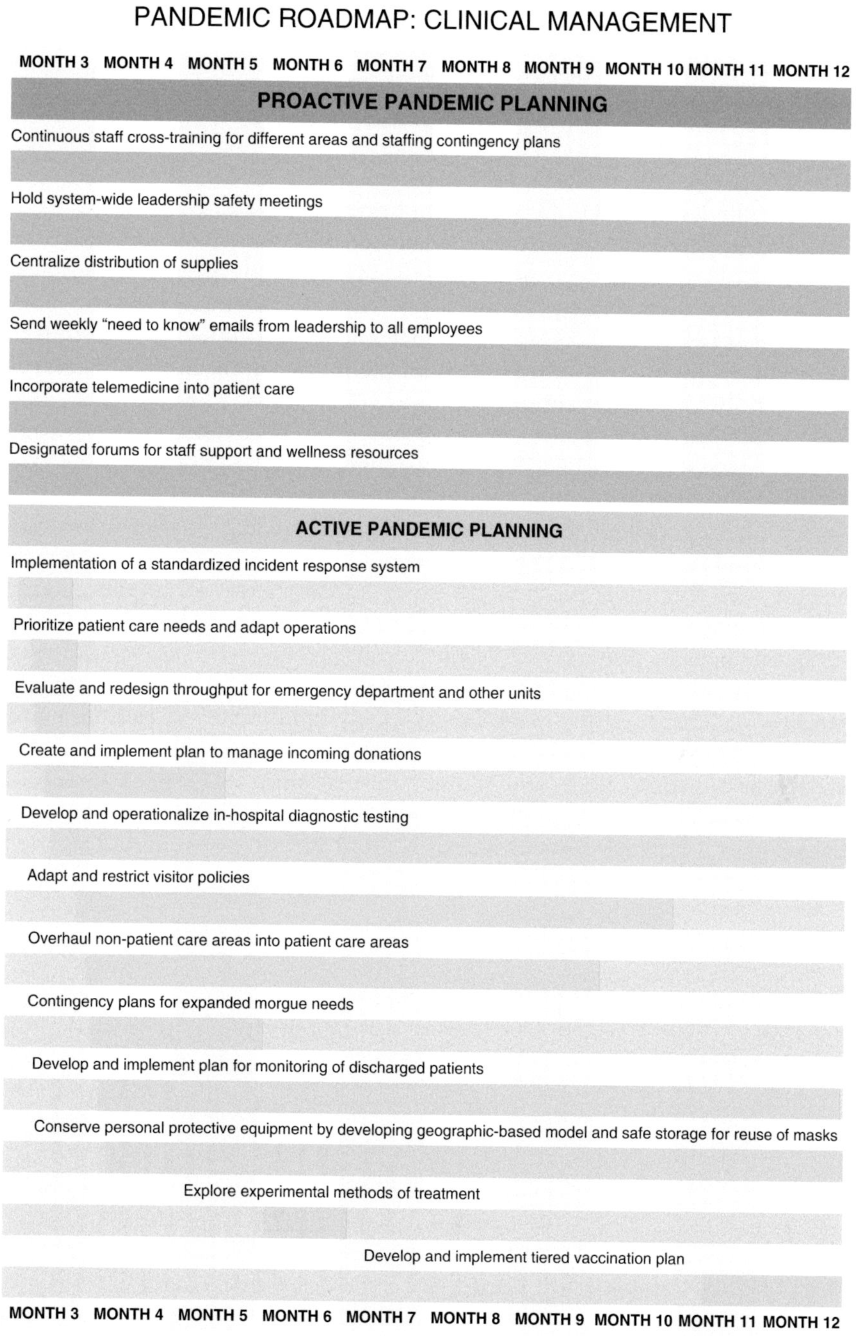

PANDEMIC ROADMAP: CLINICAL MANAGEMENT

MONTH 3   MONTH 4   MONTH 5   MONTH 6   MONTH 7   MONTH 8   MONTH 9   MONTH 10 MONTH 11 MONTH 12

PROACTIVE PANDEMIC PLANNING

Continuous staff cross-training for different areas and staffing contingency plans

Hold system-wide leadership safety meetings

Centralize distribution of supplies

Send weekly "need to know" emails from leadership to all employees

Incorporate telemedicine into patient care

Designated forums for staff support and wellness resources

ACTIVE PANDEMIC PLANNING

Implementation of a standardized incident response system

Prioritize patient care needs and adapt operations

Evaluate and redesign throughput for emergency department and other units

Create and implement plan to manage incoming donations

Develop and operationalize in-hospital diagnostic testing

Adapt and restrict visitor policies

Overhaul non-patient care areas into patient care areas

Contingency plans for expanded morgue needs

Develop and implement plan for monitoring of discharged patients

Conserve personal protective equipment by developing geographic-based model and safe storage for reuse of masks

Explore experimental methods of treatment

Develop and implement tiered vaccination plan

MONTH 3   MONTH 4   MONTH 5   MONTH 6   MONTH 7   MONTH 8   MONTH 9   MONTH 10 MONTH 11 MONTH 12

Figure 3.1 This roadmap depicts the vital activities, their chronology, and an estimated time frame in months. In the case of the SARS-CoV-2 pandemic, month 1 was December 2019, the month in which the virus was isolated, sequenced, identified, and published.

the pandemic in the United States. While each of the seven hospitals in our health system had a local incident command center, on March 13, 2020, the Mount Sinai Health System activated a system-wide hospital incident command system (HICS), a standardized incident response system utilized in hospitals to assess and operationalize disaster strategies.

Responding to the Surge: Emergency Management Response

Activation of the HICS forced the seven facilities in the Mount Sinai Health System to function as a true health system instead of as individual hospitals. This approach permitted load balancing of patients across our health system, thereby preventing one hospital from becoming overburdened. During this time, New York State mandated the cessation of all elective surgical cases, procedures, and outpatient practice appointments. While this created its own set of challenges, it also freed essential health-care workers from the ambulatory setting to help with inpatient care.

The Mount Sinai Health System implemented twice daily, system-wide safety huddle calls for key leadership to virtually "gather" around the same table to discuss the latest information from the WHO and the Centers for Disease Control and Prevention (CDC), as well as bed capacity, clinical management, facility and staffing challenges, material and supply levels, and any other pertinent information.

Changes were frequently made to the safety huddles across all Mount Sinai Health System sites, and the structure for reporting out changed. Most notably, as hospitals became inundated with patients with COVID-19, the language around mortality was changed from patient "expirations" to "casualties," signifying the true war-zone atmosphere that health-care workers were experiencing every day. Mortality rates increased, and the number of patients, staff, and their family members lost to the pandemic was sobering.

In addition to HICS, leadership realized that visibility was crucial to successfully providing high-quality care to patients. Staff watched in disbelief as COVID-19 numbers rose daily (Figure 3.2), and leadership quickly realized that increased efforts were needed to

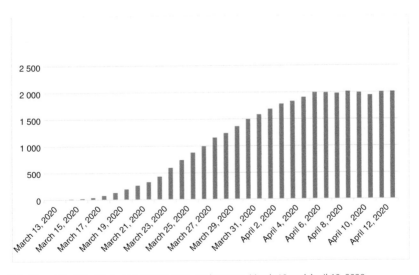

Figure 3.2 Mount Sinai Health System COVID-19 cases between March 13 and April 13, 2020.

support staff with the emotional toll that the pandemic was taking on all of us. Consistent rounding efforts were made in all units during all shifts to provide a forum to check in with staff and distribute the latest information regarding COVID-19. Leadership pivoted frequently, as messages provided in the morning had often changed by the afternoon.

Our staff members were anxious, to say the least. Not only were they afraid of becoming infected, but they also did not want to take the disease home to their families. One looming question at the beginning of the pandemic was how the virus spread; it was unknown whether the virus was airborne or spread through respiratory droplets. The overwhelming consensus at the time was that spread occurred through respiratory droplets, and surgical masks worked "just fine" as personal protective equipment (PPE). However, the staff wanted N-95 masks and we knew that, if our staff did not feel safe, our patients would not get the care they deserved. The supply levels of this PPE were a major concern.

Evolution of PPE

At the beginning of the pandemic, there was much confusion regarding masking versus non-masking and which mask provided the best protection, adding additional stress to our staff. In addition, the supply of masks was limited. Staff felt more comfortable using N-95 masks during patient interactions, and we quickly realized that we would need to find a safe way to effectively extend the use and reuse of N-95 masks to stabilize our inventory. The Infection Prevention and Control (IP) Team developed methods for stretching our PPE supply in new ways. Each staff member utilized an individual paper bag to safely store their masks between shifts, providing a sense of security without completely depleting our N-95 supply. Staff were allowed to reuse their masks if they were not soiled or visibly dirty. When seeing patients, staff placed a new surgical mask over their N-95. This was an evolution in our practice, responding to the dynamic changes in masking requirements and supplies. One of the characteristic visuals from the pandemic was that of brown paper bags filled with N-95 masks, marked with staff names, lined up on folding tables outside the main emergency department (ED) (Figure 3.3).

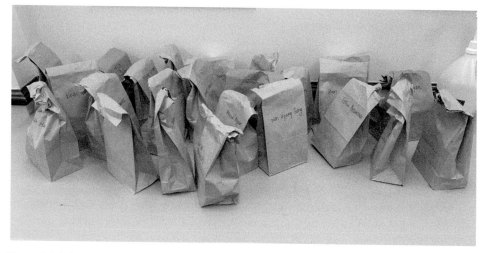

Figure 3.3 Individual staff members' bags containing personal N-95 masks.

The IP Team was crucial in developing clinical and nonclinical guidelines for our staff to help them understand how to identify and isolate patients with symptoms of the virus, as patient placement was important when determining bed assignments. The IP Team developed guidance on how to wear PPE, outlined PPE guidelines for each circumstance, and provided recommendations for visitation policy changes. Across the hospital, efforts were made to provide refresher training sessions on donning and doffing PPE, and the Environmental Health and Safety Department coordinated additional fit-testing sessions for N-95 masks for all employees, both clinical and nonclinical. Fit-testing needs grew 100-fold, especially because we switched between different N-95 masks as they became available.

Cohorting patients with COVID-19 and changing the provider coverage model allowed us to extend our PPE supply. Prior to the pandemic, we utilized a patient-specific PPE method, requiring that clinical teams don and doff PPE between each patient; we also assigned our patients to provider teams in a nongeographic model to enhance continuity and minimize handoffs. As PPE supplies began to run low and the threat of a shortage was imminent, we switched to a geographic model of patient assignment. Patients were assigned to geographic units based on COVID status. This change allowed the hospital to conserve PPE supply levels and safely allowed staff to continue to care for patients with as few delays as possible. By removing the need to don and doff PPE between each COVID-19-positive patient encounter, staff members were able to reduce the amount of time wasted and put those minutes toward caring for patients.

Fortunately, the Mount Sinai Health System began securing PPE from both internal and external sources. In response, an administrative conference room was transformed into a centralized distribution center for supplies and a central location for departments to request PPE, including the paper bags for N-95 mask storage. The IP Team helped in the transition and evolution of new rules regarding PPE use for extenuating circumstances. For example, PPE from preestablished kits, such as Ebola kits and operating room kits, were repurposed to add to the stock. This removed all barriers, providing clear steps for obtaining PPE and helping to streamline our activities.

As many medical supply factories shut down production, we experienced significant back orders for supplies. In particular, glideslopes and tracheostomy kits became rare items. The Materials Management Department worked tirelessly to find alternatives, and MSBI was fortunate to have systemic support for retrieving the necessary materials and supplies for its excessive number of patients. Although plans to develop a way to share ventilators between patients were developed, we fortunately never needed to do so.

Emergency Department

Case Study of Harold and Danny: Part 1

Harold, an 80-year-old man, presented to the ED on March 22, 2020, complaining of right upper quadrant abdominal pain, nausea, chills, and a dry cough for three days. He had tachycardia to 110 beats per minute, a respiratory rate of 28 breaths per minute, and a pulse oxygen level on room air of 90%. He was noted to be in mild respiratory distress upon arrival and was immediately given supplemental oxygen. We ordered a battery of laboratory tests that matched the findings we had come to see so frequently in patients with COVID-19. Both his chest X-ray and chest computed tomography (CT) scan confirmed our high suspicion of COVID-19. He was found to have acute hypoxic respiratory failure due to presumptive COVID-19 pneumonia, and the decision was eventually made to admit him to our Intensive Care Unit (ICU).

This case was particularly challenging for the care team. Harold was the sole caregiver of his son, Danny, a 50-year-old man with Down syndrome. After the death of his wife, Harold had not made any contingency plans for the care of his son. Owing to the complexity of Danny's care needs, we allowed Danny to remain at Harold's bedside. In addition, Danny was not willing to leave his father's side. This clearly was an exception to our no-visitor policy, but there was no better option.

Early Testing and Diagnosis

During the early pandemic period of March 29 to April 25, 2020, the total number of ED visits in the United States was 42% lower than during the same period in 2019.[1] The pandemic altered the use of EDs by the public and had a critical impact on how we provided acute care for our communities. During this period, patients who presented to the ED were of much higher acuity and were much further along in their illnesses than previously – both COVID-19-positive and non-COVID-19 patients. It was clear that we would need frequent communication across all EDs in our health system to understand the acuity and volume.

Initially, diagnostic testing for COVID-19 was available *only* from the New York State Department of Health (NYS DOH) and required approval. An ED physician would often have to spend more than an hour on the phone to get testing approval. To make matters more complicated, testing results had significant delays, up to 14 days, due to the NYS DOH turnaround time. Later, as more testing sites became available, including using our own in-house tests, laboratory turnaround time decreased significantly.

While we felt hopeless as a result of delayed diagnosis, clinical management of patients did not change; we continued to provide supportive care. With a large amount of information still unknown about how best to treat COVID-19, clinical teams began using other diagnostic methods for suspected cases, including C-reactive protein, ferritin, D-dimer, and interleukin-6. In addition, during the time that we were unable to access testing, we obtained chest CT scans and looked for classic COVID-19 patterns. This represented a significant change in practice from using evidence-based medicine to guide clinical decision-making to experimental methods for treatment.

ED Facility Modification

In February 2020, MSBI began to create a plan to respond to the influx of patients with COVID-19. However, none of us could reliably predict the number of patients or the acuity that was coming. We quickly established a working group of clinical staff, the IP Team, and engineering experts to redesign the throughput of patients in the ED. A subgroup was also formed to develop innovative ways of keeping staff safe.

Changes in policies and procedures and constantly evolving clinical protocols supported these structural modifications. The ED created a self-contained respiratory zone, which included 18 additional negative-pressure rooms with external exhaust and filtered air expelled through high-efficiency particulate air (HEPA) filters. We minimized unnecessary traffic, which helped mitigate the spread of infection among staff and other patients. This also delineated which areas in the ED were safe zones for non-COVID-19-related presentations. The waiting room redesign helped to promote social distancing for our ambulatory patients. We were able to provide entry control and screening for COVID-19 to identify highly infectious patients, provide them with masks, and collect information to determine their appropriate routing. During the third week of March 2020, masking became mandatory for all personnel inside the hospital, including visitors.

ED Staff Support

The COVID-19 pandemic undoubtedly created continual stress for the staff, hospitals, and health system. While the shortage of PPE early on was short lived, it was clear that we needed to act quickly to create a strategy that would protect our staff. As previously mentioned, we needed to conserve PPE, so we developed protocols for reuse. We initiated PPE education and huddles three to four times a day, seven days a week, to immediately deal with the challenges that staff were facing. During our rounds, we checked that staff members were using PPE correctly, ensured the strategic location of PPE carts, and refilled sanitizer dispensers and other cleaning/disinfection materials. To protect the doctors who were intubating patients and to minimize COVID-19 exposure, staff suggested the solution of an intubation bundle, including all of the necessary supplies for intubation in one consolidated bag. Staff also created an intubation box made of PLEXIGLAS®, which provided protection for staff during the intubation procedure by decreasing exposure to respiratory secretions. Although some of these changes seem minor, these actions helped us preserve the morale of the entire staff in the ED by demonstrating that ED leadership valued their safety and was willing to make the necessary changes.

Clinical Management Challenges

During the Ebola outbreak nearly a decade earlier, we developed protocols designed to minimize the potential spread of infection. As we are a teaching hospital that trains residents, having an additional person on the care team means there is one more person who could potentially contract the infection from a patient. Given the highly contagious nature of Ebola, we decided that no residents would see any persons under investigation. As we prepared for COVID-19, we decided to take a similar approach. In the first days of the pandemic, only the attending physician and a primary nurse would enter the room with a symptomatic patient. However, this proved to quickly overwhelm our attending physicians as the volume of patients rose, and we needed to quickly modify this to an "all-hands-on-deck" approach, with larger care teams for these patients.

Innovation Through Telemedicine

Telemedicine was rapidly incorporated into the care of our patients in the beginning of April 2020. We developed a "provider in triage" model, whereby providers completed assessments and placed orders to help expedite care, reducing wait times and minimizing potential exposure of symptomatic patients to other patients and staff. Telemedicine was used to link the ED with palliative care for patients and their families. Ophthalmology residents worked in the ED to help bridge the gap between ED providers and palliative care specialists, with the latter in very limited supply owing to record-breaking demand. This enabled us to have very difficult conversations with more patients around end-of-life care. Telemedicine was utilized to complete reassessments, thereby minimizing the need to don and doff PPE each time a patient needed to communicate with their health-care team and allowing for efficient consultation with specialists to help guide patient care.

We also used telemedicine to provide music therapy to our patients: Entertainment and therapeutic services were offered to all patients via a video link. Patient liaisons continued to engage with patients virtually to make their stay more comfortable. Tablets equipped with Skype, Zoom, and FaceTime were provided to patients while in the ED so they could communicate with their families.

We were able to improve access to pediatric emergency medicine services by utilizing telemedicine for our entire health system. The MSBI pediatric emergency medicine faculty used this modality to develop school-based, acute telehealth programs, which evaluated the impact and needs of school testing and focused on quality initiatives that broadened the capabilities and scope of the Pediatric Short Stay Unit. Child Life services also utilized telemedicine and so were able to continue unabated, providing services to children and adults with developmental disabilities in the ED and throughout the hospital.

The pandemic made us reevaluate how patient care was provided and who provided that care. For example, at MSBI, we brought together the ED, the Palliative Care Department, and ophthalmology residents from the New York Eye and Ear Infirmary of Mount Sinai. These redeployed residents helped to identify patients in the ED who were at risk of admission and intubation and coordinated with the patients' families, the Palliative Care Department, and ED providers to orchestrate care, clarify goals of care, and, in some cases, say final goodbyes using the telemedicine platform. This unprecedented cooperation between institutions and departments demonstrated the power of a unified medical system and how innovations such as telemedicine help bring humanity to medicine, even during a disaster.

Despite the challenges, the ED was resilient and developed innovative solutions to help maintain the highest quality of care and ensure patient safety. As the hospital pivoted to take on more COVID-19 inpatients, the ED utilized the Pediatric Observation Unit to provide care to older, non-COVID-19 patients. The faculty, nurses, and staff worked tirelessly to provide quality care for our patients and create a safe working environment for all.

Our ambulatory practices also utilized telemedicine to connect with patients. As our experience with telemedicine continued to grow, we were able to incorporate more components of the physical examination in our assessments, allowing us to provide a higher level of virtual care to our patients. Due to its convenience, patients still prefer to utilize telemedicine services to access care today.

Sobering Reality

On the patient floors, clinical teams were dealing with multiple cardiac arrests at the same time, resulting in the largest number of patient deaths that our staff had ever seen. The faces of our staff were worn, with blistered skin around their noses and raw skin behind their ears from the N-95 masks. Feelings of absolute defeat hung in the air.

One of the most sobering realities was the fact that our hospital morgue was not equipped to handle the volume of patients who would need the space. At our peak, we had two mobile morgue trailers on-site to accommodate our decedents. The sight of these trailers, which were not far from our refuse location, was disturbing to our staff and community. One of our ED attendings was so upset by this visual that he wrote to a local journal and is still speaking today about how distressing it was for him. We eventually switched to referring to patients in the morgue as guests, which helped ease some of the trauma associated with these extenuating circumstances.

As visitor policies quickly changed per state mandate on March 23, 2020, eliminating all outside personnel from entering the hospital, the toll on patients and families became immeasurable. Patients were dying alone, without family at the bedside. Even at the height of the pandemic, leadership always attempted to make exceptions for unique cases. Of course, these visitors needed PPE, which further depleted our supply. Despite this, we wanted every patient to have a family member with them at their time of death, even if we needed to utilize video calling, such as Zoom or FaceTime. The Patient Experience Team at MSBI coordinated using staff as "runners," who would bring items from family members outside the hospital to the patients in an attempt to provide any possible connection to the outside world.

External Morale and Communications

Outside the walls of the hospital, tragedy was setting in. Patients seeking care for non-COVID-19 concerns were fearful, often avoiding medical treatment altogether to avoid the risk of being infected. Patients were delaying their mammograms and routine testing, as well as cancer care. All the while, a sense of comradery stirred throughout the city, as community members came up with ways of encouraging health-care workers to keep going. The city began a daily cheer at 7 PM every night, clapping, hooting, hollering, banging pots and pans out windows, and blasting "New York, New York" from balconies. There was not a dry eye in the house.

Evolution of Testing

During the first stages of the pandemic, the NYS DOH required approval for all testing, as testing was not widely available. Clinical teams began triaging patients into two categories: persons under investigation and persons under monitoring. These categories provided a method for determining how a patient would be assigned bedding to best contain the spread of the virus. Later, the term persons under monitoring was removed from use as the virus quickly spread and the mindset shifted to the possibility that everyone was potentially infected.

Urgent care centers and hospital EDs quickly became overwhelmed with testing needs (Figure 3.4). The typical lag time for results from external testing agencies, such as LabCorp, was three days. In-house testing became available at Mount Sinai Health System on March 22, 2020, significantly accelerating the process for testing and providing turnaround times within 18 hours.

Discussions around tracing the source of infection began swirling as external efforts were focused on tracking anyone who encountered an infected individual. New York State complied with CDC's guidelines, implementing quarantine periods for those who came into close contact with the virus. This posed significant challenges for patients requiring outside support for day-to-day tasks (e.g. visiting nurse services and aids) and eliminated all interpersonal contact. Our elderly felt isolated. Manhattan shut down. Broadway theaters stopped all performances, restaurants closed their doors, and even the Metropolitan Transit Authority shut down the subway between 1 AM and 5 AM every day.

Intensive Care Unit

Case Study of Harold and Danny: Part 2

Harold was admitted to the ICU from the ED for acute hypoxic respiratory failure and required noninvasive positive pressure ventilation and high-flow nasal oxygen (HFNO).

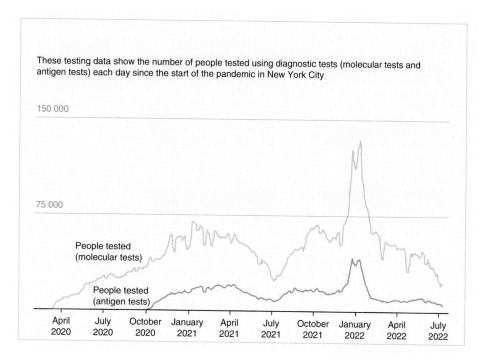

These testing data show the number of people tested using diagnostic tests (molecular tests and antigen tests) each day since the start of the pandemic in New York City

Figure 3.4 Diagnostic testing during the COVID-19 pandemic in New York City.[2]

Although he was severely hypoxic and breathing fast, he did not complain of much shortness of breath. We referred to this clinical presentation as "happy hypoxia." Under normal circumstances, this degree of hypoxia warrants endotracheal intubation and mechanical ventilator support. Based on our early experience with COVID-19, we delayed intubation as much as possible because we knew that, once intubated, many patients were unable to be liberated and died on the ventilator.

While Harold was isolated in the ICU, his son had no place to go. Due to Danny's high-risk exposure to COVID-19, group homes were unwilling to accept him as a resident. The ICU team had no choice but to allow him to remain at his father's bedside. Danny sat at his father's bedside in the ICU for several weeks. The staff adopted Danny. Despite Danny not being listed in our registry as a patient, our staff fed him, provided him with games, walked with him, and provided all of his care needs for several weeks. Unfortunately, Harold became progressively and increasingly ill and eventually expired from his illness. By this time, Danny had tested positive for COVID-19 and was admitted to one of our medical floors.

ICU Surge

Due to public fear, patients were afraid to come to the hospital, as evidenced by our decreased ED patient volume. As patients delayed care, they presented with advanced symptoms of COVID-19, resulting in higher acuity. ICUs experienced a record high in the number of admitted patients. Before the pandemic, we were able to accommodate 24

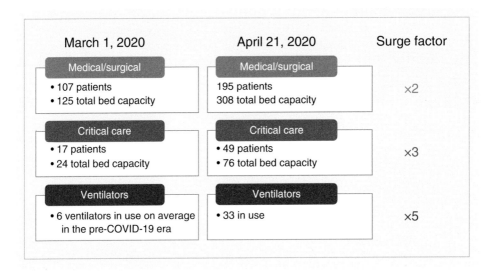

March 1, 2020	April 21, 2020	Surge factor
Medical/surgical • 107 patients • 125 total bed capacity	**Medical/surgical** 195 patients 308 total bed capacity	×2
Critical care • 17 patients • 24 total bed capacity	**Critical care** • 49 patients • 76 total bed capacity	×3
Ventilators • 6 ventilators in use on average in the pre-COVID-19 era	**Ventilators** • 33 in use	×5

Figure 3.5 MSBI side-by-side comparison of capacity by date.

critical care patients. At our peak in April 2020, we had created an additional 52 beds, giving a total of 76 critical care beds, which represented a 68% increase in bed capacity. We utilized our Post-Anesthesia Care Unit (PACU) as a non-COVID-19 ICU, closed our Post-Cardiac Catheterization Unit, and converted the Coronary Care Unit to a COVID-19 ICU. We reopened a dormant surgical ICU and eventually created an ad hoc step-down ventilator-weaning unit, all to accommodate our surge in critically ill patients (Figure 3.5).

While efforts were underway to implement testing across health-care facilities, the reality was that most test results came with significant delays, which had an impact on our ability to provide disease-specific treatment options. For the first COVID-19-positive patient in the ICU, it took nearly two weeks for the results to return, and most COVID-19 test results were delayed by 7 to 10 days.

Once patients required mechanical ventilation, they lingered. Weaning was a slow process. In order to expand our capacity, we created a ventilator-weaning step-down unit that allowed us to move intubated patients out of our ICU. As a result, we received additional ICU patient transfers to the ventilator weaning unit from other hospitals within our system to create additional ICU bed capacity across the Mount Sinai Health System.

Given that our community hospitals were overwhelmed with COVID-19 patients, we started to accept transfers. With the huge influx of cases, we stopped following our central line-associated bloodstream infections (CLABSI) policies, which resulted in three consecutive central line infections. MSBI had not had a case of CLABSI for more than an year. Fortunately, we were able to use ambulatory oncology nurses as line leaders to ensure all central lines followed protocols and processes, putting an end to the uptick in central line infections. Despite being in the middle of the pandemic, we continued to emphasize high-quality care.

Staffing Deployment and New Roles

Additional staff members were also pulled from ambulatory practices and surgical services to support the exponential needs of the ICU. A tiered coverage model was used to oversee care for patients, which assisted non-ICU staff who may have been unfamiliar with ICU patient care. The typical ICU nurse-to-patient ratio before the pandemic was one nurse to two patients, but, during the first wave of COVID-19, the ratio expanded to one to eight. One ICU nurse supervised two PACU nurses, and each PACU nurse supervised two ambulatory nurses. This same tiered model was used for physicians, advanced practice providers, and respiratory therapists. Many providers came out of retirement to assist with the surge of patients in the hospital system, refreshing their skill sets in caring for both medicine and critical care patients.

It was helpful that New York State granted emergency privileges to expedite the onboarding process. However, training posed significant challenges, including difficulty finding adequate and qualified locum staff. Onboarding took time and coordination, draining our staff even further. We also had an electronic medical record (EMR) system that was not used anywhere else in the country, further delaying onboarding.

Early Clinical Intervention Methods

Initially, China and Italy experienced the largest impact from COVID-19. Clinical information flowed from both countries through formal publications and informal forums, all attempting to pass on as much relevant information as possible. Confusion stirred around the best methods for treatment, as no specific treatment guidelines were available in the early part of the pandemic and best practices were changing constantly as the virus spread.

Some of the information gleaned from the community and social media outlets on how to manage the crisis was helpful, but often it added to the confusion rather than providing benefits. Anecdotal experiences were shared across informal platforms, and while these would typically not affect medical decision-making, desperate doctors had to use all means necessary to provide the best care for their patients.

Therapeutic Interventions

From their first day of residency, physicians are taught to follow evidence-based medical guidelines. COVID-19 made providers uncomfortable because they did not have an abundance of literature at their disposal. In the very early days, hydroxychloroquine and azithromycin were used liberally but in short order gave way to steroids, remdesivir, convalescent plasma, and monoclonal antibodies. Many patients met the criteria for remdesivir, but it was often limited in availability, causing clinicians to prioritize the most critically ill patients.

Initially, the WHO did not recommend the use of steroids based on clinical treatment failures from prior pandemics (i.e. severe acute respiratory syndrome [SARS] and Middle East respiratory syndrome [MERS]). Clinicians were faced with a contradiction between WHO recommendations and the benefits of steroids that they observed at the bedside until better evidence was available to support the use of steroids.

One ICU patient's family threatened to sue the hospital if the clinical team did not administer ivermectin to the patient as part of the treatment course. After meetings with the legal team and hospital leadership, the recommendation was to prescribe ivermectin, despite the lack of proven evidence. Other possible treatment options were circulating in the media: Significant controversy surrounded the use of hydroxychloroquine, including forceful promotion from nonmedical professionals, including the US president, despite the absence of any scientific evidence that it was beneficial. There were other reports from courts mandating the use of various unproven treatments for patients with COVID-19. This created an additional burden of stress for providers and led to mistrust between patient families and the clinical team. Despite evidence to the contrary, ivermectin continues to have stubborn champions and make news headlines.

Non-Therapeutic Interventions: Doing Less is Sometimes More

Mortality rates across hospitals in the New York metropolitan area were at an all-time high during 2020, especially for elderly patients who required intubation and mechanical ventilatory support. Many patients presented with a remarkable disconnect between hypoxemia (an abnormally low concentration of oxygen in the blood) and proportional signs of respiratory distress, at which point rapid deterioration can occur. This clinical symptom of "happy hypoxia" provided the clinical team with a high pretest probability for the disease. Severely hypoxic patients had a prolonged hospital course: intubated/extracorporeal membrane oxygenation for two to three months, and HFNO and/or nasal intermittent positive pressure ventilation for one to two months.

An elderly professor presented to our hospital with severe hypoxia. He required 100% HFNO with an additional 100% non-rebreather mask to maintain his oxygen level at 88%. The patient's hypoxia was so severe that the clinical team felt he would die without intubation. However, the patient strongly refused intubation and signed a do-not-resuscitate/do-not-intubate order. To everyone's surprise, the patient slowly but eventually improved without intubation and ultimately was discharged. From this experience, the concept of delayed intubation was developed.

Delayed intubation went against best practices taught in medical training but could potentially save a patient from prolonged intubation and a prolonged hospital stay, high sedation requirements, and critical illness myopathy, and provided the ability to save resources for the hospital at a time when resources were already lacking.

Clinical literature supports placing patients with acute respiratory distress syndrome in the prone position for improved oxygenation. We created a Proning Team of orthopedic surgeons who routinely use the prone position during spinal surgeries. We also created a Procedure Team, utilizing surgeons who ceased their elective surgeries to assist with tracheostomies, central lines, arterial lines, and dialysis catheter placements.

Staff Support Initiatives

Overhead announcements began daily around noon from the Chief Medical Officer with words of encouragement, accompanied by uplifting music to keep both staff and patients hopeful and provide a sense of connection for those in isolation. We announced when COVID-19 patients were being discharged, signifying how many lives were being saved. Weekly "need to know" emails were also sent from the Chief Nursing Officer to all employees, highlighting crucial information about changes to protocols, testing, and resources for staff who were overwhelmed.

Regular town halls were held to provide a forum for leadership to communicate with staff about our strategy and for leadership to understand the needs of our teams. We quickly adapted to a conversational question-and-answer approach, rather than a presentation approach, whereby staff were encouraged to ask questions, and hospital leadership and the IP Team provided guidance and answers. Our health system experts communicated with media and news outlets to provide guidance to the broader community as well. We also educated leadership partners from skilled nursing facilities on how to care for COVID-19 patients.

The Patient Experience Team developed two "recharge rooms," equipped with audio and visual calming displays and additional staff resources to combat the newly named "pandemic PTSD." The fitness center remained open throughout the pandemic. Free mental health services were developed for all employees and their families, and a 24/7 hotline was provided for staff to talk with a peer about their experiences as a health-care worker on the front lines of a pandemic. Many departments developed a buddy system, whereby two staff members were paired together to check in and support one another.

When possible, employees were encouraged to work from home, as this became more acceptable for both administration and staff. This helped staff who were experiencing child-care issues, as well as those attending to sick and elderly family members.

As donations began pouring in, a team was developed to manage all incoming donations and sort and distribute them in a fair manner across the hospital. Donations included masks, health-care supplies, scrubs, restaurant-prepared meals, beverages, haircuts, massages – anything to keep spirits high. These were so greatly appreciated by staff.

Hospital Medicine

Case Study of Harold and Danny: Part 3

Danny was admitted to the medical service on March 22, 2020. His blood pressure was 120/68, his heart rate was 82 beats per minute, his respiratory rate was 18 breaths per minute, his temperature was 98.2°F, and his pulse oxygen level was 98% on room air. His course was much less severe than that of his father, and he eventually recovered. Unfortunately, we were waiting on guardianship for Danny, which tends to be a lengthy process. Article 81 of New York's Mental Health Hygiene Law "authoriz[es] the court to appoint a guardian to manage the personal and or financial affairs of a person who cannot manage for himself or herself because of incapacity."

Danny lived at our hospital for over three months and, along the way, many of our multidisciplinary colleagues bonded with him. They helped him grieve the loss of his father and discover his love of Latin music. Eventually, we were able to place him in a group home in the Rockaways, where he lives and flourishes to this day.

Operational Changes

As it became clear that nearly every patient who presented to the ED had COVID-19 and needed admission, our capacity was quickly overwhelmed. In bizarre fashion, we became a specialty hospital, but for a specialty that no one wanted: pandemic management. Our census transformed from a robust mix of routine medical cases (e.g. heart failure, cirrhosis, complications of opioid-use disorders, and complications of diabetes) to a single-issue service: COVID-19 and its many emerging complications. As most patients presented as acutely ill and were admitted to the ICU, the inpatient medicine and surgical census dropped briefly. However, this changed very quickly. Prior to the COVID-19 pandemic, our inpatient medical/surgical units could accommodate 125 inpatients and 24 observation patients. To care for the influx of COVID-19 patients, we made several operational changes, including reopening old, shuttered units.

We closed the Observation Unit and deployed its staff to assist in treating COVID-19 inpatients. MSBI's census was 95% COVID-19 from the middle of March through May 2020. We also needed to create a COVID-19 dialysis unit, which was easier than transporting patients to the separate building that housed our Dialysis Unit.

With the capacity of our ICUs surging by nearly 300%, we triaged patients with a higher acuity to a newly created step-down unit. Given that this unit was not initially equipped for continuous monitoring, we utilized Masimo machines to monitor patient oxygen saturations outside the rooms. This allowed staff to monitor patients without physical entry or additional exposure. Given that critical care staff were overwhelmed, hospitalists assumed care for these higher acuity medical patients using a tiered model of care, with intensivists comanaging.

Fortunately, ambulatory practices remained closed, and hospital medicine recruited and trained multiple cohorts of providers already credentialed within our system (i.e. cardiology attendings, gastroenterology fellows, outpatient internal physicians, and family medicine physicians). These colleagues eagerly and generously pitched in and developed new hospitalist skill sets to help manage our patient volume. As patient numbers climbed relentlessly, it became clear that redeployed faculty were not going to be enough, and we partnered with a locums agency, AMI, and an international volunteer agency, Samaritan's Purse, to help manage additional patients. In one aspect, New York was lucky to be the initial epicenter for COVID-19, as many volunteers came to us from other states that had yet to experience their own surge in COVID-19 cases. This led to the credentialing of more than 500 new staff who were trained on our EMR system. We also assigned hospitalists to round with these contracted groups to ensure a high quality of care.

Within our health system, Brooklyn and Queens were being hit the hardest in terms of both the number of patients presenting and disease severity. We partnered with our system transfer center and created the role of the "triagist," a hospitalist who would quickly analyze clinical data and discuss with transferring sites which patients should be transferred to our facility, which patients would need a potential higher level of care at our facility, and which patients seemed well enough to be discharged home from the sending facility. This helped to unburden the staff at our sister sites in the boroughs being hit the hardest.

Convalescence from COVID-19 is a long and slow process, and it quickly emerged as a challenge for patient placement. Patients would often have significant oxygen requirements but could not go home to family, either because the family was not equipped to manage these new needs or because they were hesitant to allow COVID-19-positive family members into the home. Additionally, patients often shared their apartments and homes with multiple family members. Nursing homes were under fire and scrutiny for their management of internal outbreaks and were unable to accept patients. When they finally began to accept patients, they instituted strict admission requirements of two negative COVID-19 tests at least 24 hours apart. This delayed the discharge process anywhere from three to five days.

External Efforts for Decanting Hospitals

A 68-bed field hospital was opened by Mount Sinai in Central Park, with staffing support from Samaritan's Purse. Mount Sinai also partnered with the United States Army, which opened a stand-alone hospital in the Javits Center in midtown Manhattan. This stand-alone hospital was able to take convalescing patients who required up to six liters of oxygen and helped to decant our inpatient census. The United States Navy sent the USS Comfort to dock on the Hudson River, but this had far more limited use, as it was unable to take individuals with COVID-19 and patients had to be relatively able-bodied to meet the criteria for admission, which included the patient's ability to climb onto a top bunk bed. We were unable to identify any patients who met the criteria for admission to the USS Comfort during the first wave of the pandemic.

We partnered with local oxygen delivery companies for patients requiring fewer than four liters of oxygen who were able to be discharged home. The discharge team sent these patients home with a pulse oximeter and monitored oxygen connection, which would identify early warning signs of hypoxia and signal if a patient needed to return to the hospital.

Internal Morale

During the first wave, as information about the virus was updated continuously, staying on top of the latest guidance was a daunting task. The continuously changing and inconsistent recommendations from the WHO, CDC, and NYS DOH led to mistrust and fear. Many of our staff moved away from their families or sent their families away from the city to decrease their risk of acquiring the virus at work and transmitting it to their family members. For families, the fear of the unknown was even worse than for our staff. Not being able to hold a loved one's hand, caress a cheek, or kiss a forehead drove many families to desperation. Some families kept their Zoom feed on continuously so as not to miss anything. Bearing witness to family members saying goodbye to loved ones via electronic devices was haunting for many staff members. However, despite the overwhelming feelings of sadness, we found ways to celebrate successes. For our 500th discharge – an elderly man who loved Johnny Cash – we escorted him out of the hospital and into his family's car with "Walk the Line" playing jubilantly.

External Morale

As the first pandemic wave in New York City was tapering, another uprising was emerging. Protests occurred around the city at all times of the day in the wake of George Floyd's murder and in support of Black Lives Matter. There was a curfew. The city still felt partially empty – stores remained boarded up and the absence of both tourists and New Yorkers was evident. Families were unable to bury their loved ones and mourn properly, gather jointly with other loved ones, or celebrate and comfort each other. As all of this was happening outside the hospital, it was also happening in the daily lives of our staff who brought a complexity of emotions – grief, rage, and despair – with them to work every day.

Subsequent Waves and the Introduction of Vaccines

In the months following the initial surge, there was significant growth in the number of testing sites across New York City. The timeliness of testing improved, making it easier for the public to receive results and track exposures. People lined up all over the city, six feet apart, to get tested.

Then came a quiet lull. During this time, staff were encouraged to take early retirement, traveling teams were let go, and volunteers returned to their own states to help with their

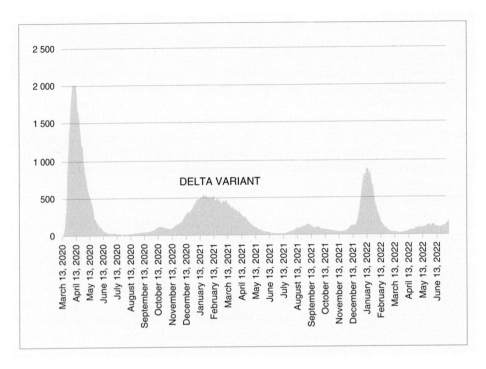

Figure 3.6 Mount Sinai Health System COVID-19 cases from March 2020 to June 2022.

own crises. Teams who had worked so successfully during the first wave were dismantled. There were no more accolades, no more donations.

So, when the second wave hit in October 2020, we did not have the staff we needed to care for our patients. This wave peaked from January to April 2021, mainly due to the delta variant, see Figure 3.6.

This was a much longer wave and felt more like a marathon than the "sprint" of the first. The delta variant seemed much more contagious, and many of our staff members became ill, creating more staffing challenges. The remaining staff had to cover for their colleagues and work over the major holidays. This, coupled with the loss of public support, caused morale to hit rock bottom. The public cheering stopped and health-care workers in scrubs were targeted and attacked on public transportation. Fortunately, the volume of patients was less than during the previous wave, providing some reprieve for our staff.

In July 2021, our hospital transitioned from our antiquated EMR system to the Epic EMR system, which, although providing significant benefits, also created a large amount of stress. Training all staff on the new EMR system while still caring for patients during a pandemic was an additional burden, but it was necessary to maximize efficiency. Switching to Epic was integral in shortening the staff onboarding process, as Epic is a widely utilized EMR system across the USA.

As vaccines from Pfizer and Moderna were successfully developed and made available (Table 3.1), "Operation Warp Speed" was put underway to distribute the vaccines across the United States.

Table 3.1 COVID-19 vaccine development

Vaccines	Date	Details
Pfizer BioNTech COVID-19 vaccine	December 11, 2020	The US Food and Drug Administration (FDA) issued the first Emergency Use Authorization (EUA) for the use of the Pfizer BioNTech COVID-19 vaccine in persons aged 16 years and older for the prevention of COVID-19.
Moderna COVID-19 vaccine	December 18, 2020	The FDA issued the second EUA for the use of the Moderna COVID-19 vaccine in persons aged 18 years and older for the prevention of COVID-19.
Janssen COVID-19 vaccine	February 27, 2021	The FDA issued the third EUA for the use of the Janssen COVID-19 vaccine in persons aged 18 years and older for the prevention of COVID-19.
Pfizer BioNTech COVID-19 booster	September 22, 2021	The FDA amended the EUA to allow a single booster dose of the Pfizer BioNTech COVID-19 vaccine to be administered at least six months after completion of the vaccine's primary series in certain populations.
Moderna and Janssen COVID-19 boosters	October 20, 2021	The FDA amended the EUAs to allow a single booster dose of the Moderna COVID-19 vaccine and Janssen (Johnson and Johnson) COVID-19 vaccines. The FDA also authorized the use of a heterologous (or "mix-and-match") booster dose of an available vaccine in eligible individuals following completion of primary vaccination with a different COVID-19 vaccine.
Pfizer BioNTech and Moderna COVID-19 boosters	March 29, 2022	The FDA authorized the second booster dose of either the Pfizer BioNTech or Moderna COVID-19 vaccine for adults aged 50 years and older and for certain immunocompromised individuals.

In December 2021, MSBI opened a COVID-19 Vaccine Pod providing vaccines for frontline health-care workers in alignment with the categories provided by NYS DOH. Staff were divided into groups based on their risk of COVID-19 exposure. We could not get the vaccines out fast enough. Staff were pulled from ambulatory sites to work in all areas of vaccination provision (including administering vaccines, scheduling appointments, and organizing supplies) and, at the peak, provided vaccines to approximately 750 staff and patients per day.

As vaccination numbers increased, the number of COVID-19-related hospitalizations slowly began to decrease. Figure 3.7 shows the number of vaccine doses administered in New York City over time. Figure 3.8 shows how vaccination and boosters impacted subsequent waves, hospitalizations, and deaths, with a sharp contrast seen between vaccinated and unvaccinated patients admitted to the hospital.

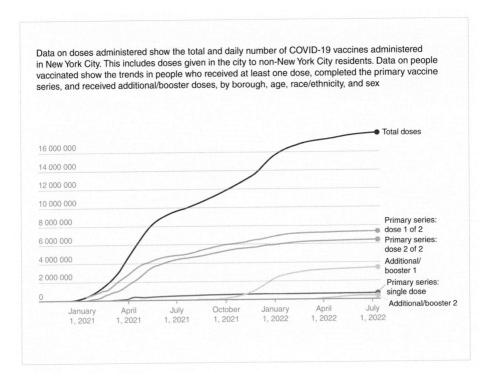

Figure 3.7 Vaccination trends in New York City.[2]
Data do not distinguish between boosters and additional doses for people who are immunocompromised. Additional/booster 1 includes the first booster dose or third dose for people who are immunocompromised. Additional/booster 2 includes the second booster dose or first booster dose of the three-dose primary series for people who are immunocompromised.

When the omicron variant struck, from December 2021 to January 2022, testing demand reached an all-time high. We created a testing pod in a separate building to offload asymptomatic staff and patients from the ED. Despite being asymptomatic, the positive testing rate in this pod was as high as 40%. Our hospital test-positivity rate for all comers reached as high as 43.7%; both numbers were remarkably high.

Conclusion

As we look back on the early days of COVID-19 with the benefit of hindsight, it seems unfathomable to think that our initial strategies for managing inpatients with COVID-19 included setting aside a select, but small, number of airborne rooms; that we would be able to limit which staff would care for these patients; and that we would be able to spare house staff from interacting with and treating these patients. And yet, those were the initial plans.

Given the lack of available testing for COVID-19, the clinical staff relied on the testing that was available, such as testing a viral panel that included influenza and respiratory viruses. If such testing gave a positive result, staff were falsely reassured that the patient's symptoms were from influenza or a respiratory virus and not COVID-19. This proved to be

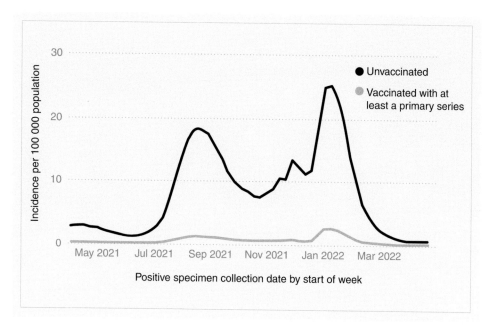

Figure 3.8 Rates of COVID-19 by vaccination status in ages 5 and up, April 4, 2021 to April 30, 2022 (30 US jurisdictions).[3]

a false assumption, as we later learned that patients with COVID-19 often tested positive for more than one virus at a time.

Never in our careers had we been asked to restrict visitors to dying patients, yet that is what we did. Refrigerated morgue trucks on the curbside were a constant reminder to staff of the horrors of this disease, an unavoidable sight as staff traveled to and from work. Not only were our staff dealing with the loss of patients, but they also suffered the loss of their colleagues and family members. Everyone was affected by COVID-19. No one was spared.

Despite the incredible amount of stress and hardship, one common theme across many staff members was the feeling of a heightened sense of purpose. Many felt that they were able to be "more useful" and were less worried about operational metrics. Staff were more focused on the purity of medicine. They were "essential health-care workers."

The pandemic forced us to function as a true health system and allowed us to establish processes for centralized distribution of materials and supplies. Resources were made more readily available to the entire health system, and we developed methods for estimating our future needs. Our current strategy is to keep an inventory that can adequately support both current and future needs.

We also had daily meetings that addressed the clinical needs of our critically ill patients. We read the literature, shared lessons learned from our patients and our challenges, and learned quickly from each other. We developed system-wide clinical guidelines that dramatically improved patient care and decreased mortality by standardizing the way we delivered care.

Recently, we came across an article about MSBI's management of the influenza pandemic from 1918 to 1920 (Figure 3.9).[4] The similarity between the two pandemics was startling. In 1918, the Department of Health advised the use of masks (albeit gauze) and the

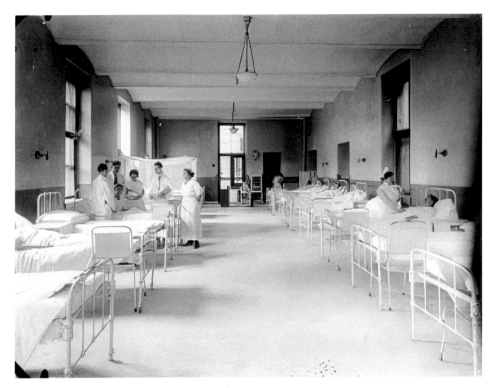

Figure 3.9 MSBI and the 1918 influenza epidemic.[4]

Founded in 1892, the early history of MSBI hospital was decorated with a series of success stories in the treatment of disease. Against the background of Manhattan's Lower East Side – then affected by poverty, close living quarters, and dangerous working conditions – its residents, largely recent Jewish immigrants, were made vulnerable to many of the contagious diseases of that era. In its first years, MSBI provided research to combat the typhoid epidemic of 1906–1907, established an after-care clinic to children affected by the 1916 polio epidemic, and is credited with finding the cure for trachoma, which had previously been a reason to turn away new immigrants at Ellis Island.

Only 25 years after MSBI's opening, the United States was embroiled in World War I. The hospital encouraged its medical staff to join the Medical Reserve Corps, with approximately half of its doctors signing up. The hospital had also encouraged its nurses, physicians, and other staff to join the war effort.

This left MSBI in a precarious position when the 1918 influenza epidemic reached New York City. Being chronically understaffed, the hospital's Medical Board contacted the Department of Health for advice. The response was simply "There is nothing to advise except the use of gauze masks which did not always prevent the disease." In November 1918, the hospital eliminated visiting hours, curtailed teaching hours, and turned the male medical ward over to the Department of Health to use as an isolation facility for the pandemic. (The Department of Health never used the facility because it was similarly understaffed.)

Female ward of MSBI, Jefferson and Cherry Street, circa 1910

hospital eliminated visiting hours and turned a medical ward into an isolation unit. Staffing shortages were a problem, and incentive pay was offered. Staff were trained to become nurses on the job. The second wave hit, which was more deadly than the first, and significantly reduced the staffing pool, making patient care more challenging than ever.

Fast forward to 2020, and the same issue of staffing shortages was still present. One valuable lesson from the COVID-19 pandemic has been the importance of cross-training staff and having contingency plans for when staff are sick. MSBI utilized third-party agencies to provide staffing, which helped significantly with the patient load per provider but still posed significant training challenges.

While it has always been thought that a pandemic is a once-in-a-lifetime event, we continue to be vigilant in our strategies to prepare for future infections. Although not a pandemic, we are now managing patients with mpox infections, using the same isolation and PPE practices that we utilized for COVID-19. Due to the advancements in testing capabilities during the COVID-19 pandemic at Mount Sinai, we are currently in the process of quality control verification of a newly developed assay for *Orthopoxvirus*.

Lessons Learned

Since the start of the pandemic, leadership teams in health care have learned, through the process of trial and error, which management approaches are most successful for patient care and for optimizing resources during a time of strain. The following steps were crucial in the success achieved in navigating the COVID-19 pandemic at MSBI:

- Streamlined information through a standardized incident response system ensured that all resources were allocated to the site that was the most in need
- System-wide leadership safety meetings provided a forum to feed information upstream from local incident command centers to the system command center
- The development of testing transformed the way that we care for our patients, impacting bed placement and appropriate precautions for infection prevention. In-house testing decreased turnaround times, and pop-up testing sites made testing available nationwide. The eventual development of home testing kits was game-changing in terms of preventing the spread of the virus
- Continuous evaluation and adaptation of visitor policies allowed us to keep our patients and staff as safe as possible during surges of the virus. We continue to evaluate visitor policies on a routine basis to ensure that our policy is doing what is best for both our patients and our staff
- Centralizing the distribution of supplies at the start of the pandemic allowed us to keep a closer eye on supply levels and determine contingency planning as we noticed items beginning to run low. Without a centralized plan for supplies, we may have run out of PPE, like many other hospitals in the United States
- One of the early steps in managing patient throughput was the evaluation and redesign of our ED. By transforming the unit to include negative pressure rooms, we were able to mitigate the spread of infection between patients and staff
- While the "pause" on elective surgeries lasted longer than we could have ever imagined, it was a necessary step in prioritizing patients with higher acuity. The additional staff members who were previously involved in elective cases were retrained to support services internally for both COVID-19 and non-COVID-19 patients
- Telemedicine bridged the gap between patients and providers, allowing patients outside the hospital to receive care from ambulatory providers and for hospitalized patients to communicate with their clinical teams without prolonging exposure time
- Fortunately for us, our hospital had previously decommissioned several units in preparation for our new campus plans. We were able to reallocate these spaces to build units from scratch to support the surge of patients from our community. The Facilities and Engineering Teams overhauled non-patient care areas, transforming and equipping the spaces to accommodate more patient care units

- Town halls for staff proved to be successful and continue to be held on a rotating basis. The use of weekly "need to know" emails from leadership to all employees gained positive feedback and is something that continues today. Additionally, these town halls and leadership emails help to provide a designated forum for staff support and to spread awareness about wellness resources available to our Mount Sinai community
- As we tragically learned, our morgue was not equipped to handle the volume of patients needed during the COVID-19 pandemic. We utilized mobile trailers during this time, but we are now aware of the need for contingency plans in the case of another surge
- All staff, at some point since March 2020, have stepped into another role's "shoes" to help keep our hospital operational. We utilized third-party vendors and partnered with our clinical teams to provide additional staffing. As part of this process, we identified the need for continuous cross-training for staff to be able to cover different areas successfully
- Conservation efforts for PPE may have saved our hospital from running out of supplies. By developing a geographic-based model and safe storage for the reuse of masks, we were able to extend our supply until we had the reassurance that supplies would be replenished
- In a time of unprecedented clinical management, we explored experimental methods to treat our patients. While some experimental methods failed, others were successful, such as delayed intubation and the use of steroids
- Keeping up with the amount of donations proved to be overwhelming. Through trial and error, we found success in managing donations through one centralized team that was able to document and appropriately distribute the donations equitably
- Discharging our patients with monitoring equipment aided in communication between patients and providers, even after their hospital stay. We sent patients home with pulse oximeters and methods for monitoring patients remotely to ensure a successful recovery. This allowed us to discharge patients sooner, shortening the length of stay and freeing up more beds for additional patients
- NYS DOH mandated the distribution of vaccines through a tiered system, prioritizing the distribution to essential health-care workers. Our staff in the ED and critical care units were included in one of the first tiers, followed shortly by immunocompromised patients and patients with multiple comorbidities. This tiered distribution plan allowed for vaccines to be given to those with the highest risk of infection first, giving providers a fighting chance to continue to care for patients with a significantly reduced risk of developing COVID-19. In the beginning stages of our COVID-19 Vaccine Pod, we struggled with the logistical needs of the vaccine. Refrigeration at subzero temperatures and time-sensitive doses that had to be given from an open vial were just some of the challenges that we had to overcome

Through all of this disruption, it would have been easy to take our eyes off our quality metrics, given the hardship and stress that the pandemic brought. We are proud that we were able to hold steady while also improving on hospital metrics, including length of stay, excess days, readmissions, and mortality. When adjusted for case complexity – our observed and expected rates in these realms were the best in the Mount Sinai Health System. It was also very important that we limited the acquisition of hospital-acquired infections. Reporting agencies and regulatory bodies suspended some of the reporting from the first half of 2021 due to the pandemic, and we are pleased that we were able to beat set targets for hospital-acquired infection rates in nearly all realms, particularly for *Clostridium difficile* infections, catheter-associated urinary tract infections, and CLABSI.

As we move toward the next phase of the post-COVID-19 experience, we strive to deliver the highest value care. Given the new requirements for hospitals in the post-COVID-19 world, our leadership team recognizes that previous plans to develop a new campus will no longer fit that need. As the world has learned to adapt, we too are learning to pivot in a new direction – to redesign, renovate, and transform our current campus to meet the needs of our community.

References

1. CDC, Impact of the COVID-19 Pandemic on Emergency Department Visits – United States, January 1, 2019–May 30, 2020 (June 12, 2020). www.cdc.gov/mmwr/volumes/69/wr/mm6923e1.htm (accessed January 27, 2023).

2. City of New York, COVID-19: Data (2023). www.nyc.gov/site/doh/covid/covid-19-data-totals.page (accessed January 27, 2023).

3. CDC, Rates of COVID-19 cases and deaths by vaccination status (2023). https://tinyurl.com/yckw32wb (accessed January 27, 2023).

4. Icahn School of Medicine at Mount Sinai, Mount Sinai Beth Israel and the 1918 influenza epidemic (June 4, 2020). https://tinyurl.com/38phz76v (accessed January 27, 2023).

Contribution of RADx® Tech to the Rapid Development of COVID-19 Diagnostic Tests

Steven C. Schachter, John M. Collins, Michael K. Dempsey, Laura L. Gibson, Matthew L. Robinson, and Paul Tessier

Introduction

This chapter is an overview of the processes used by the Rapid Acceleration of Diagnostics (RADx®) Tech program during the COVID-19 pandemic. RADx Tech was conceived by the US government to be the diagnostics component of a three-pronged national strategy, including vaccines and therapeutics, that aimed to significantly reduce the impact of COVID-19 on the US public. The goals of RADx were to improve clinical laboratory tests and identify, evaluate, support, validate, and commercialize innovative point-of-care and home-based tests that directly detected the presence of the severe acute respiratory syndrome coronavirus 2 (SARS-CoV-2) virus. As described throughout this book, many aspects of RADx Tech were unprecedented for an initiative of the National Institutes of Health (NIH) – the scale of its mission, the budget, the accelerated time frame, the extent of cross-government agency collaboration and information exchange, and the blending of business, academic, and investment best practices.

US Senator Lamar Alexander, the former Chair of the Senate Committee on Health, Education, Labor, and Pensions, described RADx Tech as "at least a mini-Manhattan Project."[1] Senator Alexander framed his view in an opinion piece with Senator Roy Blunt (Chairman of the Senate's Health Appropriations Subcommittee), proposing a "shark tank" approach.[2] They recognized that the urgency of the situation required not only an entrepreneurial approach akin to that of the reality TV show "Shark Tank," but also the utilization of the full capacity of the government itself, in coordination with the academic and private sectors, to "pull out all the stops" and create new technologies. Numerous processes designed and implemented specifically for RADx Tech were instrumental to its success, including cloud-based software platforms that enabled the program's infrastructure and processes, expert review panels, and the unique facilitation and mentoring provided to the funded projects.

Inception of the RADx Tech Processes

In close collaboration with the NIH's National Institute of Biomedical Imaging and Bioengineering (NIBIB), RADx Tech was designed and implemented by CIMIT (www .cimit.org), which served as the Point-of-Care Technologies Research Network (POCTRN: www .poctrn.org) Coordinating Center.[3] POCTRN was established in 2007 by NIBIB to advance the development of technologies that address unmet medical needs at the point of care, rather than in centralized health-care settings.

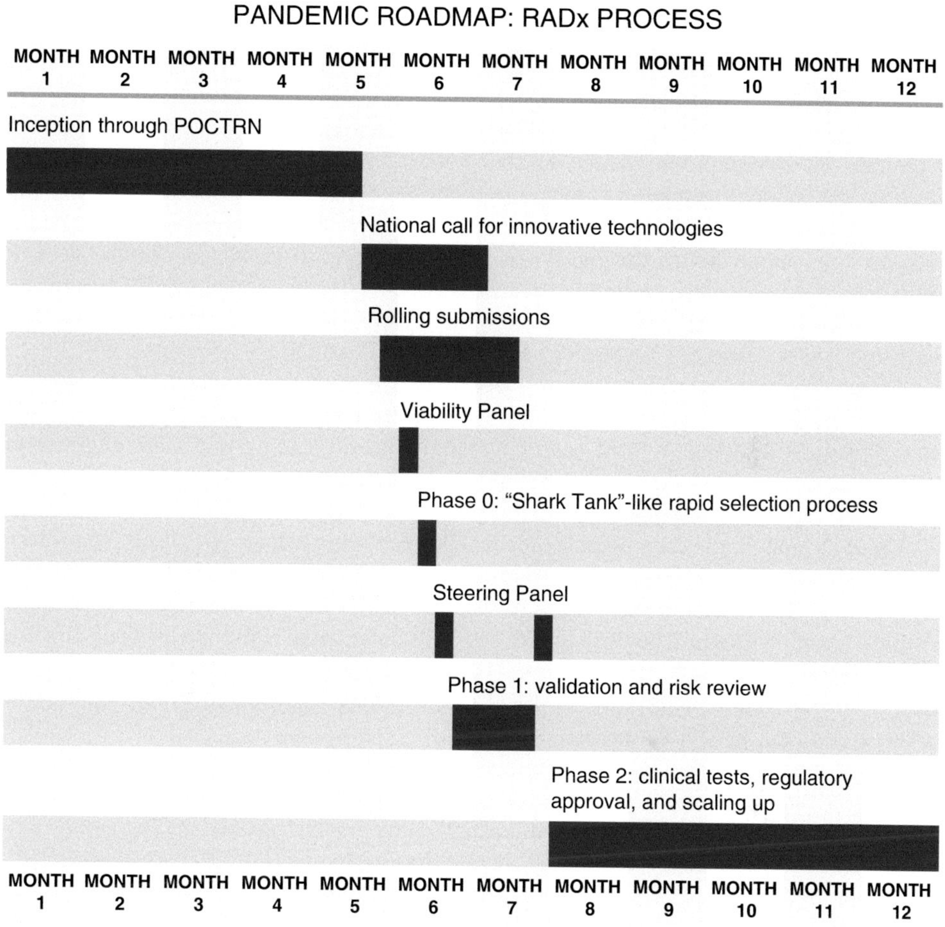

PANDEMIC ROADMAP: RADx PROCESS

Figure 4.1 This roadmap depicts the vital activities, their chronology, and an estimated time frame in months. In the case of the SARS-CoV-2 pandemic, month 1 was December 2019, the month in which the virus was isolated, sequenced, identified, and published.

Each task, starting with the Viability Panel, repeats with each new RADx project.

POCTRN, Point-of-Care Technologies Research Network.

Since its launch, POCTRN has created a national research network of academic sites (POCTRN centers) to foster multidisciplinary, multi-institutional partnerships and expertise in the development of integrated point-of-care systems using a variety of technologies for a wide range of clinical applications.

POCTRN's centers, with the help of the POCTRN Coordinating Center, annually fund teams of engineers, physicians, and scientists to advance early-stage technology development projects toward commercialization. POCTRN's new partnership-based model supports and facilitates collaborations across disciplines, institutions, and geographic regions to successfully drive innovative solutions through the early stages of translation toward commercially viable products for further investment.

In response to the COVID-19 pandemic, the US Congress appropriated $500 million to the NIH "to accelerate research, development, and implementation of point of care and other rapid testing related to coronavirus" (fourth congressional supplement, Public Law 116–139, April 24, 2020).[4] As a result, the POCTRN Coordinating Center was tasked by NIBIB Director Bruce Tromberg to establish a program to accomplish the goals set forth by Congress. The program was named RADx by NIH Director Francis Collins to reflect the need for the "rapid acceleration of diagnostics" into practice and as an homage to the "Rad Lab" at the Massachusetts Institute of Technology, where radar was further developed to support the United States during World War II. It was later named RADx Tech to differentiate it from sister programs sponsored by the NIH to address COVID-19 testing priorities, including RADx Underserved Populations (RADx-UP), RADx Radical (RADx-rad), and RADx Advanced Technology Platforms (RADx-ATP).

Fortunately, just before the pandemic began, two of the four actively funded centers in the POCTRN network were internationally recognized for their expertise in virally mediated infectious diseases. A third center featured a world-leading academic engineering group that thoroughly assessed and often improved upon point-of-care diagnostic tests. The fourth center had considerable experience in carrying out nationwide clinical studies.

Upon its launch, the starting point for RADx Tech was a call for proposals for projects that could lead to the development of commercialized diagnostic tests to detect the SARS-CoV-2 virus. The selection criteria for funded projects were very different from those of a typical granting program because RADx Tech was designed to simultaneously de-risk and accelerate the commercialization of projects that could address the national need for SARS-CoV-2 testing. Consequently, the RADx Tech workflow emphasized speed, agility, and timely attainment of deliverables.

Together with NIBIB, the Coordinating Center implemented the RADx Tech program by building on its management of POCTRN with cloud-based infrastructure tools, leveraging the strengths of the POCTRN centers to meet its new charge, and adding several new features to the RADx Tech funnel to accelerate the development of COVID-19 diagnostic tests from the laboratory bench to clinical use. These cloud-based infrastructure tools and features of the RADx Tech funnel that were new for translational research initiatives are discussed next, followed by a description of the overall workflow.

Cloud-Based Infrastructure Tools: CoLab and GAITS

RADx Tech scaled up very quickly, comprising hundreds of people from the academic and commercial biomedical and medical technology (MedTech) communities. The initiative's infrastructure enabled them to work together on complicated projects and problems at a scale and speed that required frequent communication, as well as coordination and monitoring. Consequently, the Coordinating Center took its existing web-based and cloud-based programs, namely CIMIT's management platform CoLab and its Guidance and Impact Tracking System (GAITS), and built further capabilities to enable the work of RADx Tech to proceed smoothly.[5] CoLab was used to manage the flow of funding applications from innovator teams through multistage, interactive selection and management processes. GAITS supported, facilitated, and monitored the funded projects through the commercialization process.

The overall goal was to use a cloud-based infrastructure to support the accelerated timelines of RADx Tech, capturing a longitudinal record for each project in a consistent way and allowing for workflows to proceed smoothly. CoLab and GAITS were modified to support rigorous, secure, and scalable workflows that could be implemented quickly and modified as needed. This enabled effective collaboration across multiple institutions and regions, while providing near real-time reporting to the RADx Tech and NIBIB leadership on the progress of projects and ensuring that proper controls were in place and approvals were obtained. Both CoLab and GAITS contained records of RADx Tech funding recommendations and justifications and related NIH decisions to facilitate analytics.

The CoLab platform tracked several workflows, including the management of vendors and suppliers approved by the NIH and test platform specification development. CoLab also monitored compliance with conflict-of-interest, confidentiality, and security policies and procedures. It offered the ability to easily communicate with users and affirm adherence to these requirements with a date stamp and digital signature while easily tracking those not in compliance. CoLab was linked to other security-related documents and recorded when an individual confirmed they had read and accepted the guidelines, such as information security overviews and security guidelines for project team members. A partner organization provided the virtual infrastructure to monitor, track, and approve the time spent by everyone involved outside the NIH in supporting funded projects.

The GAITS platform helped project teams successfully move MedTech projects toward commercialization by assessing and tracking the maturity of a project in four domains – clinical/workflow, market/business, regulatory, and technology – along the continuum from proof of concept to established clinical practice and by identifying deliverables for each stage of maturity and each domain. Funded teams, with the help of RADx Tech facilitators, embedded work plans in GAITS, including deliverables and go/no-go milestones. Importantly, GAITS provided a common framework that allowed hundreds of people from different organizations and backgrounds to work together efficiently.

Data and Communications Security

In its work for RADx Tech, the Coordinating Center followed all applicable NIH security guidelines and required POCTRN centers' staff, project subcontractors, and consultants to abide by NIH standards for confidentiality, conflict of interest, and data security. These measures protected the interests of innovators and resource providers and mitigated cybersecurity risks, such as data theft.

The Coordinating Center maintained a system security plan for its web-based systems that was based on National Institute of Standards and Technology (NIST) special publication 800-171, revision 2, on protecting controlled unclassified information in nonfederal systems and organizations. The security requirements for protecting the confidentiality of data processed by the systems were based on requirements derived from NIST 800-53 controls. An authorization-to-operate package (made up of the system security plan, a security assessment report, and a plan of actions and milestones) was developed to ensure that system security posture was maintained. Penetration testing, security control assessment by an independent third party, and regular vulnerability assessments of the underlying platform were conducted. Risk management of the plan of actions and milestones involved tracking and mitigating any risks identified.

Developing Expertise and Infrastructure

One of the key aspects that made RADx Tech successful was the recognition that, in addition to requiring funding, most teams that applied to the initiative did not have all of the resources and/or expertise they would need. It was determined that the missing resources would be the same for many teams. Rather than have each team try to establish its own resources independently, which would waste time and money, support infrastructure was developed to assist teams as needed. The following is an overview of the key infrastructure made available to project teams.

Clinical Studies Core

To field test the funded SARS-CoV-2 diagnostic testing and screening technologies in real-world settings with diverse populations, RADx Tech established the Clinical Studies Core at the Center for Advancing Point of Care Technologies in Heart, Lung, Blood, and Sleep Diseases, one of the POCTRN centers operating when the pandemic began.[6] Each diagnostic test was developed to address one or more specific use cases. The Clinical Studies Core evaluated test platforms on their usability in the populations and settings for which they were intended, such as communities with a high burden of COVID-19. These communities included Native American/American Indian populations, African Americans, and Latinx communities, who all bore a disproportionate share of the morbidity and mortality of COVID-19.

Within several months of the launch of RADx Tech, the Clinical Studies Core had leveraged expertise in clinical study design, biostatistics, human subjects research, study logistics, and community engagement to establish its infrastructure. The infrastructure for clinical studies included a master protocol approved by a single Institutional Review Board (with amendments for specific devices and sites), digital study platforms, data management systems, and multisite partnerships, including other POCTRN centers. Data from some of the studies were used to support applications for US Food and Drug Administration (FDA) Emergency Use Authorizations.

Many studies were executed, with NIH support, through the Eureka digital study platform developed at the University of California San Francisco. Potential research participants used Eureka to assess their eligibility for a study, provide consent, and complete digital health history surveys. After samples were collected at study sites or participants' homes, a second survey asked about result interpretation and device usability.

Study protocols, materials, and Eureka web content were also developed with attention to literacy levels and cultural sensitivities with guidance from the Community Health Equity and Engagement Team to evaluate whether RADx Tech-supported technologies were usable and deemed acceptable by diverse populations. All study participant interfaces were available in English and Spanish.

Through its innovative design and streamlined operations, the Clinical Studies Core reduced the typical time and cost of conducting clinical studies as part of medical device development. Timely studies conducted by the Clinical Studies Core answered practical questions regarding the use of SARS-CoV-2 rapid antigen tests, including the relative performance of antigen tests for emerging variants and optimal strategies for serial testing.[7, 8]

Clinical Review Committee

A key lesson learned through the POCTRN was that early and granular feedback on the intended use case for a device by experts and prospective end users is crucial. Such feedback lessens the risk of subsequent development bottlenecks created by unanticipated clinical challenges, systems engineering and technical usability flaws, cumbersome workflows, and insufficient validation.[9]

Because many of the RADx Tech-funded companies did not have ready access to experts who could provide a granular level of feedback while the test prototypes were under development, a Clinical Review Committee comprising clinicians, bioengineers, regulatory experts, and laboratorians was created to provide structured feedback to innovator teams about their funded SARS-CoV-2 diagnostic projects. Each company was offered a one-hour facilitated meeting with the Clinical Review Committee soon after it was funded in RADx Tech. Company representatives at these meetings included CEOs and the leaders responsible for engineering, marketing, product development, and regulatory strategy.

Over the course of dozens of meetings, the Clinical Review Committee identified common barriers to device design finalization, including issues related to biosafety, workflows, result reporting, regulatory requirements, sample types, supply chains, limits of detection, a lack of relevant validation data, and an inappropriate retail price considering a test's performance characteristics and intended use. The structured feedback from the Clinical Review Committee allowed device companies to identify common design challenges and improve their assays before design finalization.

Building a Network of Experts

Two partner organizations with long track records in managing translational research worked with the Coordinating Center to identify and engage hundreds of people in roles in the non-NIH components of RADx Tech. Extensive vetting was used to identify and retain the best experts in all fields relevant to the RADx Tech mission, whose depth of experience and proven productivity allowed for effective and timely decision-making without the usual bureaucratic delays of large organizations.

RADx Tech Workflow: From Submitted Applications to Funded Projects

A funnel process to narrow down the applications for funding to choose which projects to fund is common for organizations that award grants – including for POCTRN prior to the pandemic, managed by the Coordinating Center. For RADx Tech, the Coordinating Center added several new innovative features to the funnel process, as described in this section and in Chapters 8 and 11.

As already mentioned, the starting point for RADx Tech was a call for proposals for projects that could, within months, lead to commercialized diagnostic tests to detect the SARS-CoV-2 virus. In their proposals, applicants provided an overview of the solution, the development and implementation plan, partnerships and/or collaborations, key risks and mitigations, the support requested from RADx Tech, and a high-level schedule and budget. Less detailed information about the proposed work plan was required in the proposals than in a typical NIH small business innovation research (SBIR) application, as the work plan was revised at a later point in the funnel called the deep dive.

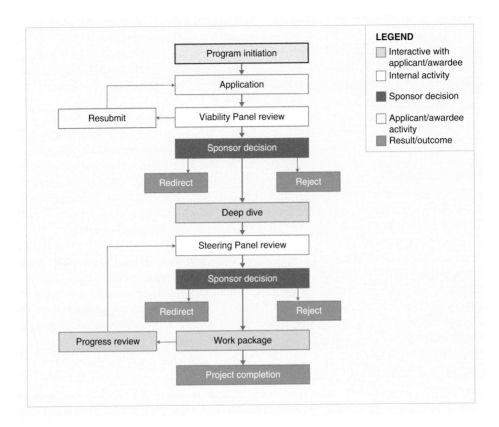

Figure 4.2 RADx Tech workflow.

Submitters were from large and small companies, start-ups, and academic groups. Their proposals entered the funnel workflow, which consisted of several unique features designed to blend best academic and business practices while moving projects through the evaluation and funding stages as quickly as possible.

The Coordinating Center developed a unique, multistage review process for proposals with two review panels – a Viability Panel and a Steering Panel – separated by a deep dive evaluation (Figure 4.2). Panel members were selected who had decades of commercialization and business experience or extensive scientific and technical knowledge. The breadth and depth of experience of the panel members fostered detailed discussions on projects during facilitated panel meetings, resulting in the selection of projects that were most likely to be successful, considering the goals of RADx Tech.

Viability Panel

The Viability Panel determined if a proposal was a good fit with the RADx Tech program and should therefore move into the deep dive.[10] Of the eight panel members, four had extensive business and technical expertise and were serving in senior technical and management roles in large companies and/or start-up operations. Two were physicians with many years of clinical, managerial, and business experience, including in retail clinic settings. Two represented the NIH.

The Viability Panel evaluated each proposal against the performance criteria stated in the RADx Tech solicitation and assessed its likely clinical use case(s) if it advanced to the market, such as doctor's and dentist's offices, pharmacies, manufacturing facilities, business offices, schools, and traditional testing locations (i.e. hospitals and laboratories). The goal was to advance meritorious projects that addressed a wide variety of use cases, which was further assessed at later stages in the funnel.

After reading proposals in CoLab, Viability Panel members made comments and recommended one of the following actions:

1. move the proposal to the deep dive phase
2. request that the applicant resubmit the proposal with additional information
3. send the application to a subject matter expert for their opinion
4. redirect the application to another funding mechanism
5. reject the application

The Viability Panel then met as a group to reach a consensus recommendation on each proposal, with actions 1, 4, and 5 sent to the NIH for its decision. While panel members could modify their comments and recommendations in CoLab after the panel discussions, they were encouraged to express their individual perspectives and opinions for the NIH to consider when making its decisions.

To keep the process moving as fast as possible, proposals were reviewed by the Viability Panel within one or two days, on average, after submission. The review process consumed well over 40 hours a week for many consecutive weeks.

Deep Dive

When the NIH agreed that a proposal could proceed in the funnel to a deep dive, a highly experienced team of experts from RADx Tech was selected to engage with the applicant team for one to two weeks. The deep dive resulted in a much more comprehensive understanding of the potential of and risks associated with the projected work than was apparent based on the proposal submitted. Using this approach, the deep dive team could provide a well-informed recommendation to the Steering Panel.[11]

The deep dive team for each proposal comprised a portfolio executive, a team lead, and project facilitators, with further support provided by subject matter experts as needed.[11] Portfolio executives and team leads typically had over 20 years of C-level management experience with in vitro diagnostics or in medical device companies. Nearly all had founded their own companies, and most had previously invested in start-up companies. Many team leads had designed and implemented tests during the HIV pandemic in the 1980s.

The team leads were matched to a project based on their individual business and technical skills. For example, if the proposal was led by an academic-based researcher with limited business experience, a team lead with very strong business experience would be selected.

Project facilitators were skilled project managers with 20 or more years of experience in diagnostics or other aspects of the MedTech industry. Assistant project facilitators were baccalaureate or master's students in biomedical engineering who helped coordinate meetings, create presentations, and take meeting minutes while gaining valuable experience with product development.

The initial contact for the deep dive team was typically the proposal's lead applicant, but given the breadth of information that was needed, the interactions regarding the application often expanded to include the CEO, the sales and marketing team, the regulatory affairs team, the manufacturing team, and company scientists. The applicant received $25 000 from the NIH for its team's time in meeting with the deep dive team.

Deep dive teams assessed projects against the performance and timeline criteria outlined in the RADx Tech solicitation, with particular attention paid to the GAITS framework, made up of the following four components:[5]

1. Technical: Can the technology be developed to the highest levels of analytical performance (e.g. sensitivity, specificity, dynamic range, limit of detection, reliability, accuracy, speed, and throughput) and operational performance, such as patient- and user-friendly design, alternative sampling strategies (saliva, exhaled breath, etc.), optimization of swab materials and test reagents, mobile-device integration, increased accessibility, and home-based use? Do these technical/design advances reduce barriers to expanding national testing capacity and provide clear advantages over current approaches?
2. Clinical: Does the proposal provide a realistic approach to increasing SARS-CoV-2 testing in a way that can be rapidly integrated into and adopted by the health-care system?
3. Commercial: Assuming the technology works as anticipated, can it be implemented and made available/manufactured at scale in an economically viable way?
4. Regulatory: Are there feasible plans to perform the studies required to obtain FDA Emergency Use Authorization and to subsequently obtain FDA clearance?

In addition to assessing the strengths and weaknesses of proposals and applicants, deep dive teams worked with applicants to develop the fastest commercialization plans possible by reworking the budget, refining or adding deliverables and milestones, or changing the timeline for review by the Steering Panel and the NIH. The revised work plans were captured in GAITS. Approximately 50% of the deep dives resulted in increases in the requested budget, signifying that the deep dive team felt the applicant had underestimated the magnitude of the work required.

Deep dive teams were assisted by RADx Tech cores and consultants who provided expertise such as benchtop performance verification (the Clinical Validation Core), clinical studies planning (the Clinical Studies Core), work plan development (the Workplan Review Panel), usability and use case fit (the Clinical Review Panel), and regulatory pathways. These inputs helped the deep dive team determine which RADx Tech resources the project would need during the performance period to be successful.

Deep dive team members were not personally invested in the success of any specific RADx Tech project in which they were involved. Strict conflict-of-interest rules prohibited any member of the deep dive team members from being an employee of or a consultant to any of the applicants during and for a period after the RADx Tech performance period.

The management of budgets and administrative project oversight for the deep dives was the responsibility of the Coordinating Center and its partner organizations that monitored time spent by non-NIH personnel.

Steering Panel

Once the deep dive was complete, the deep dive team uploaded summary information and a presentation into CoLab. This information was conveyed to the Steering Panel by the team lead during Steering Panel meetings without the applicant being present to maximize objectivity of the review.[10]

There were 19 members on the Steering Panel, whose experience included extensive business and technical expertise, which was gained through serving in senior technical and management roles. They had considerable experience in scaling up operations and implementing national clinical testing programs, in clinical settings and translational research, and in obtaining regulatory approvals and working with regulatory agencies; they also had extensive knowledge of clinical testing and included representatives of NIH. To provide consistency with the Viability Panel stage and the inputs of the RADx Tech cores during the deep dive, Viability Panel members also served on the Steering Panel and four Steering Panel members represented the RADx Tech cores. Unlike typical NIH review panels, each member of the Steering Panel reviewed every application, thereby providing consistency.

After hearing the presentation from the deep dive team lead, followed by a facilitated discussion, the Steering Panel voted to recommend to the NIH that the project:

- enter one of two funded stages – either work package 1 (WP1) or work package 2 (WP2)
- be redirected to another funding mechanism
- be rejected from further consideration

WP1 was comparable to SBIR phase 1 and WP2 was comparable to combined SBIR phases 2 and 3. In addition, the Steering Panel judged whether the proposed work plan for a recommendation to proceed to WP1 would provide sufficient evidence to eventually justify proceeding forward to WP2 and whether the proposed work plan for projects recommended to proceed to WP2 was appropriate for bringing the product to market.

If the NIH agreed to move a project into WP1, the same team that conducted the deep dive continued to work with the applicant team. This allowed consistency in terms of mentoring and the execution of the work plans.

WP1

Once the NIH approved a project to advance to WP1, the deep dive team (hereafter called the RADx Tech team) and the project team began to implement the work plan that was developed during the deep dive, improved upon by the Steering Panel, and approved by the NIH, with budgets that typically ranged from $1 to 5 million.[11]

The RADx Tech team coordinated all of the resources for every project and provided direction and support, typically spending up to 50 hours a week working with the project teams during WP1. They decided what additional resources from RADx Tech were needed and provided scientific, business, or other strategic advice. Working closely with project teams, the RADx Tech teams were able to troubleshoot and solve problems as they arose, often with the assistance of portfolio executives. The key resources that they brought to the project teams were experience, judgment, and contacts. They could help applicants understand what to do and in what order and they knew who were the "best in class" contacts that could provide help.

A large amount of responsibility, creative thinking, and authority was given to RADx Tech teams because of the depth of their experience and proven productivity. This allowed for timely decision-making and immediate action assignments without the requirement of several layers of approvals.

The RADx Tech teams advocated for projects in WP1 when there were technical difficulties or schedule slips. Each week, the RADx Tech teams presented the progress of their projects in WP1 to RADx Tech and NIH leadership, as well as to their peers. Often, this led to questions that needed to be answered to move past hurdles (e.g. Why is this taking so long? Are you sure the technical problem is really solved? Will this really be a competitive product?). If a project was not meeting milestones or could not be appropriately de-risked during WP1, funding for the project was terminated, with the approval of the NIH. The management of budgets and administrative project oversight for WP1 was the responsibility of the Coordinating Center, the POCTRN centers, and the organizations that monitored the time spent by non-NIH personnel.

WP2

If the Steering Panel recommended that a project proceed to WP2, an NIH Funding Panel reviewed the comments and recommendations from the Steering Panel. If the proposal was selected for WP2 support, a funding memo was sent to the relevant NIH contract staff to initiate the negotiation and execution of a WP2 contract.

The deep dive process served as market research in support of the contract request for proposals and provided input to the contract technical review to expedite the contracting process. This was an atypical order of operations for contracting, and a sole-source request for proposals was issued to selected organizations. The streamlining of acquisition processes for RADx contracts was authorized by the declaration of a national emergency. This enabled unprecedented time savings in preparing acquisition plans and executing contract awards.

A standard NIH commercial contract template was used to ensure consistency and efficiency in negotiating final terms and conditions for the contract awards. Commercial contracts were intended to support regulatory approval, product launch, and manufacturing scale-up. Milestones, deliverables, timelines, and payment schedules developed during the deep dive process were refined prior to final award.

A cross-functional team of NIH program officers, contract officers, and RADx Tech consultants formed around each contract to manage the projects, review the progress made toward deliverables, and approve/disapprove milestone payments. Frequent interactions with WP2 awardees aided in reviewing progress and enabled the provision of commercialization support. WP2 contracts ended with successful completion of all milestones or termination due to a lack of progress toward milestones.

Collaborations Across the US Government

To achieve the NIH's target for commercially available COVID-19 diagnostic tests within the desired time frame, RADx Tech established close working relationships with several other government agencies, including the FDA, the Department of Defense, the Department Health and Human Services, and the Biomedical Advanced Research and Development Authority, to expedite regulatory decisions and provide logistical support for deployment. Bidirectional FDA engagement enabled RADx Tech to deliver accurate and timely regulatory advice to device manufacturers in the context of a rapidly changing regulatory framework and to present real-world evidence to the FDA to guide best practices for COVID-19 test use.[12]

Educational Aspects of RADx Tech

The COVID-19 pandemic arrived with little known about the SARS-CoV-2 virus or the illness resulting from human infection. Consequently, RADx Tech launched a webinar series[13] to provide current information by leading experts to the scientific, medical, and technology communities. Topics included:

- pathogen surveillance for emergent epidemics
- the evolution of SARS-CoV-2 variants and its effects on viral detection tests, including the creation of the Variant Task Force genotyping assay
- the epidemiology of omicron
- vaccine immunology – pandemic response and preparedness
- developing a COVID-19 vaccine during a pandemic
- an overview of long COVID
- the intersection between COVID-19 vaccination and testing
- the RADx Pooling Task Force
- the acceleration of sustainable kindergarten to 12th grade (K–12) school reopenings for in-person learning
- a global view of COVID-19
- returning to in-person instruction for K–12 schools
- the epidemiology of COVID-19
- a path to in-person instruction – on-campus "pooling in a pod" testing for COVID-19

As the US public had never conducted self-testing at the large scale envisioned for home COVID-19 diagnostic testing, and to help ensure that the unprecedented achievements of RADx Tech had the intended maximal impact on ending the pandemic, RADx Tech launched web-based educational tools, called "When To Test" (www.WhenToTest.org) and "My COVID Toolkit" (www.mycovidtoolkit.org). These tools focused on the optimal usage of test kits and the importance of strategies to mitigate the risks of becoming infected and infecting others in different social settings.

Overall Outcomes

RADx Tech launched its call for proposals on April 29, 2020, and nearly 400 proposals were received in the first 24 hours. A total of 716 completed applications were received before the funnel was closed to new applications on August 11, 2020.

Of these completed applications, 142 (20%) moved from the Viability Panel to the deep dive process. Of the projects that underwent a deep dive, 34% (48/142) moved forward: 26 to WP1 and 22 to WP2.

The average time from receipt of a completed application to a funding decision was 35 days. Within eight months, RADx Tech had funded 30 projects, resulting in 31 FDA Emergency Use Authorizations covering five over-the-counter/home tests, 12 point-of-care tests, and 12 central laboratory tests. At that time, and in the same year that RADx Tech was launched, 1 million FDA-authorized tests supported by RADx Tech were shipped per day. As of November 10, 2022, just over 2.5 years after the launch of RADx Tech, 5 billion tests and test products had been produced under 46 FDA authorizations.

Summary

RADx Tech proved to be a new and productive model for accelerating translational MedTech projects through development, commercialization, and distribution to end users.[14] The RADx

Tech model has begun to be utilized at the NIH for other initiatives, including diagnostic tests for mpox, HIV, and hepatitis C, as well as mitigating maternal and fetal mortality.

The achievements of RADx Tech were unprecedented, yet significant logistical constraints imposed by the pandemic – such as challenges associated with quarantine workers and supply chain shortages – presented hurdles that could potentially be avoided in future pandemics.

Lessons Learned

- The RADx Tech processes are applicable to future pandemics
- Future efforts to accelerate the development and distribution of point-of-care and home-based diagnostic tests will benefit from:
  - o close coordination with vaccine and therapeutics development
  - o close engagement with public health authorities to enhance the public's acceptance of self-testing and reporting of test results
  - o harmonization with international diagnostic development efforts
  - o working with governmental authorities to inform national policies

Acknowledgments

This work was supported by NIBIB under grant 5U54EB015408-06. The views expressed in this manuscript are those of the authors and do not necessarily represent the views of NIBIB; the National Heart, Lung, and Blood Institute; the NIH; or the US Department of Health and Human Services.

RADx Tech Collaborators

Chad Achenbach, Bruce Barton, Allison Blodgett, Oliver Brand, John P. Broach, Bryan Buchholz, Elias Caro, William Clarke, Rebecca Cleeton, Marshall R. Collins, Denise R. Dunlap, Nisha M. Fahey, Jennifer K. Frediani, Charlotte Gaydos, Nathaniel Hafer, Claudia Hawkins, Lisa R. Hirschhorn, Yu-Hsiang Hsieh, Wilbur A. Lam, Stephenie C. Lemon, Yukari C. Manabe, Mark Marino, Greg S. Martin, Sally McFall, Tamara McKenzie, David D. McManus, Robert L. Murphy, Risha Nayee, Jared O'Neal, Jeffrey E. Olgin, Richard Rothman, Adam Samuta, Cheryl Stone, Barbara Van Der Pol, Miriam B. Vos, Leona Wells, and Lea E. Widdice.

References

1. R. Taylor, Health officials Senate testimony transcript on new tests for COVID-19 (May 7, 2020). https://tinyurl.com/fk9txwm7.

2. L. Alexander and R. Blunt, Opinion: we need more covid-19 tests. We propose a "shark tank" to get us there, *Washington Post* (April 20, 2020). https://tinyurl.com/bdf3ecma.

3. P.F. Carleton, S. Schachter, T. B. Lash, et al., Point-of-Care Technology Research Network: an evolving model for collaborative translational research in biomedical engineering. *Curr Opin Biomed Eng*, **11** (2019), 145–148.

4. B. J. Tromberg, T. A. Schwetz, E. J. Pérez-Stable, et al., Rapid scaling up of Covid-19 diagnostic testing in the United States – the

NIH RADx initiative. *N Engl J Med*, **383**, 11 (2020), 1071–1077.

5. J. M. Collins, M. R. Collins, T. McKenzie, and M. Marino, The role of CoLab and GAITS in enabling the RADx Tech program. *IEEE Open J Eng Med Biol*, **2** (2021), 119–124.

6. L. Gibson, N. Fahey, N. Hafer, et al., The RADx Tech Clinical Studies Core: a model for academic based clinical studies. *IEEE Open J Eng Med Biol*, **2** (2021), 152–157.

7. A. Soni, C. Herbert, A. Filippaios, et al., Comparison of rapid antigen tests' performance between delta and omicron variants of SARS-CoV-2: a secondary analysis from a serial home self-testing study. *Ann Intern Med*, **175**, 12 (2022), 1685–1692.

8. A. Soni, C. Herbert, H. Lin, et al., Performance of rapid antigen tests to detect symptomatic and asymptomatic SARS-CoV-2 infection. *medRxiv* (2022), https://doi.org/10.1101/2022.08.05.22278466.

9. M. Robinson, C. Gaydos, B. Van Der Pol, et al., The Clinical Review Committee: impact of the development of in vitro diagnostic tests for SARS-CoV-2 within RADx Tech. *IEEE Open J Eng Med Biol*, **2** (2021), 138–141.

10. P. Tessier, M. Dempsey, J. Collins, and S. Schachter, RADx Tech Viability and Steering Panels: a model for MedTech translational grant review. *IEEE Open J Eng Med Biol*, **2** (2021), 125–130.

11. M. Dempsey, P. Tessier, J. Collins, and E. Caro, The RADx Tech deep dive and work package 1 process. *IEEE Open J Eng Med Biol*, **2** (2021), 131–137.

12. FDA, At-Home COVID-19 Antigen Tests-Take Steps to Reduce Your Risk of False Negative Results: FDA Safety Communication. Updated November 17, 2022 (2022). https://tinyurl.com/5bdn25y4.

13. POCTRN, RADx Tech webinar series 2023. www.poctrn.org/radx-webinars (accessed January 29, 2023).

14. M. Akay, S. Subramaniam, C. Brennan, et al., Healthcare innovations to address the challenges of the COVID-19 pandemic. *IEEE J Biomed Health Inform*, **26**, 7 (2022), 3294–3302.

Coordination of Resources for the Manufacturing and Deployment of COVID-19 Diagnostic Assays

Maren Downing, Mia Cirrincione, Adam Samuta, Kevin Leite, Sam Dolphin, Emily Muth, Jose Valdesuso, and Brian Walsh

Introduction

The success of Rapid Acceleration of Diagnostics (RADx®) Tech would have been significantly diminished without its strategic focus on identifying and providing the resources necessary to bring in vitro diagnostic tests to market. Within the RADx initiative, the Deployment Core was established to identify and provide these necessary resources. The role of the core was especially pertinent during the severe acute respiratory syndrome coronavirus 2 (SARS-CoV-2) pandemic, as timelines were greatly reduced and market demand was constantly changing. The Deployment Core was formed in May 2020 in response to the need for consultant expertise and various resources to support the development and scale-up of diagnostic tests.

Deployment Core Inception and Process

The Deployment Core established processes to ensure that there were no gaps in coverage for getting a product to market for any company. A successful process needed little to no oversight, and systemization is required for each process to ensure reproducibility across multiple projects, given the sheer volume of projects in the RADx Tech portfolio. Systemization involved Deployment Core team members assessing the purpose of the process and who was going to benefit, and anticipating how the resulting information would be used. Many of the processes put in place at the beginning of the program had to be adapted as the program grew and different needs arose.

An example of a successful systematized process that adapted throughout the program was mitigating supply chain risk. At the outset of RADx Tech, many companies came up against roadblocks related to extensive lead times for or a lack of materials. The Deployment Core accelerated these lead times and closely monitored supply chain patterns among companies. This led to the inception of a supply chain forecast form that was given to each project to anticipate risk and provide both quantitative and qualitative information for a better plan.

Anticipating Needs, Expanding Our Network

The mission of the Deployment Core was to provide these projects with whatever resources they needed. After interactions with several companies, a convergence of needs was identified. Additional needs were identified for meeting the demands of the pandemic as the program evolved. These needs fell into one of two categories, as shown in Figure 5.3.

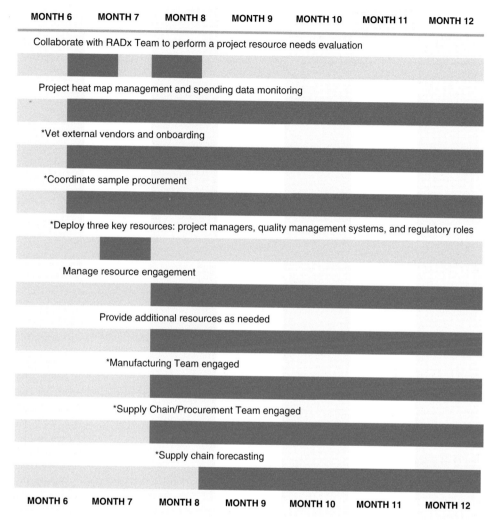

Figure 5.1 This roadmap depicts the vital activities, their chronology, and an estimated time frame in months. In the case of the SARS-CoV-2 pandemic, month 1 was December 2019, the month in which the virus was isolated, sequenced, identified, and published.

Each task is facilitated on an as-needed basis.

* These tasks repeat as necessary with each new RADx Tech project.

We vetted resources and onboarded them with the expectation that they would be utilized in multiple projects. As we interacted with more projects and maintained continual communication, we recognized patterns and gaps among companies and paired them with these newly onboarded resources. As more projects came into the program and we continued to expand our network, we were better able to support requests. We frequently made the RADx

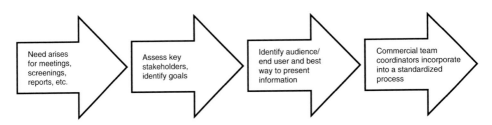

Figure 5.2 Process development workflow.

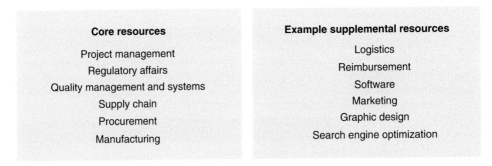

Figure 5.3 Deployment Core resources supplied throughout the pandemic.

Tech team leaders aware of resources that were available across the initiative, ensuring that everyone was aware of the capabilities of the program and how they could benefit, this process is shown in Figure 5.2.

Core Resources

The Deployment Core was introduced to RADx projects by their assigned commercial team coordinator (CTC) through an introductory meeting at the start of their engagement (work package 1) and sometimes in the deep dive phase. This was the start of the relationship between the RADx Tech project and the CTC, which would continue throughout the program, allowing communication with the Deployment Core.

We identified three key resource areas as critical for test development and commercialization: project managers, quality consultants, and regulatory consultants. These individuals followed each company throughout the RADx Tech program. Other core capabilities related to the supply chain, procurement, and manufacturing, among others, were also offered at no cost to the companies. Written intake forms followed by detailed conversations were used to assess current resource gaps, many of which the companies had yet to recognize on their own.

Project Management

Project management support was invaluable to the project teams, especially to smaller companies and academic institutions. Many larger companies also benefited from project management support. The project manager often became a part of the project team, at varying levels of engagement. RADx Tech's detailed project milestones and checklist requirements made these resources invaluable to teams.

Regulatory Affairs

Regulatory consultants were imperative to the success of the initiative. Emergency Use Authorizations (EUAs) were a new event with which most companies were unfamiliar, making our regulatory personnel essential and highly valued by project teams. Some companies required full analyses and document drafting, while others needed only ad hoc advice. Regulatory affairs are discussed in further detail in Chapter 10.

Quality Management and Systems

Quality management consultants were offered to each project. While many start-up companies and academic institutions assumed that they would not need a quality management system (QMS) because a separate entity would be manufacturing their product, this is often not the case. These teams needed to quickly document their design controls and development processes. The quality management consultants worked closely with existing quality personnel on the project team and/or alongside team members in other roles to establish a functioning QMS.

At the beginning of the RADx Tech program, the Deployment Core identified a QMS tool that would be funded and used by companies if desired. Utilizing one QMS platform across companies allowed the core to quickly and efficiently align QMS capabilities and consultants, resulting in standardized measures and better performance across companies.

Supply Chain

The pandemic introduced an unprecedented demand for raw materials needed for diagnostic test manufacturing. For example, swabs used to collect patient samples had never been required at such volumes before. Manufacturing plants experienced production slowdowns and/or complications in scaling as a result of labor challenges brought about by the virus and the concomitant shutdowns and quarantines. Offshore manufacturing posed a significant supply chain risk due to potential bans on imports and exports. US imports became increasingly congested due to COVID-19-related labor shortages at the ports, increasing both the cost of freight and the time to receive product.

Within the RADx Tech initiative, large companies producing millions of tests per month and small companies seeking to procure a few components for small-batch manufacturing competed for the same limited raw material supply. Large companies struggled to secure sizeable allocations of materials, while small companies struggled to ascertain any allocation at all.

Procurement

To combat the procurement challenges of companies within the RADx initiative, the Deployment Core established a team of procurement professionals. The Procurement

Team worked to help companies place one-time orders with raw material manufacturers, to improve delivery dates of purchase orders already placed, to find alternative suppliers for critical components, to help those attempting to scale up establish a relationship and long-term supply agreement with high-demand suppliers, and to negotiate terms, pricing, and conditions as needed. Each project team completed a procurement request form so that the level of support required could be identified. This form collected all of the pertinent information required for the Procurement Team to establish meetings with suppliers to negotiate on behalf of (or with) the RADx project team. Each request was then characterized and prioritized for daily discussion and action within a matrix to help manage the high volume of requests.

Manufacturing

Initial interactions with the project teams regarding manufacturing needs identified a much broader and more extensive set of needs, ranging from assay development to commercial distribution. In May 2020, there were no suppliers identified to provide project-specific or overall program support. As project teams completed initial deep dive activities and moved into work package 1, the need for supplier resources was increasing by the hour.

All efforts were focused on connecting with as many suppliers as possible that were well positioned to provide appropriate and necessary levels of support. The pace and scale of the RADx Tech program were like nothing suppliers had previously been associated with, which created multiple challenges. Typical manufacturing scale-up durations of 18–24 months were requested to be completed in 5–6 months. Typical daily production targets of thousands were requested to be hundreds of thousands. Many suppliers were not comfortable with the pace and scale, and as such declined to engage, increasing the challenge of building the supplier pool.

Supplier connections were accomplished by leveraging internal RADx resources and internet research. From June to November 2020, a wide portfolio of resources was identified and made available to provide project and program support. From June 2020 to June 2021, numerous direct supplier engagements were conducted. A growing number of suppliers and supplier engagements have continued to meet the evolving needs of the RADx Tech program.

Suppliers engaged with project teams as either a RADx supplier, which was the preferred method for RADx-funded activities, or through a direct connection to the project team, which was preferred when the timing and/or funding of the project work was unclear.

Suppliers included:

- design and development firms specialized in assay development, including lateral flow assay development, molecular assay development, and microfluidic assay development
- design and development firms specialized in component design to provide the packaging around the assay
- design and development firms specialized in electronic analyzer development
- contract manufacturers with capabilities for high-volume manufacturing of the consumable test kits and low-volume manufacturing of the reusable analyzer devices
- reagent manufacturers of both bulk and specialty reagents
- injection molding contract manufacturers with capabilities for high cavitation tooling and high-volume manufacturing
- design and fabrication firms specialized in fully custom, high-volume, high-complexity automated manufacturing assembly equipment, capable of achieving RADx scale volumes

- technical resources with expertise in operations consulting, information technology, microfluidics, quality testing, wafer fabrication, etc.
- logistics companies with capabilities to move scaled up volumes of commercial products internationally – initial logistics support also included low-volume material movement to support design, development, and clinical trial activities

The Manufacturing Team assisted with the selection of commercial partners, drove early engagement, ensured activities moved forward per the timeline, and facilitated a smooth transition at the point that the company assumed supplier responsibility.

Additional Resources

A critical part of the Deployment Core was anticipating company needs before they were realized. We categorized potential areas of concern and sought resources as early as possible to meet those needs. Some of these additional resource areas included logistics, reimbursement, software, marketing, graphic design, and search engine optimization support. The Deployment Core and other members of RADx Tech vetted these resources to ensure that they could work with companies of all sizes at all stages of development, ranging from academic institutions to large, established industry partners.

RADx Tech companies were not spared logistical challenges during the pandemic. Companies that were shipping materials internationally often experienced delays at US customs. These holds could last days or even weeks, which would delay device analyses at RADx-designated laboratories within the United States. Resources were identified for working with customs and resolving any outstanding conflicts, helping to accelerate the delivery of devices to testing locations.

As the sale of COVID-19 tests increased and insurance providers became more involved, the need for reimbursement support became evident. The Deployment Core onboarded a reimbursement specialist to help. Additionally, smaller companies (with fewer than 50 employees) often have little to no personnel dedicated to software, and many requested additional support for development. We provided individual consultants and company vendors to aid in software development. If a company was expanding and did not already have a human resources department, the Deployment Core connected them with recruiting assistance.

Variant Task Force

As SARS-CoV-2 variants became a concern in the United States and around the world, the RADx Variant Task Force (VTF) was created. Members from the Deployment Core were integrated into the VTF from its inception to manage logistics and processes. The core also established criteria, vetted entities, and found resources to create a bioinformatics platform and conduct *in silico* analysis of COVID-19 tests on emerging variants. In parallel with these efforts, the Deployment Core managed the process of more than 50 companies sending tests to a central laboratory for in vitro analysis. Please refer to Chapter 9 for more information on the sequencing, tracking, and surveillance of variants.

Clinical Studies and Analytical Studies

As teams progressed through the RADx Tech process, they were expected to complete analytical studies listed in an EUA template provided by the US Food and Drug Administration (FDA). These studies could be completed internally, externally, or through

RADx, depending on their RADx position and contract. The Deployment Core worked to onboard analytical testing laboratories with sufficient capacity and the ability to rapidly complete a full set of analytical studies. Once these laboratories were onboarded, the Deployment Core managed the process – from study requests and funding approval to study completion and report delivery.

In parallel with analytical studies, RADx teams completed clinical studies. To initiate their clinical study, each team had the option of working with the Deployment Core protocol-writing resources. With a completed protocol, the team could request clinical study quotes from clinical research organizations (CROs) – CROs were reviewed, interviewed, and onboarded by the Deployment Core – or could choose to proceed with the National Institutes of Health (NIH)-funded POCTRN research center at Emory University, the Atlanta Center for Microsystems Engineered Point-of-Care Technologies (ACME POCT), or the Center for Advancing Point of Care Technologies (CAPCaT), the latter also being a POCTRN Center and partnership between UMass Medical School and UMass Lowell. In situations in which a CRO was the desired path, the RADx team reviewed various quotes from several CROs and chose the one best suited for the company. As studies progressed, it was the responsibility of the Deployment Core to track and report weekly on the progress of each clinical study until EUA submission to the FDA.

Government Entity Support and Relations

The risk associated with establishing supply chain roots overseas encouraged a shift among all diagnostic manufacturers to begin purchasing from US raw material suppliers. US suppliers often did not have the same manufacturing capacity as overseas competitors. Government connections became imperative to help provide the Procurement Team with additional leverage on top of the RADx Tech project's government contracts. The Procurement Team met weekly with program managers and program logisticians from both the US Department of Defense (DOD) and the US Department of Health and Human Services (HHS). The DOD specifically drew individuals from its Joint Project Manager Office for Chemical, Biological, Radiological, and Nuclear Defense – Medical Office (JPM CBRN Medical) and the Joint Rapid Acquisition Cell (JRAC; formerly known as the Joint Acquisition Task Force [JATF]), whereas HHS provided support through the Office of Assistant Secretary for Preparedness and Response (ASPR). Both government organizations provided teams in an effort to support the nation in rapidly acquiring medical supplies and materials to combat the pandemic and to mitigate the supply chain risk outside RADx.

A shared spreadsheet was tracked by the Procurement Team and discussed with representatives from the HHS and the DOD. It was populated with those RADx Tech procurement requests requiring additional leverage and support. The Procurement Team, along with DOD/HHS support, established meetings with the supplier to continue to negotiate on behalf of the project, often achieving a greater degree of success than the project had previously been able to achieve. This support was very influential and was critical in establishing credibility and priority with US suppliers.

Defense Production Act Ratings

When faced with extreme supply constraints, some RADx Tech projects were unable to receive any allocation of critical raw materials and components. The refusal of allocation to these projects was often the result of suppliers having other government-mandated obligations to supply certain manufacturers' products. Such government-mandated obligations stem from test manufacturers that have a Defense Production Act (DPA) rated order, namely a purchase order from a company that has received a DPA rating, stating that the supplier must prioritize the rated order and fulfill said order before any other non-rated orders. A DPA rated contract is awarded to select government-contracted suppliers after receiving approval from the DPA Emergency Response Authorities (DPA-ERA) branch under the HHS. This branch evaluates a manufacturer's qualifications, the supply constraint, and the implications of awarding a DPA rating. The Procurement Team, with the support of the NIH, prepared a memo to submit to the DPA-ERA for review, discussion, and potential DPA rating award when appropriate.

Forecasting Future Needs and Risk

Forecasting became an important exercise for RADx Tech projects and involved outlining the demand for raw materials and components for each month as product manufacturing escalated. When compiled across all RADx projects, forecasting enabled us to set expectations when the Procurement Team and government entities negotiated allocations to government projects. The Procurement Team helped projects understand how to anticipate future needs through forecast forms. Later, a supplier risk management analysis was completed, which identified the types of risk that each device component could carry and its potential mitigation strategy. The Procurement Team compiled component requirements across projects after collecting the forecast forms and supplier risk management analysis documents. This allowed valuable data to be provided to raw material suppliers and government supply chain expansion programs.

Troubleshooting Ongoing Scale-Up Issues

Throughout the course of each project, the Manufacturing Team was asked to assist with vendor challenges that were identified. The nature of the requests varied. Some included meeting with vendors to request raw material supply prioritization, expediting vendor timelines to meet RADx Tech timeline goals, or working with logistics companies to expedite and move materials. Others included reaching out to local planning authorities to expedite building permits. The Deployment Core assisted projects in resolving challenges at any stage of the scaling up process.

There was a willingness by most contract manufacturers to support the RADx initiatives for the betterment of the country; however, the engagement of contract manufacturers became increasingly challenging as the pandemic continued. There were increasing concerns regarding the aggressive timelines, high volumes, uncertain future demand, and ability of RADx Tech projects to fund the capacity. Manufacturers referenced return on investment and floor space utilization decisions, for example, as justifications for passing on engagement requests. While the Deployment Core was able to satisfy project team requests, it proved more difficult than initially expected.

Independent Test Assessments

In October 2021, the RADx Tech program was expanded to include the Independent Test Assessment Program (ITAP) to accelerate regulatory review and the availability of high-quality, accurate, and reliable over-the-counter COVID-19 tests to the public. The objective was to quadruple the supply of at-home tests by the end of 2021, equating to up to 200 million at-home tests per month.

The Manufacturing Team supported the ITAP process by completing manufacturing capability evaluations for all ITAP projects. Because these high-volume manufacturing facilities were located outside the United States and travel was not an option, remote paper evaluations were necessary.

The Manufacturing Team developed a checklist that requested detailed information regarding:

- raw materials, including identified suppliers, inventory levels, material lead times, sole versus single-sourced suppliers, the existence of supply agreements, confirmation of scale volume supply, and vendor approval status
- manufacturing facility details, including relevant manufacturing experience related to the project product, FDA registration, inspection status, International Organization for Standardization (ISO) certifications, European conformity (CE) marks, floor plans, facility videos, personnel, and manufacturing methods (manual versus automated)
- transportation experience, including moving high volumes of product internationally, the use of air and sea methods, planned US entry points, and the strategy to finance significant logistics activities
- distribution experience and strategy (the distributor model, the third-party logistic model, or both) and evaluation of the relevant capabilities of the distributor(s) to handle the significant volumes associated with the ITAP companies
- post-market support, including an evaluation of the project company's strategy to ensure that products approved for commercial distribution remain in commercial distribution, as well as an evaluation of the internal and/or external capabilities of the responsible party

The evaluation of the documentation and information received drove a manufacturing risk ranking, which provided a recommendation to the ITAP for inclusion and/or remediation efforts.

Sample Procurement

To facilitate the VTF's activities in the RADx portfolio and FDA-requested testing of COVID-19 products, RADx and partners negotiated sample procurement contracts with key sample providers to conduct sequencing on their sample inventories, with the aim of building a biobank of well-characterized samples reserved for use in RADx variant testing. Contracts were set to a defined quantity or value of samples, but the limits were increased through contract amendments as needed when fulfillment approached those limits.

The Deployment Core provided ongoing support for sample procurement by tracking sample inventory versus contracted limits. When order fulfillment totals approached a given contract limit (within 500 samples of the limit), the recontracting process was initiated to increase the limit well before sample needs surpassed the existing contract allowance. Additionally, per-order tracking and sample quantity data were used to validate supplier invoices on an ongoing basis.

In this arrangement, sample suppliers provided detailed inventory lists on a weekly basis, which included data such as the sample collection date, cycle threshold values from original comparator test results, specific SARS-CoV-2 lineage, and Global Initiative on Sharing All Influenza Data (GISAID) identifiers. In addition, FASTA files (a text-based format for representing either nucleotide sequences or amino acid sequences) were also provided, describing the exact ribonucleic acid (RNA) sequence of all samples for bioinformatics. Using the FASTA files and publicly available resources, RADx was able to quickly analyze the sequence data of available samples and purchase only those with relevant mutations characteristic of variants of concern with minimal additional mutations and sufficient cycle threshold values. See Chapters 7 and 8 for more details on the sample selection, storage, and testing processes.

Project Tracking and Organization

As a central part of RADx Tech, the Deployment Core provided organizational and scheduling support to projects to ensure that each was completing project milestones (referred to as gates) and utilizing all that the core had to offer. CTCs managed the calendar for and scheduled meetings with the Clinical Review Committee (see Chapter 7). CTCs managed the logistics related to the weekly FDA meetings and ensured that each project had its appropriate documents ready. The Deployment Core was also in the unique position of setting up processes to develop workflows for planning clinical studies, as well as verification planning for projects to take their technologies to the Verification Core. By managing these workflows, our team was able to appropriately allocate scheduling times and priorities and communicate clearly with all parties. This oversight prevented chaos, such as scheduling mistakes, projects falling through the cracks, and miscommunications.

Heat Map

A heat map – which expressed the state of each project in a single snapshot with regard to the gates that needed to be addressed in the EUA process – was reported to the NIH on a regular bases, an example heat map is shown in Figure 5.4. The goal of the heat map was to anticipate the need before it was expressed. The heat map included every gate through which companies had to pass (e.g. analytical testing and design freeze). Color coding created a concise visual representation of companies' status in RADx. Most importantly, the heat map helped the Deployment Core understand if more or different resources were needed and if those resources were needed across multiple projects.

Spend-to-Date Reports

Metrics were frequently requested to assist in reports and evaluations, including spend-to-date reports. This information and careful monitoring were imperative for good financial stewardship. Because the Deployment Core had direct contact with every RADx Tech company, we served as a point of contact to obtain these reports and distribute them to the companies. This process minimized additional work for the contracting offices; instead, only one member of the Deployment Core handled all of the requests, streamlining the process.

Case Study

A critical component of the Deployment Core was our ability to anticipate a company's need before it was voiced. As examples of this approach, we will examine a case study of two in vitro diagnostic test manufacturing companies: company Y (fewer than 50 employees) and company Z (more than 500 employees). A CTC was assigned to each team and presented the same set of resources to each company.

Prior to beginning work package 1, company Y had one dedicated employee who filled both the regulatory and the quality roles. It had no previous regulatory submissions and did not have an operating QMS. Considering these gaps, the company accepted the services of

Priority	Company name	CLIA class	Asymptomatic/ symptomatic	Sample type	Design lock	Preliminary LoD	Formal LoD	Analytical testing	Triage complete	Clinical study	Clinical pathway
H	A	OTC	Both	Saliva	Yes	Complete	Complete	Complete	Yes	30 positive samples, > 150 total subjects, > 10 asymptomatic patients Usability; 100 participants (50 test themselves, 50 tested an other)	CRO-1
H	B	Moderate complexity	S	MT swab	Yes	Complete	August	Incomplete	No	30 positive/30 negative samples, 10–20% low positives (Ct > 30) or within 2–4 Ct of comparator LoD. Natural prospective or banked samples	Internal test
H	C	POC W	Both	MT swab	Yes	Complete	Complete	Complete	Yes	30 positive/30 negative samples, 1–2 sites, 5–6 untrained operators, 10–20% low positives (Ct > 30), 10 low negatives/10 low positives required per site. Add 20 positive/100 negative samples from a diverse prospective asymptomatic population	CRO-2
H	D	POC W	S	MT swab	Yes	Complete	Complete	Complete	Yes	30 positive/30 negative samples, 1–2 sites, 5–6 untrained operators, 10–20% low positives (Ct > 30), 10 low positives/10 low negatives required per site	CRO-3
H	E	High complexity	S	Saliva	Yes	In progress	Incomplete	Incomplete	No	30 positive/30 negative samples, 10–20% low positives (Ct > 30) or within 2–4 Ct of comparator LoD. Natural prospective or banked samples. Add study comparing saliva to nasal sample type	TBD
H	F	OTC	Both	AN swab	Yes	Complete	Complete	Complete	N/A	Complete	Internal test
H	G	Moderate complexity	S	NP swab	Yes	Complete	Complete	Complete	Yes	30 positive/30 negative samples, 10–20% low positives (Ct > 30) or within 2–4 Ct of comparator LoD. Natural prospective or banked samples	CRO-2
H	H	High complexity	S	NP swab	Yes	Complete	Complete	In progress	August	30 positive/30 negative samples, 10–20% low positives (Ct > 30) or within 2–4 Ct of comparator LoD. Natural prospective or banked samples	CRO-2
H	I	POC W	S	AN swab	Yes	Complete	Complete	Complete	No	30 positive/30 negative samples, 1–2 sites, 5–6 untrained operators, 10–20% low positives (Ct > 30), 10 low negatives required per site	CRO-2
M	J	POC W	S	AN swab	Yes	Complete	Complete	Complete	Yes	30 positive/30 negative samples, 1–2 sites, 5–6 untrained operators, 10–20% low positives (Ct > 30), 10 low positives/10 low negatives required per site	CRO-2
M	K	POC W	S	AN swab	August	Incomplete	Incomplete	Incomplete	No	30 positive/30 negative samples, 1–2 sites, 5–6 untrained operators, 10–20% low positives (Ct > 30), 10 low positives/10 low negatives required per site	TBD
M	L	POC W	S	Saliva	Yes	Complete	Incomplete	Incomplete	No	30 positive/30 negative samples, 1–2 sites, 5–6 untrained operators, 10–20% low positives (Ct > 30), 10 low positives/10 low negatives required per site. Add study comparing saliva to nasal sample type	TBD
M	M	POC W	S	Saliva	August	Incomplete	Incomplete	Incomplete	No	30+ / 30–; 1–2 sites, 5–6 untrained operators, 10–20% low positives (Ct > 30), 10 low positives/10 low negatives required per site. Add study comparing saliva to nasal sample type	TBD
L	N	POC W	S	MT swab	Yes	August	Incomplete	Incomplete	No	30+ / 30–; 1–2 sites, 5–6 untrained operators, 10–20% low positives (Ct > 30), 10 low positives/10 low negatives required per site	TBD
L	O	POC W	Both	AN swab	August	Incomplete	Incomplete	Incomplete	No	30 positive/30 negative samples, 1–2 sites, 5–6 untrained operators, 10–20% low positives (Ct > 30), 10 low positives/10 low negatives required per site. Add 20 positive/100 negative samples from a diverse prospective asymptomatic population	TBD
L	P	POC W	S	AN swab	Yes	Complete	Incomplete	Incomplete	No	30 positive/30 negative samples, 1–2 sites, 5–6 untrained operators, 10–20% low positives (Ct > 30), 10 low positives/10 low negatives required per site	TBD

Figure 5.4 Heat map utilized to report to NIH leadership.

Heat map key

Priority — NIH assigned priority rating with respect to advancing to a clinical study. H, highest priority; M, medium priority; L, low priority. Projects were addressed and funneled through the Triage Approval Panel according to priority

Company name — Company name, deidentified for this example

Clinical Laboratory Improvement Amendments (CLIA) class — Indicative of the use-case environment in which the project intended to receive FDA authorization. POC W, point of care waived; OTC, over the counter

Asymptomatic/symptomatic — Indicative of the regulatory claim for which the company intended to receive FDA authorization relative to patient symptom status. A, asymptomatic; S, symptomatic

Sample type — Sample type that the company's assay uses for virus detection

Design lock — Completion status or date when the company intends to make no future changes to the device. Design lock is required to complete formal FDA-required studies and remain in compliance with FDA design control regulations

Preliminary limit of detection (LoD) — A preliminary assessment benchtop (laboratory) study done to observe the relative LoD or relative lowest viral load that the assay can detect. This was performed to predict success in the formal LoD

Formal LoD — An FDA-required benchtop (laboratory) study done to confirm the LoD or relative lowest viral load that the assay can detect. Required for EUA

Analytical testing — FDA-required benchtop (laboratory) studies that must be completed in addition to LoD studies for EUA. Examples include cross-reactivity, inclusivity, stability, and flex studies

Triage complete — The EUA Triage Panel reviews the project's status relative to clinical study preparedness, the proposed study, and the proposed CRO pathway. Recommendations from the panel are reviewed by NIH leadership for approval. The clinical study may proceed after the decision of NIH leadership

Clinical study — The project's proposed clinical study to validate the device's performance with real patients – this field includes the number of patients, sites, sample requirements, etc. The fields in the table provided are not comprehensive in capturing all clinical study details and are not reflective of all FDA requirements. Ct, cycle threshold

Clinical pathway — The organization that will conduct the clinical study on behalf of the company. The company could pursue support through CROs. TBD, to be decided

RADx-provided regulatory and quality consultants. The regulatory consultant served as a bridge between the company and the FDA and could field questions to the FDA at weekly meetings. The quality consultant implemented a RADx-funded QMS and was highly active in providing and populating quality templates. These resources worked in partnership with the company's in-house employees. Company Y's lead scientist was filling the role of project management and gladly accepted support from a RADx project manager due to time constraints on managing deliverables. Company Y frequently had questions and utilized many other RADx Tech resources, such as reimbursement and graphic design. As the company grew, it eventually utilized a RADx-provided recruitment specialist to hire its own quality management professional. The CTC was heavily involved and attended weekly meetings.

Company Z was an established company that had previous success with in vitro diagnostic regulatory submissions and a functioning QMS with established quality and regulatory departments and personnel. It did not request the services of a RADx-provided quality management consultant, but it did frequently interact with a regulatory consultant due to the new EUA landscape for COVID-19 diagnostics. The company had an in-house assigned project manager dedicated to working with RADx, and therefore did not request the services of a RADx-provided project manager. It also did not request any other resource assistance beyond procurement. The CTC used a much lighter touch for this company and only attended meetings every other week.

While the process of utilizing resources and deploying COVID-19 tests greatly differed between these two companies, both were ultimately successful in deploying their COVID-19 tests to the market.

Applying Our Experience to Other Programs

The principles demonstrated in this chapter could be modeled and applied to further extensions of RADx and future initiatives regarding global health challenges. For instance, the RADx Accessibility Program focuses on creating accessible design changes for the low vision, no vision, low dexterity, and aging populations. The Deployment Core supports this effort by recruiting subject matter experts (including visually impaired subject matter experts) and design firms. Then, the in vitro diagnostic test manufacturing companies follow a process outlined in Figure 5.5, iterating their designs accordingly and addressing the accessibility concerns of current SARS-CoV-2 product lines. Standardizing a process creates a uniform practice for companies to follow that not only creates transparency for projects, but also streamlines the work for the Deployment Core. As more companies went through the process, the efficacy of the work grew exponentially. Templates were created for

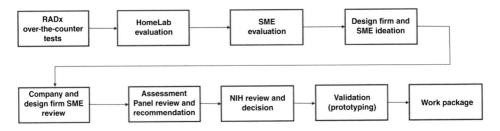

Figure 5.5 Design review process flowchart for the RADx Accessibility Program.
SME, small or medium-sized enterprise. Homelab is a center for usability evaluations of the novel technologies

reporting to government agencies, and each member of the team had responsibilities that transferred from one company to the next.

Conclusion

The Deployment Core was critical in ensuring consistency across dozens of RADx Tech projects and in enabling these teams to bring their tests to market and scale up their companies. The processes we created required little oversight and enabled our team to stay small. The resources we engaged were consistent and predictable, which reduced the amount of monitoring and minimized sources of risk. The systemization of processes allowed the team to quickly identify potential risk factors. Overall, the Deployment Core and its functioning are integral to the RADx success story, and its continual ability to evolve and adapt to changes contributed to the successful deployment of COVID-19 tests to the market.

Lessons Learned

- **Resources should be assigned gradually.** Through working with varying sizes of companies of different backgrounds, we quickly realized that "companies didn't know what they didn't know." If we worked with a small company (fewer than 10 employees) and started to provide them with resources, the company's management could quickly become overwhelmed: Providing resources could literally double the size of these smaller companies within a week. We learned to assign resources gradually and at a pace that was commensurate with growth.
- **Forecasting can help prepare for unforeseen events.** While it is impossible to anticipate every shortage or complication that may arise within the supply chain, proper forecasting, supplier relationships, and supplier contracts can mitigate unanticipated shortages.
- **US suppliers can reduce material lead times.** It can be more difficult to expedite products with long lead times coming from offshore suppliers than for those from US suppliers.
- **Government prioritization should be sought when possible.** If companies have a US presence, government services such as a DPA rating from the DOD can be utilized to help prioritize products.
- **Cost savings in the supply chain should be pursued.** General Services Administration (GSA) pricing is sometimes available with suppliers, but only if you are a government agency or under a government contract that includes GSA pricing eligibility. We have seen some success in lowering prices by negotiating on behalf of the company, using the NIH government contract number, and leveraging other agencies that are using the same product. In addition, setting up supplier contracts with forecasting and placing blanket orders to leverage yearly usage can result in lower prices for each product. The most effective strategy is to include a flow-down statement for GSA pricing within the contract between the government entity and the awardee.
- **Design experts should be included from the start.** In hindsight, a product design expert would be a highly utilized team member by all projects. Through manufacturing assessments and meetings with the Clinical Review Committee, it became apparent that many assay workflows required design adjustments. Having a design expert as part of the Deployment Core would have been beneficial.

- **Money can't buy time.** Project timeline reduction did not correlate with the amount of money supporting that project. As was learned, there is still a minimum amount of time required for design firms, automation companies, and contract manufacturers to understand, design, and execute a project, many of which were extremely complex. Vendors were still utilizing pre-pandemic internal processes that had not been optimized to provide substantially expedited timing. There was an unwillingness to overpromise and under-deliver. With that said, there were many examples of significant project acceleration, although not to the degree initially envisioned by RADx.
- **Accessibility efforts should be implemented early on in test development to improve the level of access across the entire population.** Making changes to a test in the middle of development poses challenges that could have been mitigated earlier in the development process.

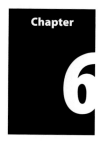

Quality and Risk Management Processes for Diagnostic Assays during an Emergency Pandemic Response

Devon C. Campbell and Christie Johnson

Introduction

Quality management systems (QMSs) and risk management are the two most fundamental elements and are woven into the very fabric of all successful medical devices and diagnostic development. In this chapter, we will establish a common understanding of quality and risk management as a mindset and then explore how those perspectives influence diagnostic development. We will provide an overview of the predominant regulations that guide the application of quality and risk management thinking. We will also share key terms that the industry uses to describe core quality and risk management deliverables to establish a strong understanding of how these concepts are ordinarily handled. This grounding in the status quo will serve as the backdrop for our examination of how quality and risk management had to evolve in order to support the Rapid Acceleration of Diagnostics (RADx®) Tech initiative, which was aiming to accelerate innovation in the development, commercialization, and implementation of technologies for COVID-19 testing during the severe acute respiratory syndrome coronavirus 2 (SARS-CoV-2) pandemic.

What Is Quality Management?

The US Food and Drug Administration (FDA) has a set of regulations that outlines the current good manufacturing practice requirements that medical device manufacturers bringing products into the US market must follow: the Code of Federal Regulations Title 21, Part 820 (21 CFR 820). These current good manufacturing practice requirements ensure that medical device companies establish a QMS that enables the delivery of safe, effective, and compliant products.

As stated by the FDA, these regulations cover "the design, manufacture, packaging, labeling, storage, installation, and servicing of all finished devices intended for human use."[1] In 21 CFR 820, quality is defined as "the totality of features and characteristics that bear on the ability of a device to satisfy fitness-for-use, including safety and performance."[2] Additionally, it defines a quality system as "the organizational structure, responsibilities, procedures, processes, and resources for implementing quality management."[2]

In terms of the scope and reach of 21 CFR 820, it covers nearly *every single aspect* of diagnostic development. The ideas of quality management and its peer risk management are quietly present in the background of all other chapters in this book describing the development, verification and validation, clinical testing, manufacturing, scale-up, distribution, and use of COVID-19 diagnostic tests.

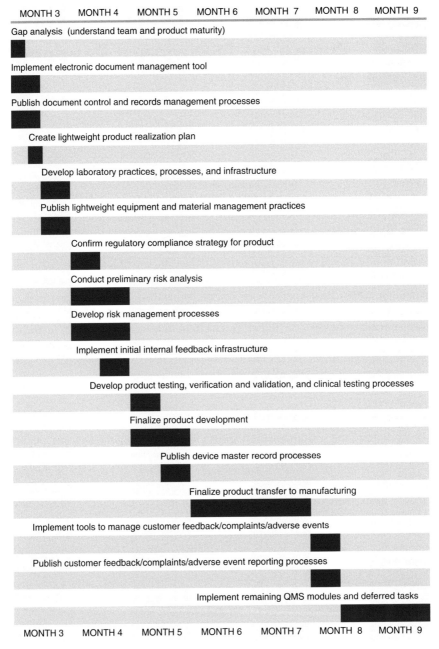

PANDEMIC ROADMAP: QUALITY AND RISK MANAGEMENT

MONTH 3   MONTH 4   MONTH 5   MONTH 6   MONTH 7   MONTH 8   MONTH 9

Gap analysis (understand team and product maturity)

Implement electronic document management tool

Publish document control and records management processes

Create lightweight product realization plan

Develop laboratory practices, processes, and infrastructure

Publish lightweight equipment and material management practices

Confirm regulatory compliance strategy for product

Conduct preliminary risk analysis

Develop risk management processes

Implement initial internal feedback infrastructure

Develop product testing, verification and validation, and clinical testing processes

Finalize product development

Publish device master record processes

Finalize product transfer to manufacturing

Implement tools to manage customer feedback/complaints/adverse events

Publish customer feedback/complaints/adverse event reporting processes

Implement remaining QMS modules and deferred tasks

MONTH 3   MONTH 4   MONTH 5   MONTH 6   MONTH 7   MONTH 8   MONTH 9

Figure 6.1 This roadmap depicts the vital activities, their chronology, and an estimated time frame in months. In the case of the SARS-CoV-2 pandemic, month 1 starts in December 2019, the month in which the virus was isolated, sequenced, identified, and published.
The tasks repeat with each new RADx Tech project.

A Note about Organizational Size

The RADx Tech initiative supported many different types and sizes of organizations. The National Institute of Biomedical Imaging and Bioengineering created a RADx Tech advanced technology platform (ATP)/independent test platform dashboard to help share summary data on proposals submitted to the RADx Tech and ATP programs. The number of submissions by organization illustrates the diversity of the cohort applying for RADx support, as shown in Figure 6.2.

Organizations with fewer than 50 employees dominate the application pool, with more than 50% of all proposals originating from companies classified as "small businesses" on the dashboard. Together with academic organizations and start-ups (companies in business for less than one year), the three populations make up over three-fourths of all applications. Granted, this represents the pool of applications, and not every application in this pool entered the RADx Tech program, but many did. In fact, the RADx Tech response to the pandemic was, by design, a healthy blend of organizations both large and small. The two extremes complemented each other and contributed to the pandemic response in different and important ways. This would likely be the case in the future should a similar response need to be mounted again and, as such, both organizational types will play a role.

Mid-sized and large diagnostic businesses generally already have strong and robust QMSs and risk management processes in place. They also are well staffed with knowledgeable and experienced employees and have the infrastructure required to effectively implement compliant quality and risk management processes throughout the life cycle of their products and services. Small businesses, academic institutions, and start-ups, however, are unlikely to have the resources for such strong internal teams and infrastructure. In many cases during the pandemic, those organizations needed to tackle the creation of quality and

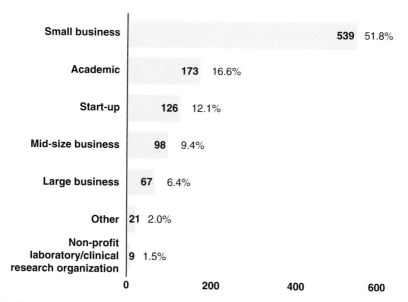

Figure 6.2 Number of RADx proposals by organization type (as of November 29, 2022).[3]

risk management infrastructure *while* they were working furiously to develop, test, and commercialize their diagnostic products.

This chapter is written more with small businesses, academic institutions, and start-ups in mind – namely organizations that may lack the depth of knowledge, experience, and mature processes that their larger counterparts enjoy. Nevertheless, the recommendations shared in this chapter are equally applicable to organizations of all sizes. The difference in our recommendations lies in prioritizing the creation of new documentation or processes for small businesses, academic institutions, and start-ups versus prioritizing the application of existing documentation or processes for medium-sized and large companies. The roadmap associated with this chapter considers smaller teams needing to create and implement quality and risk processes from scratch. Larger, mature teams will likely be able to accelerate through the roadmap more quickly, as they have much of the processes and resources required in place already.

Quality and Risk Management Are Mindsets

As noted in the chapter introduction, quality and risk management are not "stand-alone" deliverables that a team might create, nor are they specific phases of any given project. Often, quality and risk management are thought of as tasks that an organization does at the end of development, or worse, they are something thought of as only applying to manufacturing. The thinking that "we don't need quality yet; we'll get to that once we start manufacturing our test" is a recipe for a disastrous FDA audit someday. It is not the case that an organization does something and then afterward does the "quality" part or the "risk" part. Instead, quality and risk management are mindsets and represent a collection of best practices that are highly integrated throughout all aspects of the product realization process, including research, development, testing, manufacturing, launch, and support.

The most successful medical device and diagnostic development organizations know that it is wrong to follow regulations purely for the sake of earning the regulatory stamp of approval. Instead, they embrace quality and risk management mindsets as a way of working, in which high-performing products that meet patient needs are created. Meeting regulatory expectations is considered a direct result of having done things right. Modern quality and risk management regulations are a collection of decades of ever-evolving best practices in the industry and exist to share those best practices for safe and effective products. Adherence to these regulations results in devices and diagnostics in which patients can feel confident.

Regulations and Standards

Quality

There are two major documents that most of the world uses to guide medical device development quality. We have already introduced 21 CFR 820, which governs things in the USA. Outside the USA, many countries rely on the International Organization for Standardization (ISO) standard ISO 13485, *Medical Devices – Quality Management Systems – Requirements for Regulatory Purposes.*[4] ISO 13485 was published for the first time in 1996 by the ISO and, just like the FDA's 21 CFR 820, it describes a comprehensive QMS for the design and manufacture of medical devices. At the time of writing this chapter, the latest version of ISO 13485 was released in 2016 (and reviewed/reconfirmed in 2020) and is commonly referred to as ISO 13485:2016.

It is worth noting that 21 CFR 820 and ISO 13485:2016 are exceedingly similar. They are so similar, in fact, that the FDA has started taking steps to harmonize the two by amending the current good manufacturing practice requirements of 21 CFR 820 to align more closely with ISO 13485:2016. The new Quality Management System Regulation (QMSR) will incorporate, by reference, ISO 13485:2016, thereby aligning the two standards.[5, 6] As of June 17, 2023, the FDA timetable for QMSR final rule is December 2023.[7]

To illustrate these similarities, Table 6.1 maps several key sections of 21 CFR 820 that correspond with sections of ISO 13485:2016. The similarities in these key sections demonstrate the broad impact that both documents have across nearly all functions of a company and phases of a product's typical life cycle. We will refer to many of these quality regulations and deliverables later in this chapter.

Risk Management

ISO 13485:2016 has a more obvious and explicit integration of risk management than 21 CFR 820, but the expectations for the ISO standard and the FDA regulation are very similar in spirit. Both 21 CFR 820's preamble and ISO 13485:2016 introduce and require risk management concepts, which are now codified in ISO 14971:2019, *Medical Devices – Application of Risk Management to Medical Devices*.[8] Upon adopting ISO 13485:2016 within the FDA's new QMS regulation, there will be a stronger push from regulators for US manufacturers to comply with ISO 14971:2019.

ISO 14971:2019 is the worldwide "state of the art" standard for medical device risk management. Risk management is intentionally not given its own section in Table 6.1 (and there is also no such section in ISO 13485:2016), as nearly every section of the ISO standard has an expectation of or "nod" to risk, and emphasizing risk management is not a standalone activity. ISO 13485:2016 requires manufacturers to carefully consider risks during every step of design, development, manufacturing, and post-market processes. ISO 14971:2019 has an informative, related technical report (ISO/TR 24971:2020, *Medical Devices – Guidance on the Application of ISO 14971*),[9] which is full of decades of best practices to guide firms along their risk management journey.

ISO has gifted the medical device community with informative guidance developed specifically for diagnostics in another technical report, namely in Annex H of ISO/TR 24971:2020, "Guidance for in vitro diagnostic medical devices." This annex provides 22 pages of best practices for risk analysis tools, definitions, thought exercises, and considerations specifically for in vitro diagnostic risk management.

Human Factors

Human factors, often referred to as "usability," focuses on the interactions between people and device technologies, with the aim of minimizing use-related hazards and risks and ensuring the effective and safe use of the device. Human factors engineering has two primary sources of definition and requirements: the FDA's guidance document titled *Applying Human Factors and Usability Engineering to Medical Devices*[10] and the International Electrotechnical Commission (IEC) standard IEC 62366-1:2015, *Medical Devices – Part 1: Application of Usability Engineering to Medical Devices*[11] (reviewed/reaffirmed in 2021). Like the risk management standards, IEC 62366-1:2015 has an adjacent, supporting technical report, which contains suggestions,

Table 6.1 Similarities between 21 CFR 820 and ISO 13485:2016

| FDA 21 CFR 820 | | ISO 13485:2016 | |
Section	Description	Description	Section
§ 820.5	Quality system	QMS	4
		General requirements	4.1
		Documentation requirements	4.2
§ 820.20	Management responsibility	Management responsibility	5
§ 820.22	Quality audit	Internal quality audits	8.2.4
§ 820.25	Personnel	Resource management	6
§ 820.30	Design controls	Planning of product realization	7.1
		Customer-related processes	7.2.1
		Review of requirements related to product	7.2.2
		Design and development	7.3
§ 820.40	Document controls	Control of documents	4.2.4
§ 820.50	Purchasing controls	Purchasing process	7.4.1
		Purchasing information	7.4.2
		Verification of purchased product	7.4.3
§ 820.60	Identification	Identification	7.5.8
§ 820.65	Traceability	Traceability	7.5.9
§ 820.70	Production and process controls	Human resources	6.2
		Infrastructure	6.3
		Work environment and contamination control	6.4
		Control of production and service provision	7.5.1
		Validation of processes for production and service provision	7.5.6
§ 820.72	Inspection, measuring, and test equipment	Control of monitoring and measurement equipment	7.6
§ 820.75	Process validation	Validation of production and service provision	7.5.6
§ 820.80	Receiving, in-process, and finished device acceptance	Planning of product realization	7.1
		Verification of purchased product	7.4.3
		Control of production and service provision	7.5.1
§ 820.86	Acceptance status	Identification	7.5.8

Table 6.1 (cont.)

FDA 21 CFR 820		ISO 13485:2016	
Section	Description	Description	Section
§ 820.90	Nonconforming product	Control of nonconforming product	8.3
§ 820.100	Corrective and preventive action	Corrective action	8.5.2
		Preventive action	8.5.3
§ 820.120	Device labeling	Medical device file	4.2.3
		Identification	7.5.8
		Preservation of product	7.5.11
§ 820.130	Device packaging	Medical device file	4.2.3
		Identification	7.5.8
		Preservation of product	7.5.11
§ 820.140	Handling	Medical device file	4.2.3
§ 820.150	Storage	Planning of product realization	7.1
§ 820.160	Distribution	Identification	7.5.8
§ 820.170	Installation	Preservation of product	7.5.11
§ 820.180	General requirements	Documentation requirements	4.2
		Medical device file	4.2.3
		Planning of product realization	7.1
§ 820.181	Device master record	Medical device file	4.2.3
§ 820.184	Device history record	Control records	4.2.5
		Planning of product realization	7.1
		Identification	7.5.8
§ 820.186	Quality system record	Documentation requirements	4.2
		Planning of product realization	7.1
§ 820.198	Complaint files	Communication	7.2.3
		Feedback	8.2.1
		Complaint handling	8.2.2
		Reporting to regulatory authorities	8.2.3
§ 820.200	Servicing	Medical device file	4.2.3
		Planning of product realization	7.1
		Servicing	7.5.4
		Identification	7.5.8
§ 820.250	Statistical techniques	General	8.1
		Analysis of data	8.4

examples, and best practices for human factors/usability: IEC TR 62366-2, *Medical Devices – Part 2: Guidance on the Application of Usability Engineering to Medical Devices.*[12]

Diving a little deeper, we are going to examine a select few of these concepts and deliverables during different phases of a product's normal development life cycle.

Quality in Early Development

Early product development should be primarily focused on planning. Planning activities include, as a minimum, the following:

- product development process planning
- identification of user and product requirements
- risk management planning and preliminary risk analysis
- human factors planning

The process of planning and defining the product takes significant time, effort, and energy. A good rule of thumb is to invest approximately one-third of the total time and effort it takes to develop a product into this planning phase.

Product Development Processes

Planning in product development can be boiled down to three linked activities: product development process planning, requirements management for user needs, and requirements management for product requirements (design inputs). All of these are touched on within 21 CFR § 820.30 and ISO 13485:2016 §§ 7.1–7.3. Risk management and human factors also are best introduced early in the planning processes as they are intimately interwoven into product development, user needs, and design input.

Once a team has documented a development plan, requirements, and early risk/human factors activities, the team should review all of the documentation, adjust it where necessary, and approve transitioning into formal development. Development, risk management, and human factors activities all inform each other. Requirements often drive new product risks that must be mitigated and managed; product risks often drive new requirements that must be verified or validated.

Quality during Development and Testing

Development teams normally follow the development plan to work through several iterations of the design before identifying a candidate that they feel is ready for formal testing. At some point during the development process (ideally, very early), documentation would have been created to individually specify every aspect of the design or process. As changes are introduced during development to those parts and processes, the changes are recorded, reviewed, and approved before being introduced. The entirety of this documentation is referred to as the "design output."

The design output is then tested in several phases, ultimately resulting in "verification" testing to confirm that the product successfully meets all of the design input product requirements. This is followed by "validation" testing to confirm that the product successfully meets the user need requirements. The design output includes manufacturing processes and the validation of those processes as well.

The design output, including manufacturing process specifications, is often called the device master record (DMR), which is a term used in the current version of 21 CFR 820. The

Table 6.2 Planning activities and quality deliverables

Planning activity	Quality deliverable(s)
Product development process: The development organization carefully plans for the processes it intends to follow to design, develop, test, launch, and support the product. Generally, mature companies have a generic product development plan or new product introduction process that defines how to create a product-specific development plan.	Development plan
Requirements management – user needs: Developers should understand market, user, and patient needs to ensure the resulting product at the end of product development fully satisfies the expectations of everyone involved in delivering the best patient care. Documenting user needs is essentially part of careful planning to ensure that a product is what patients and/or users want.	User needs
Requirements management – design input: The development organization looks at user needs and specifies features that the diagnostic product or process itself will require to meet those expectations. These specifications or requirements, called the "design input," are product specific. Design input product requirements set out *how* the product will deliver what the patient and/or users want.	Design input (product requirements)
Risk management and human factors: The organization creates a risk management plan and a human factors plan and undertakes early risk analyses to support both. Risk management in early development serves to identify unacceptable risks that have design implications, inform the regulatory strategy, and ensure the safety of the device.	Risk management plan Human factors plan Risk analyses

entire process is documented and becomes part of something the FDA calls a design history file (DHF). 21 CFR 820 and ISO 13485:2016 are harmonized in terms of the spirit of the design output documentation, but they use different terminology. With the migration of 21 CFR 820 to align substantially with ISO 13485:2016, the terms DMR and DHF will no longer be listed in the regulation. The terminology that ISO 13485:2016 uses instead is "medical device file." Often, during the verification and validation testing phase of development, risks are identified. The risk management file should be updated to mitigate and manage these new risks.

As a product is developed, suppliers are selected to provide materials and components for the device. It is imperative to carefully select suppliers that are both capable of providing the type and quantities of materials/components and capable of meeting quality expectations. Once suppliers are selected, supplier quality agreements should be created to codify the expectations.

It is important to note that product development and risk management do *not* stop once a product is transferred to manufacturing. A launched product generates many questions, feedback, and complaints from users and patients. The ability of an organization to collect and respond to this feedback is critical and well described in regulatory documents. Of critical importance is the ability to assess feedback to determine if any of it represents what the FDA calls an "adverse event." Responding to feedback, assessing any new risks that it may reveal, and updating the product or process accordingly in the spirit of continuous improvement are all part of successful medical device development. The team supporting and improving a device or process may change; however, *development never really ends* until that product is finally taken off the market and is no longer used in the field.

Quality in Manufacturing

In production, the proof that a manufacturing process was followed using acceptable parts and processes is called the device history record (DHR), which is sometimes also referred to as a batch record, lot record, or similar terms. The DHR provides traceability to all the components, raw materials, tools, equipment, processes, and production records used to manufacture a specific device. The DHR can be inspected to ensure that all component/raw material inputs to the device were of an acceptable quality, everyone involved in the process was appropriately trained, the latest released documentation was used, and all equipment used was functioning properly.

DHF versus DMR versus DHR: A Piece of Cake

Consider a new diagnostic test as a new, unique kind of birthday cake. The DHF is the story of how you came up with the final cake recipe. It is all the things you considered when planning the cake, all of the requirements that the final cake has to meet, the story of your successes and failures on the way to a recipe that tasted perfect, how you tested that recipe against others, etc.

The DMR is the final recipe itself. It is the final ingredients list with the exact proportions, plus carefully worded instructions regarding how to blend those ingredients and what equipment you need to use to do so. The recipe describes the type of oven, the temperature of that oven, the time the cake is in the oven, and where to place it in the oven. It is much more than just a list of ingredients, and it must be detailed enough that you should be able to give the recipe to friends and they are able to make it correctly every time. The DHF and DMR you just created are like your medical device file in ISO 13485:2016.

Now you give the recipe to a friend. The DHR is a record of exactly what that friend did when they followed your recipe. What brand of flour did they use? Did they weigh out an appropriate amount? What was the make and model of the scale they used to weigh out the ingredients? What about the oven? How long did they actually bake it for? How long did they let it cool before spreading the icing? Who was the cook? The DHR is unique to each cake.

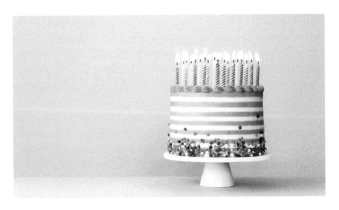

Figure 6.3 Birthday cake.

The Impact of Documentation

Returning for a moment to the holistic and all-encompassing scope of quality and risk management processes, let us consider the impact that these processes have on our development timelines. In "normal" medical device and diagnostic test development, the team marches through a well-documented product development process, as guided by the QMS. A well-known adage among quality professionals and regulatory inspectors is "If it is not documented, it did not happen." This means that you cannot just say that you did something; you must have objective evidence that you did it. As such, working within a mature QMS leads to the generation of a large, well-controlled, and immutable trail of evidence demonstrating, among many things, that the team and leadership (1) thought carefully about planning the development of the product, (2) did everything they were supposed to do as defined in their QMS, (3) considered all of the risks involved, (4) adequately tested the product, and (5) are prepared to support users, patients, and consumers once the product is launched.

Without the urgent and immediate response necessary to address a situation like the COVID-19 pandemic, experienced medical device product developers are careful to document decisions, detail analyses, review plans, consider risks, and carefully test, verify, and validate products through clinical studies and the launch. This takes time. Even though you may feel the desire to expedite product launch, *you want this to take time*. As a patient, you want to know that test developers and manufacturers are incredibly detailed and deliberate throughout the entire life cycle of the product being used to diagnose you. Therefore, the regulated development of diagnostic products can take so much longer than the development of unregulated products. It simply takes more time to weave the highest quality and risk-based thinking throughout the process and create evidence. As professionals in this field, medical device developers and manufacturers approach these responsibilities to patients and their caregivers with the utmost seriousness and with a strong aversion to doing anything less.

So, how does the industry adapt when confronted with a global pandemic in which we do not have the luxury of time? How do we evolve while still holding ourselves as product development professionals to the highest quality standards? How do we develop when we feel juxtaposed between the importance of doing things right and getting products to market to serve the public emergency?

To respond quickly and efficiently to COVID-19 demanded a different approach. The resulting nimbleness employed by many RADx Tech teams to accelerate products to market while maintaining high quality standards required a rethinking of the "quality status quo" by focusing on *re-prioritization*.

COVID-19 Pandemic Response

The RADx initiative itself is a shining example of finding a way to rapidly and nimbly develop diagnostic tests and testing capabilities when faced with an urgent situation unlike anything we have faced in modern times. Clearly, one of the most important contributions to being able to move rapidly and nimbly was the removal of barriers associated with the status quo, which included providing unprecedented access to the FDA and the FDA's willingness to allow tests to reach patients through the Emergency Use Authorization (EUA) process.

This raises an interesting question for developers regarding QMSs and if it is even ethical to "do less" to speed things up. We understand that developing products in a traditional manner compliant with 21 CFR 820/ISO 13485:2016 has, to some degree, overheads associated with adequately planning and documenting along the way. But faced with a rapidly expanding and ever-evolving global pandemic, we do not have the time or the luxury to do things in a traditional way. If we accept that the current good manufacturing practices built into 21 CFR 820 and ISO 13485:2016 represent decades of well-honed best practices and if we further accept that quality and risk management practices are a mindset, not just a task or phase, then how could we ever justify doing anything less than the regulations call for? When it comes to quality, there are no shortcuts.

The answer is to focus on the *here and now* by meeting the development teams and their new technologies where they are, with an emphasis on moving forward from there. More on this later, but we will first evaluate the FDA's approach to managing quality amidst the pandemic.

The FDA, EUAs, and QMSs

The FDA's *Policy for Coronavirus Disease-2019 Tests*[13] contains guidance for diagnostic test developers and their own staff, including a variety of EUA "templates." These templates reflect the FDA's current thinking on the data and information that developers should submit to facilitate the EUA process. A common misconception is that EUAs give developers carte blanche to avoid needing a QMS. For example, the molecular diagnostic template (October 6, 2021)[14] and antigen diagnostic template (October 6, 2021)[15] both include the following statement:

> Under an EUA, certain sections of the 21 CFR Part 820 Quality System Regulation (QSR) requirements <u>may</u> be waived for an authorized product during the duration of the EUA, but FDA recommends that test developers follow comparable practices as much as possible, even if such requirements are waived. Please see recent letters of authorization for examples of which QSR requirements have been required.

If all one remembers from that excerpt is the word "waived," then it is understandable where the misconception may have crept into our communal conversations that a QMS is unnecessary. The FDA's emphasis of the word "<u>may</u>" is a strong indication to readers that the FDA is willing to work with someone, depending on the size of their company and the maturity of their quality infrastructure, throughout the EUA process. This was key to accelerating the development of COVID-19 diagnostics to market in terms of quality management.

It is important to note how the EUA templates direct test developers toward "recent letters of authorization for examples of which QSR requirements have been required." The FDA used the letters of authorization as a means to communicate their frequently evolving quality system regulation (QSR) expectations of test developers. As of September 27, 2022, 430 distinct COVID-19 tests had been issued with EUAs.[16] As of January 12, 2023, another 59 individual EUAs had been issued for antigen diagnostic tests for SARS-CoV-2[17] and 274 had been issued for molecular diagnostic tests for SARS-CoV-2.[18] One example of the FDA prescribing QSR requirements beyond those requirements in the templates is in the letter of authorization for the Abbott Diagnostics BinaxNOW COVID-19 Antigen Self Test (EUA No 210264, sent on December 23, 2022).[19] Section III states that the FDA is waiving the following requirements for the product during the duration of this EUA:

> Current good manufacturing practice requirements, including the quality system requirements under 21 CFR Part 820 with respect to the design, manufacture, packaging, labeling,

storage, and distribution of your product, but excluding Subpart H (Acceptance Activities, 21 CFR 820.80 and 21 CFR 820.86), Subpart I (Nonconforming Product, 21 CFR 820.90), and Subpart O (Statistical Techniques, 21 CFR 820.250).

The list of subparts H, I, and O is then called out again identically in Section IV, "Conditions of authorization" (see condition N).

The letter of authorization for Mesa Biotech's molecular Accula SARS-CoV-2 Test (EUA No200028/S006, sent on August 17, 2022)[20] includes the same Section III waiver and Section IV conditions of authorization (see condition M) as they relate to 21 CFR 820 QSRs.

In both cases, the letters of authorization include many other conditions of authorization including, but not limited to, conditions related to labeling and lot release procedures, These conditions ensure that the tests released for distribution have the same clinical and analytical performance claimed in the authorized labeling.

What do these and other letters of authorization tell us about the FDA's willingness to deviate from the status quo? They all squarely put the emphasis on ensuring that diagnostic tests can be produced reliably and can perform well.

It is also important to note that any QSR waivers are only applicable if the EUAs are still active. It is not enough for a product to only meet the required QSRs – they also need to be moving toward a fully compliant product and quality management system once the EUAs are eventually terminated. The FDA publicly updated its COVID-19 guidance on September 27, 2022, to encourage developers to seek traditional premarket review (i.e. *de novo* classification or clearances under Section 510(k) of the Food, Drug and Cosmetic Act) for most test types, which will allow their diagnostics to be sold after the US government's COVID-19 public health emergency declarations expire.

The takeaway is that developers will eventually need a fully compliant quality system to support traditional premarket reviews, so it is important to start building it right away – maybe just in a different order from how they normally would do it.

Building a Solid Foundation

There are a few quality fundamentals and best practices that should never be taken for granted and that every team needs to have in place, regardless of size or maturity. Larger teams will already have processes to support the following best practices, but smaller teams and start-ups should first deploy quality processes and tools to introduce the following four fundamentals.

Create a Single Source of Truth

No matter what, teams need a strong, undeniable single source of information that is accessible to them always. In practice, this means that all quality system processes and product documentation (the design input, design output, test protocols, test results and data, etc.) must exist in only one place at one time.

It makes good business sense to make it easy for teams to quickly find exactly what they need and know it is the most up-to-date version. All modern collaboration tools reinforce this importance.

Document Early and Revise Often

When you have a single document repository, you need to make changes to those documents and ought to have some processes by which you can process those changes and evaluate their impact. Documentation that is to be created early and revised often may include procedures, plans, protocols, reports, and bills of material.

Both 21 CFR 820 and ISO 13485:2016 stress the need to change process and product documentation in a manner that is well controlled, peer reviewed, and holistically considered (i.e. implementation planning) before the change is implemented. However, as stated earlier, the best-performing companies and teams do not implement document and change management processes only because the regulations say so – they do it because it expedites product development and post-launch support.

Many smaller teams and start-ups in the RADx program did not come into the program with all of their documents in a single location, let alone one with change controls. The RADx program strove for rapid implementation of infrastructure and processes as a first port of call when teams did not yet have this capability in place.

The electronic QMS platform developed by Greenlight Guru (a provider of QMS software for the RADx initiative)[21, 22] is a great example of using modern tools to collaborate around a single source of information and manage changes robustly.

Embrace Feedback

Eventually, the developer of diagnostic tests or processes needs to meet regulatory requirements to accept, review, and react to feedback from users and patients. Generally, this takes the form of some sort of ticketing system for a new product plus many internal business and quality processes to effectively react to external feedback.

However, during rapid development, our experience has shown that *internal* experiences are key to tracking if a team wants to move nimbly. As such, developing tracking mechanisms for RADx teams and encouraging their use during internal development, verification, validation, and clinical testing is important. Teams will need this infrastructure *and* some associated quality processes before they launch anyway, so it is best to develop and use those building blocks early.

Note, one of the post-launch QSR requirements that the FDA clearly lists in the EUA templates is that all companies must have processes in place to evaluate feedback and report on "adverse events." This infrastructure is not optional.

Generate Trustworthy Data

It is imperative to create laboratory and operational systems to instill confidence in the data being generated, especially while moving quickly. To accomplish this, there are several "laboratory fundamentals" that require attention. If teams are not already working within a mature laboratory operations framework, then taking steps to implement the following controls will help ensure that the data generated are trustworthy:

1. Raw materials and samples used to perform the experiment or test must be of known, documented quality (not expired, labeled, stored appropriately, etc.)
2. The equipment used is maintained and calibrated appropriately
3. Laboratory personnel are trained
4. Experimental protocols are written down and reviewed before execution

The goal is not to slow down the scientists, but to empower them to report confidently that their data are reliable and that pivotal company decisions can be confidently made based on their results.

QMS Re-prioritization

Reflect for a moment on the structure of the sections of 21 CFR 820 and ISO 13485:2016. The order in which the QSRs are listed generally follows the traditional life cycle of a product, and QMS processes are typically deployed in a similar manner when being created from scratch for new companies. Using the FDA's EUA templates and FDA letters of authorization as guides, RADx quality "content experts" often opted to re-prioritize the order in which the quality processes occurred, especially for small companies and start-ups, to move at the pace required to respond to the pandemic while still ensuring that high-quality products were produced.

Often, during the initial introduction of a quality content expert to a new RADx team, perhaps a small company or start-up, we would find ourselves having to interrupt the introduction, saying something along the lines of the following:

> You've got something really cool here and this diagnostic testing capability would clearly make a difference. I love it and applaud the science behind it but let's stop talking about how you got here. Instead, let's talk about how you are going to prove to us and yourselves that it works well time and time again, then tell me about your plans to scale it up.

Let us tease that apart using some of the phrases introduced earlier in the "Regulations and Standards" section.

"Let's stop talking about how you got here" represents a *de*-prioritization of the DHF. It should be recalled that the DHF is really a collection of everything you did to get here so far. Spending time playing catch-up and documenting what was done and why somehow does not seem all that important when there is a pandemic raging. If you have a useful diagnostic test that can be deployed, let us focus on the present and future, not the past.

"Prove to us and yourselves that it works well time and time again" speaks to the high prioritization of processes associated with strong *assay development practices* and *testing* (especially verification and validation, as well as clinical testing), all of which are concepts that are well explored within other chapters of this book. The QMS infrastructure necessary to support these efforts includes the development of strong quality processes around the documentation, review, and approval of the design output (documenting what you are testing) and testing protocols and reports (documenting how to test and the results of those tests). Therefore, putting in place, if they are not already there, QMS processes associated with later development and especially testing all become important.

"Tell me about your plans to scale it up" represents a strong *prioritization of the DMR and DHR*. The DMR is more than just the design output, as it includes how to manufacture the diagnostic test (and the validation of those processes) and quality assurance procedures (how to test it in the factory). When we discuss the DMR, the commercialization topics explored in Chapter 11 of this book become relevant. As such, QMS processes associated with supplier management and everything that goes into the DHR are necessary.

A Note on Supplier Management and "Scaling Up"

Large, mature teams already know that they can never take their suppliers for granted, and they must work hard to earn their suppliers' business. This means that suppliers, especially contract manufacturing organizations, often need to have their own robust quality pro-cesses in place, are open to being audited regularly, and are willing to participate in process validation exercises. The QMS processes associated with the robust, thorough supplier qualification and auditing necessary to support the creation of an approved supplier list and supplier quality agreements need to be put in place for smaller teams if they do not have these processes in place already. In many cases, smaller teams need to learn how to visit suppliers on-site to audit them. It is never enough to presume that suppliers are doing the right thing; one often needs to go there to see it and *know* they are doing the right things.

Table 6.3 illustrates the general re-prioritization efforts and those QMS standard operating procedures (SOPs) that RADx Tech experts helped put into place for supported teams if they did not already have the necessary infrastructure and resources. The SOPs are listed in the typical order that a company might normally

Table 6.3 Suggested QSR re-prioritization for small businesses creating new quality systems

Tier	SOP	Description
3	Quality manual	General policies governing a company's QMS
1	Document control and records management	Document control and change management processes, as well as record management
	Management responsibility and review	Processes to ensure that the responsibility, authority, and interrelation of all personnel who manage, perform, and verify work affecting quality is defined and that they set out how the quality system is to be reviewed by management to ensure its continuing suitability, adequacy, and effectiveness
4	Design and development	Design control process used by the company throughout all stages of the design and development of its products
1	Product testing, verification, and validation	Processes to define how the company should plan, document, and execute product testing, including verification and validation
1	Clinical testing	Process that defines how the company should plan, document, and perform clinical testing
1	Risk management	Process that defines the risk management activities required, including criteria for risk acceptability
	Human factors engineering	Process that defines the human factors activities required, including use specifications and human factors testing
4	DHF	Document that sets out how to compile and maintain DHFs for products
2	Supplier evaluation	Process that defines the criteria and methods for selecting, evaluating, and monitoring suppliers for addition to or disqualification from the approved supplier list

Table 6.3 (cont.)

Tier	SOP	Description
2	Purchasing	Procurement of materials, supplies, and services
2	Receiving and incoming inspection	Receiving and inspection of materials, including work in progress, finished goods, components, and raw materials
	Customer order	Customer order process and collection of relevant records associated with each order (such as the DHR)
1	DHR	Document that sets out how to compile and maintain DHRs (including, but not limited to, product assembly reports, product test reports, certificates of conformance/compliance, and product packing reports)
1	DMR	Document that sets out how to compile and maintain DMRs containing the procedures and specifications for a finished device manufactured at the company
	Nonconforming materials	Processes and responsibilities for documenting and addressing nonconforming materials
	Corrective action	Processes and responsibilities for identifying the causes of nonconformities, initiating corrective action(s), and performing follow-ups to ensure that the corrective action(s) have been effective in preventing the reason for the nonconformance
	Preventive action	Processes to be used to identify potential nonconformities in medical devices/products/tools and services and determine actions to prevent their occurrence
	Complaint handling	Receipt, review, and evaluation of complaints
1	Customer feedback	Processes to document and implement methods for monitoring and controlling the product using data to detect quality problems, determine satisfaction, and identify opportunities for improvement
	Adverse event reporting	Processes and responsibilities for reporting an adverse event in accordance with the requirements of external regulatory bodies
	Corrections and removals	Processes and responsibilities associated with reporting product corrections and removals (21 CFR 806)
	Master validation	Process that defines the validation processes for all product manufacturing processes requiring validation, including any processes for which 100% verification is impractical
	Software validation	Process that defines software validation processes for all software used for QMS and in the manufacturing, engineering, quality, and regulatory processes of a medical device (does not pertain to software being developed for use in a finished medical device)

Table 6.3 (cont.)

Tier	SOP	Description
	Preventive maintenance	Processes and criteria for preventive maintenance of key process and manufacturing equipment
	Calibration	Calibration requirements for all equipment, gauges, measuring devices, test fixtures, etc., used to take measurements and ensure quality criteria are met
	Analysis of data	Processes and responsibilities for the analysis of data to demonstrate product conformity and determine the suitability and effectiveness of the QMS
	Training	Process that defines the training requirements and processes for the company
	Internal auditing	Process that defines the quality system internal auditing process for the company
	Post-market surveillance	Processes, responsibilities, and activities required to monitor and assess device performance and safety
1	Labeling	Processes associated with product labeling
	Traceability	Process that defines the traceability requirements and documentation
	Post-market clinical follow-up	Planning, conducting, and documenting post-market clinical follow-up evaluations
1	Regulatory compliance policy	Company strategy for regulatory compliance

develop and implement them. The numbers 1–4 to the left of the SOPs help demonstrate the RADx Tech prioritization (i.e. create and implement the tier 1 SOPs first, then the tier 2 SOPs, and so on). SOPs with no number are important to put into place once the top-four tier SOPs are implemented. Of course, every company in the RADx program was unique, and this prioritization was not necessarily the same in each case. However, the focus on what is most important to implement first generally stands.

It is worth noting the recommendation not to skip any sections of the QSR. The entire QSR is important. Instead, in response to the pandemic, it was recommended that the timeliest items be worked on first, namely those that support the confident production of a well-performing test, then the earlier stage items that were deferred can then be returned to and developed.

If looking *only* at tier 1 SOPs, it is clear that the *highest* prioritization was given to document controls (including change management), product documentation (the DMR, the DHR, and labeling), and product testing (including clinical evaluations). Bear in mind that this prioritization presumes that a team entered the RADx Tech program with a core diagnostic technology or process that was strong enough to gain access to the program in the first place (i.e. the bulk of early development had already happened).

In review, the RADx Tech QMS re-prioritization efforts involved deferring documenting the past and instead ensuring quality processes were in place so that the diagnostic test or process was (1) well documented, (2) capable of performing reliably in the field, and (3) able to be confidently scaled up to large volumes.

Risk Management Considerations

In developing products to serve the pandemic response, RADx content experts and the teams they were supporting often used risk management tactically by closely studying ISO/TR 24971:2020, Annex H. Although many tools are commonly used in early development for risk management (see ISO/TR 24971:2020, Annex B, for more details on suggested tools), the following were prioritized to be completed first and placed into a matrix for easy reference.

Preliminary Hazard Analysis

Preliminary hazard analysis identified hazards and hazardous situations that could lead to harms in single and multiple fault conditions. ISO/TR 24971:2020, Annex A, provided a starting place for identifying hazards and characteristics related to safety, along with the guidance for risk analysis in Annex H, section H.2. Priority was given to identifying hazards that needed design mitigations, with the purpose of avoiding costly design iterations later. Adverse events listed in the FDA's medical device reporting database were studied to ensure that teams considered and learned from the adverse events experienced with other, similar, diagnostics. Finally, relevant international safety standards (such as IEC 61010-1) were consulted to identify risks related to electrical and mechanical safety and electromagnetic compatibility.

Fault Tree Analysis

Fault tree analysis, used sparingly on the most severe risks, helped teams to identify all of the foreseeable events and hazardous situations that could lead to the highest risks. Fault tree analyses for biohazard contamination, loss of sample integrity, false negatives, and sample loss were the most useful.

Use-Related Risk Analysis

Use-related risk analysis identified the severity of use errors, which highlighted to the teams if there were any critical tasks (critical tasks are those that, if omitted or completed incorrectly, could cause serious harm). Critical tasks were then flagged as needing risk reduction, control, and verification/validation. Risk control for all other tasks was also de-prioritized for later product improvements to minimize the human factors testing efforts needed.

Other widely used tools, such as design and process failure modes and effects analysis, could also have been confidently de-prioritized, as such tools are primarily single-fault reliability tools. Risk management files were further developed and expanded as the development cycle progressed, with frequent iterations throughout verification, validation, and commercialization.

Summary

Developing diagnostics for the pandemic allowed the typical order of QMS implementation to be rearranged to make it more nimble for development efforts. Infrastructure was created to ensure that a digital, single source of documentation existed; this gave the entire team access to relevant documentation, even if they were in isolation or quarantine. Using those tools, the early creation and frequent revisioning of documentation were possible and highly encouraged. Importance was placed on the lightweight management of materials and equipment to ensure that the data being generated were trustworthy. As most teams already had a working prototype on entering the RADx initiative, developing the DHF was de-prioritized; instead, focus was placed on ensuring that the assays were adequately tested to the FDA's requirements and that manufacturing processes were scalable. Finally, risk management was used strategically as a decision-making tool to identify risks very early, which required design controls and testing to avoid costly redesign efforts.

To help ensure applicability in the future, the pandemic response roadmap for quality was developed to best illustrate the re-prioritization efforts employed in a manner that did not precisely call out aspects of 21 CFR 820 (as they are expected to be harmonized with ISO 13485:2016), but stayed true to the intent of the QSRs that are already highly aligned. The roadmap was developed with smaller teams in mind, so it includes time to write and implement QMS processes and time to execute or follow those new processes. Larger developers and manufacturers will already have QMS processes implemented and may likely skip the "creation" steps.

QMS resources provided by the National Institutes of Health to support all RADx Tech diagnostic teams made it possible to accelerate product development while creating strong quality infrastructure. Small teams and start-ups benefited from bringing in seasoned experts to advise on and develop infrastructure, and larger or more established teams were able to advance their technology more quickly using the extra human effort. The entire RADx program taught us all amazing new ways to collaborate and bring impactful diagnostic tests to market. This is true across the board, including in the way we look at quality and risk management. Future development efforts, even those undertaken outside the hyper-urgency of a pandemic, would do well to closely consider the novel product development, quality, and risk management approaches that RADx introduced and to look for opportunities to adopt these approaches.

Lessons Learned

- A digital document repository/electronic QMS platform should be implemented quickly to give all team members access to documentation and create a single source of information, even when being physically together is impossible.
- QMS processes should be re-prioritized (in contrast with what is typically done) to ensure that, first, the specifications for how to make the device and how to scale up manufacturing are established quickly; the balance of the QMS should be deployed later.

- Infrastructure for accepting feedback from internal users should be created to allow rapid identification and implementation of improvements.
- Trust the data generated from prototypes, lightweight equipment and materials management processes and laboratory practices/training should be created.
- Risk management should be utilized tactically to find and mitigate risks early.

References

1. FDA, CFR – Code of Federal Regulations Title 21, Volume 8, Section 820.1, Scope (2022). https://tinyurl.com/39bfw37y (accessed January 12, 2023).

2. FDA, CFR – Code of Federal Regulations Title 21, Volume 8, Section 820.3, Definitions (2022). https://tinyurl.com/6bj4whbc (accessed January 12, 2023).

3. National Institute of Biomedical Imaging and Bioengineering, RADx Tech/ATP/ITAP Dashboard (2023). https://tinyurl.com/y6xuets8 (accessed January 12, 2023).

4. ISO, ISO 13485:2016, *Medical Devices – Quality Management Systems – Requirements for Regulatory Purposes* (2022). www.iso.org/standard/59752.html (accessed January 12, 2023).

5. FDA, Quality system (QS) regulation/medical device good manufacturing practices (February 23, 2022). https://tinyurl.com/24vcvjt8 (accessed June 21, 2023).

6. Federal Register, Medical devices; quality system regulation amendments (February 23, 2022). https://tinyurl.com/yc27nsdk (accessed June 21, 2023).

7. Reginfo.gov, View rule: medical devices; quality system regulation amendments (2022). https://tinyurl.com/33hmsc33 (accessed June 21, 2023).

8. ISO, ISO 14971:2019, *Medical Devices – Application of Risk Management to Medical Devices* (2019). www.iso.org/standard/72704.html (accessed January 12, 2023).

9. ISO, ISO/TR 24971:2020, *Medical Devices – Guidance on the Application of ISO 14971* (2020). www.iso.org/standard/74437.html (accessed January 12, 2023).

10. FDA, *Applying Human Factors and Usability Engineering to Medical Devices: Guidance for Industry and Food and Drug Administration Staff* (2016). www.fda.gov/media/80481/download (accessed January 12, 2023).

11. ISO, IEC 62366-1:2015, *Medical Devices – Part 1: Application of Usability Engineering to Medical Devices* (2021). www.iso.org/standard/63179.html (accessed January 12, 2023).

12. ISO, IEC/TR 62366-2:2016, *Medical Devices – Part 2: Guidance on the Application of Usability Engineering to Medical Devices* (2016). www.iso.org/standard/69126.html (accessed January 12, 2023).

13. FDA, *Policy for Coronavirus Disease-2019 Tests (Revised): Guidance for Developers and Food and Drug Administration Staff* (2023). https://tinyurl.com/2s3bse7u (accessed January 12, 2023).

14. FDA, *Molecular Diagnostic Template.* www.fda.gov/media/135900/download.

15. FDA, *Antigen Diagnostic Template.* www.fda.gov/media/137907/download.

16. FDA, *Coronavirus (COVID-19) Update: FDA Updates COVID-19 Test Policy, Encourages Developers to Seek Traditional Premarket Review for Most Test Types* (2022). https://tinyurl.com/yckpw2w7 (accessed January 12, 2023).

17. FDA, *In Vitro Diagnostics EUAs – Antigen Diagnostic Tests for SARS-CoV-2* (2023). https://tinyurl.com/yn9nna4t (accessed January 12, 2023).

18. FDA, *In Vitro Diagnostics EUAs – Molecular Diagnostic Tests for SARS-CoV-2* (2023). https://tinyurl.com/229wpmmd (accessed January 12, 2023).

19. FDA, BinaxNOW COVID-19 antigen self-test – letter of authorization (2022). www.fda.gov/media/147251/download (accessed January 12, 2023).

20. FDA, Accula SARS-CoV-2 test – letter granting EUA revision(s) (2021). www.fda.gov/media/145700/download (accessed January 12, 2023).

21. National Institute of Biomedical Imaging and Bioengineering, Greenlight Guru named premier QMS software for NIH RADx initiative (2021). https://tinyurl.com/59m72c6m (accessed January 12, 2023).

22. Cision PRWeb, Greenlight Guru named premier QMS software for NIH RADx initiative (2021). https://tinyurl.com/3s59vkch (accessed January 12, 2023).

Development of Assays to Diagnose COVID-19

Yukari C. Manabe and William Clarke

Introduction

When a new viral pathogen emerges in humans, a critical race begins – one that will help determine whether this new pathogen will be managed and controlled or potentially evolve into a pandemic that will create a surge of morbidity and death. When we isolate and identify (or sequence) the new virus, the race to develop a diagnostic test ensues; without this diagnostic test, we cannot specifically treat patients or control the spread. This diagnostic test must be sensitive and specific, but, to be globally effective, it must also be developed quickly and at a reasonable price, and it must not require cold-chain shipping and storage.

For antigen diagnostic test development, antigen-specific targets need to be identified along with the corresponding antibodies (or equivalents) that bind to these targets. Once the target and antibody are identified, appropriate sample types, internal and test controls, a workflow, and curated patient samples must be determined and acquired. Likewise, for molecular diagnostic test development, the full genetic sequence of the virus needs to be identified along with the corresponding relevant ribonucleic acid (RNA) sequence that binds to essential transmission or pathogenic targets. Again, once the targets and RNA sequence are identified, appropriate sample types, internal and test controls, workflow, and curated patient samples must be determined or acquired. A key output of Rapid Acceleration of Diagnostics (RADx®) Tech was the creation of its Clinical Review Committee, which bridged the gap between diagnostic device developers and clinical users, providing real-time feedback on usability. These and other critical aspects of assay development will be discussed in this chapter within the context of severe acute respiratory syndrome coronavirus 2 (SARS-CoV-2); the lessons learned which can be applied in future pandemics, will also be discussed.

General Considerations

Definitions

According to the US Food and Drug Administration (FDA), in vitro diagnostic devices are "tests performed on samples taken from the human body to detect diseases or other conditions and can be used to monitor a person's overall health to help cure, treat, or prevent diseases."[1] COVID-19 diagnostic tests are the subject of this chapter. These tests directly detect parts of the SARS-CoV-2 virus and can be used to diagnose infection with the SARS-CoV-2, that is, COVID-19.

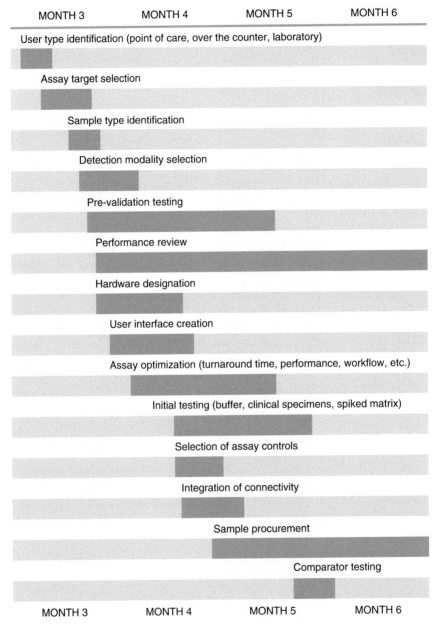

Figure 7.1 This roadmap depicts the vital activities, their chronology, and an estimated time frame in months. In the case of the SARS-CoV-2 pandemic, month 1 was December 2019, the month in which the virus was isolated, sequenced, identified, and published.

The tasks repeat with each new RADx Tech project.

Classifications

Diagnostic tests include molecular tests and antigen tests. In general, assay development should be informed by unmet needs and, ultimately, should inform the intended use – that is, what the manufacturer puts on the label and the instructions for use.

Molecular tests are those that amplify a portion of the RNA in the virus and then detect that amplicon. Most of these tests amplify more than one region of the virus and, in general, target viral genes that have the least likelihood of developing new mutations (e.g., ORF1ab and parts of the nucleocapsid [N] gene) to decrease the risk of non-detection with new variants. In general, assays that first extract the RNA and then amplify a large proportion of that extract volume are the most sensitive. Isothermal amplification takes less energy, because it does not require cycling through very hot temperatures to melt DNA duplexes, and it tends to be simpler – often isothermal amplification can be performed in a single tube and does not require much manipulation; there is often a trade-off, with slightly lower sensitivity due to a higher limit of detection. It includes approaches such as loop-mediated isothermal amplification (LAMP), helicase-dependent amplification, nucleic acid sequence-based amplification (NASBA), clustered regularly interspaced short palindromic repeats (CRISPR), and recombinase polymerase amplification. Several LAMP assays have been granted FDA authorization (e.g., Abbott ID NOW and Uh-Oh Labs). Some have even been granted over-the-counter (OTC) Emergency Use Authorizations (EUAs) (e.g., Mesa Biotech, COVID Detect, and Cue) because of their simplicity.

Antigen tests usually use antibodies against specific parts of the virus (usually the nucleocapsid, although a few tests have targeted the spike (S) protein) and use different readouts to show specific binding. Samples are put into a buffer that has two purposes: (1) lysis of the virus to release the N protein that is contained inside the viral coat and (2) viral killing, which is important for biosafety. That buffer is then applied to a lateral flow assay, whereby the immobilized antibody binds to the viral antigen. A secondary antibody that also binds to the viral antigen is linked to a detector molecule that undergoes a chemical colorimetric change that can be read by eye or with a reader. Readers tend to be more sensitive than the naked eye, although ultimately the sensitivity of the assay is more dependent on the quality of the capture antibody. Although rapid (10–15 minutes), the sensitivity of antigen assays is much lower than that of molecular methods (80–97%),[1, 2] although their specificity is relatively high (96–100%). Because the N protein from the original severe acute respiratory syndrome (SARS) virus is nearly identical to that from SARS-CoV-2, all antigen assays that target the N protein cannot distinguish between the two.

Assay Design and Development

Designing and developing an assay and deciding how the tests will be used by patients and clinicians is a crucial process that will benefit from the following questions.

Who Will Perform the Test and Where?

Tests vary in complexity; with increasing complexity, increasing levels of skill are required. Reference laboratory tests are usually moderately or highly complex and require a trained laboratorian to perform the assay. Training may also be required to perform such tests accurately and reproducibly. Point-of-care (POC) assays that are Clinical Laboratory

Improvement Amendments (CLIA)-waived[3, 4] are performed by paraprofessionals and are simple enough to be performed by anyone who reads and understands the instructions for use. Once the user has read the instructions, they should be able to reliably perform the test without training. CLIA-waived POC tests must be performed at sites that have obtained a CLIA waiver certificate, which can be a barrier to adoption. Finally, OTC tests can be performed by a layperson at home by following the written instructions. Such tests can be obtained by prescription (prescription OTC tests) or purchased directly by the consumer. Prescription OTC tests require a health-care professional to help the consumer to interpret the results, whereas OTC tests do not. Many OTC tests will not be connected to any laboratory information system. Therefore, the test result is often not reported to public health officials unless the consumer reports the result to their physician or to a public health agency. Prior to COVID-19, there was only one self-test OTC available for the diagnosis of an infectious disease, the OraQuick HIV self-test.[5] At the time of writing this chapter, there were 30 OTC COVID-19 tests commercially available.

What Is the Sample Type?

For molecular tests, the most common sample type is a clinician-collected nasopharyngeal (NP) swab (flocked) that is put into viral transport media (VTM) or universal transport media that stabilizes the live virus.[6] Flocked swabs are the swab type most often used because data from molecular assays for sexually transmitted infections have shown that flocked swabs have a superior ability to capture a sample and then release the sample in buffer. Another sample type is a mid-turbinate swab, which does not go all the way back to the NP space. Although slightly less sensitive than NP swabs, they are better tolerated by patients. Mid-turbinate specimens can be used for reference laboratory testing and for POC CLIA-waived assays. Finally, bilateral nasal (anterior nares) swabs (with and without nose blowing prior to collection) are the most common sample type for OTC tests, as these can be easily and safely self-collected by users. In a meta-analysis comparing sample types, nasal plus oral swabs were the most comparable in terms of sensitivity to NP swabs.[7, 8] Interestingly, this led the United Kingdom to suggest swabbing both the throat and the nose in guidance for lateral flow assays.[9] In a recent publication of a SARS-CoV-2 human challenge model,[10] granular information in young volunteers showed that the viral loads in the throat increased more rapidly than in the nose, but the viral load peaked higher in the nose and persisted longer, such that the area under the curve for the nose was larger.

Some data suggest that saliva reverse transcription polymerase chain reaction (RT-PCR) can be positive slightly earlier than NP swab RT-PCR.[11–13] Most of the assays that use a saliva sample type require heat inactivation prior to testing, which increases the turn-around time of the test.[14] No saliva antigen tests have been granted an EUA.

Blood is often used to measure the humoral antibody response in people who have been exposed to and/or infected with SARS-CoV-2. There is one reference laboratory antigen assay that uses plasma or serum to measure SARS-CoV-2 antigens (i.e., Quanterix). In general, this is a rare sample type for the direct detection of a virus.

Who Will Collect the Sample?

Clinician-collected samples for the detection of SARS-CoV-2 are generally processed in reference laboratories or in POC laboratories under a CLIA waiver. Patient-collected samples can be submitted or mailed to reference laboratories or tested immediately at either

CLIA-waived POC laboratories or OTC. Therefore, who collects the specimen is important and should be considered, as it will inform the design of the sample collection device. For self-collected samples, guides may be necessary to ensure that the user does not insert a swab too deeply into the nose, for example.

Does It Need to Be Tested Right Away?

For assays that allow samples to be mailed or delayed testing, the stability of the sample will need to be documented, as will the maximum allowable time and the conditions of transport. In general, viruses in NP swabs in VTM, in dry flocked swabs, and in saliva have been very stable in transport with little decrement in sensitivity with SARS-CoV-2 assays.

What Biosafety Issues Need to Be Considered?

For assays that will be used at POC in laboratories with CLIA waivers, buffers that inactivate the virus are helpful to avoid complicated waste disposal instructions. These are not an issue for OTC tests, as it is assumed that the person performing the test is the person who is suspected of being ill. However, for OTC tests, all reagents must be shown to be safe if accidentally ingested.

How Long Does the Test Take to Generate the Result and How Many Tests Can Be Done Simultaneously?

There are two aspects of an assay that are important to consider when deciding on use case: turnaround time and throughput. For assays in which a single device runs a single test, the throughput is low, but each test may be rapid (e.g., lateral flow tests). Throughput could also be fast if many users test simultaneously, but keeping specimens organized and matched to the right user can be complicated, as can reading the test at the correct time after initiation. If a reader is used, however, the throughput may be much lower if the cartridge must stay in the reader for the entire time, for example. For tests that are done at home, a longer turnaround time may be acceptable for some use cases. If OTC tests are to be used to screen people for entry into a public area, even 15 minutes may not be fast enough. For POC CLIA-waived testing in a medium-throughput clinic, having a more sensitive molecular assay might be the most desirable, but each test should occur within the time period of a clinical encounter. If the patient submits a sample and then leaves to be contacted at home, the turnaround time of the test may not be as important. Some manufacturers attempt to increase throughput by suggesting that multiple machines be purchased or "daisy-chained." Although this does increase throughput, it also increases cost and maintenance time and uses valuable bench real estate, which small POC laboratories may not have.

How Is the Test Being Used?

In terms of this question, the following options are considered: use for asymptomatic screening, use for symptomatic testing, and use in recent contacts of known cases of COVID-19. The kinetics of SARS-CoV-2 have been studied and great heterogeneity has been shown across individuals.[11, 15] Transmissibility varies based on the variants of concern (e.g., omicron to delta to ancestral strain). After exposure, most people who are productively infected will have viral replication within two to three days, although there is great heterogeneity in the timing, magnitude of viral burden, and length of time that people

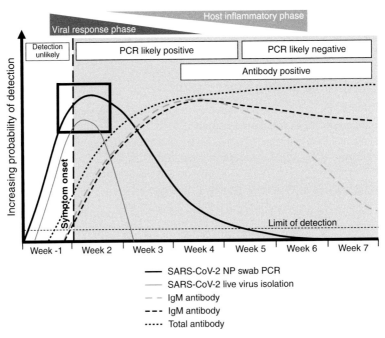

Figure 7.2 Trajectory of molecular test positivity from infection through symptom onset. The box shows the period during which antigen tests have the highest sensitivity because the viral burden is highest. Notably, it can start slightly before symptoms. Diagram is for illustrative purposes only. Adapted from Siddiqi and Mehra (2020)[26] and Sethuraman et al. (2020).[27]

shed virus. In the literature, infectiousness is measured by the ability of a patient's NP sample in VTM to have virus that can be propagated in cell culture (e.g., Vero E6 or Vero E6 TMPRSS2). By approximately 10 days, most people will no longer have a culturable virus,[10, 16–20] although viral RNA can be detected for longer periods of time.[21] Unlike SARS and influenza, patients with COVID-19 can have infectious transmissible virus prior to the onset of symptoms[22–24] – this is SARS-CoV-2's superpower, which has allowed it to propagate for so long across the globe. Although viral burden peaks with symptom onset, SARS-CoV-2 can be spread to others during the presymptomatic phase of infection. Therefore, screening by symptoms alone is inadequate for interrupting transmission.

In symptomatic illness when viral burdens are high, antigen tests can detect most infections. In addition, such tests will detect the majority of patients with a transmissible virus, as there is significant overlap between viral burden and infectiousness.[25] After five to seven days, most patients will become antigen-negative.[25] Although viral RNA is often detectable in saliva one or two days prior to NP swabs, viral RNA clears faster in saliva specimens.[12, 13]

For asymptomatic screening, serial antigen testing is recommended.[10, 28] For example, if a patient is in the presymptomatic phase after contact with a person with SARS-CoV-2, serial testing allows confirmation of infection by maximizing the likelihood of testing when viral burden is high enough to be detected.[28] In household contacts where the chance of transmission is high, even molecular testing that is more sensitive can be negative if performed too early – that is, a single negative test may not be enough to assure that transmission has not occurred.[29]

There are trade-offs between turnaround time and test accessibility. If molecular tests may take more than three days to return, serial antigen testing may be preferable to molecular testing, even if less sensitive.

Clinical Review Committee

The Johns Hopkins Center for Innovative Diagnostics for Infectious identified a critical gap in diagnostic device development in the area of clinical use cases over three cycles of National Institutes of Health (NIH) funding.[30] Many companies fail to narrow development to a clinical use case that best matches their technology. Within RADx Tech, we assembled a Clinical Review Committee (CRC) comprising infectious disease, emergency medicine, and ambulatory, pediatric, and adult clinicians; medical directors of College of American Pathologists-certified laboratories and diagnostic testing developers; and marketing experts with real-world bedside and clinical laboratory COVID-19 experience. Every RADx Tech-funded company at any stage beyond proof of concept was offered a one-hour facilitated meeting with the CRC to provide structured feedback. The previous experience of the Johns Hopkins Point-of-Care Technology Research Network (POCTRN) in shepherding novel POC tests for sexually transmitted infections – including HIV – from proof of concept to FDA approval was leveraged to provide SARS-CoV-2 diagnostic developers with the infectious disease and use-case expertise necessary to understand how a test would be used for decision-making by clinicians and other end users. Such concepts of clinical usability and feasibility are as important to success as test performance and accuracy. Detailed written feedback including recommendations from the 60-minute CRC meeting was prepared by the committee chairs and sent to each participating company and the NIH within one week.

More than 70 companies participated in a clinical use-case discussion. Diagnostic tools were intended to be used at the POC (with or without a device), in reference laboratories, in a mobile van, or for sample collection and preparation. Detection modalities included antigen detection, nucleic acid tests, concentration and capture, and others. (Once live, you will be able to visit pandemicresponseroadmap.org to view related graphics.)

Process

Between 4 and 12 committee members attended each meeting. Device company representatives included leadership (CEOs, marketing personnel, scientific developers, and personnel involved in regulatory aspects) and RADx Tech programmatic leadership (including the team lead, the portfolio executive, the FDA liaison, the NIH representative, and other RADx Tech support team members).

The majority of the meeting time was used for discussing the device use workflow and suggestions for process improvement, rather than the use case and preclinical pilot studies. For most of the assays discussed, insufficient data on device performance characteristics for clinical specimens led to uncertainty around the viability of some of the devices. There were some common barriers to design finalization:

1. **Complex workflow:** Many developers overestimated how much specimen-handling reference laboratories were willing to do. One device type that we found struggled to find a market was one that performed amplification after a nucleic acid extraction step.

Most of these devices targeted medium-throughput laboratories, which may not want to invest in a large reference laboratory machine. Unfortunately, few laboratories have personnel that can do a careful extraction and PCR with appropriate controls. These kit-device assays often did not fare well. For assays that were aimed at POC CLIA-waived laboratories, developers would expect precise pipetting or a pipette that was not intuitive to use. In addition, expectations for users to move very small amounts of liquid into small ports precisely was another commonly encountered workflow issue.

2. **Poor sensitivity due to the assay or workflow:** Several assays had lower-than-expected sensitivity for one of two reasons: (1) too much diluent (needed for microfluidics) or (2) too little sample input (devices that had pivoted from blood sampling with microfluidics optimized for 10–100 μl of sample were immediately disadvantaged in terms of the limit of detection compared with devices that accepted 500 μl–1 ml of sample).

3. **Inappropriate sample types:** In mid-2020, some papers using saliva as a sample type for centralized molecular testing were published, and developers decided that saliva was a better sample type for POC and OTC tests. There were no data at the time to support or refute this. Since that time, sample heat inactivation has been recognized as an important step in sample processing to optimize performance, but this is time-consuming and increases the turnaround time of POC tests. As an antigen sample type, saliva was not suitable for a sensitive test. Finally, saliva could be provided as spit, passive drool, sputum, or other sample types, which often led to poor clinical study results.

4. **Lack of internal and test controls:** Some innovative assays (e.g., lollipop antigen tests) never made it across the EUA finish line because developers did not consider the internal controls needed to show that the test had been performed correctly. Debates regarding sensitive process controls versus human DNA controls occurred often, especially with sample types likely to have inhibitors to amplification assays. Human gene controls are the most useful when the adequacy of the sample type is in question. For the most part, this has not been an issue with COVID-19, as most users try hard to obtain a good specimen (and not an air swab) because they are interested in getting a good result. To detect to mpox, however, dry swabbing has resulted in inadequate samples and the need for a human gene control has become clear.

5. **Lack of validation data:** In large programs like RADx Tech, developers are eager to please and often overestimate the performance of their assay. Having an independent validation of performance and limit of detection was very important for determining the likelihood that a particular assay would be granted an FDA EUA (see Chapter 8 for more information).

6. **Supply chain bottlenecks:** Early in the pandemic, there was a shortage of flocked swabs due to the large amount of surveillance and the volume of testing nationwide. Understanding the performance of assays with other swab types was challenging and costly from a clinical studies point of view. Some novel swabs including injection molded swabs (which appeared uncomfortable but were not when tested for usability) are interesting innovations that may be useful in future pandemics.

7. **Mismatch between the cost of goods sold and the use case:** It is important to remember the end goal at the beginning of the process. Some devices were ingenious but so complicated that manufacturing costs, assembly, and components led to a cost of goods that made them unattractive at POC or for OTC home self-tests. Antigen tests were approximately $5–15, and while molecular tests may have higher sensitivity, they exceeded the willingness-to-pay threshold.

8. **Not ecofriendly:** As consumers become more concerned with "green" technology and their plastic footprint, the size of and amount of plastic in consumables should be considered at the time of initial design. Although not frequently raised as an issue by the CRC, this is likely to become a larger issue in the future and may limit the platform potential of some devices.

These one-hour meetings were appreciated by both team leads and companies for the opportunity they provided for in-depth review and feedback on critical areas (Table 7.1).

The workflow was the most frequently discussed topic area followed by the use case, market strategy, clinical studies, biosafety, sample type, CLIA classification, and internal assay changes (controls, etc.). The various combinations of topics that were discussed and the number of companies that had similar topics of conversation are shown in Figure 7.3.

Assay Design

There are many important considerations for assay and instrument design. These factors range from the design of the assay to how things are detected to the user interface and how data are moved around. All factors must be carefully considered for a device to be both useful and impactful. The intended use of the assay will drive performance targets during the design, development, and validation processes.

Nucleic Acid Amplification Tests (Molecular Assays)

The most sensitive assays are those that test for the presence of RNA from the virus. These tests are so sensitive because they are amplification-based tests; they reproduce the nucleic acids of interest during the assay so that there is more material to detect. The two most

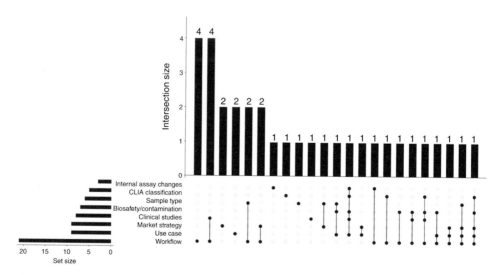

Figure 7.3 UpSet plot showing the most important CRC discussion content areas from a company perspective and the number of companies that valued the same topical areas. Listed in ascending order of importance: internal assay changes, CLIA classification, sample type, biosafety/contamination, clinical studies, market strategy, use case, and workflow.

Table 7.1 Sample meeting feedback

Feedback area	Common pitfalls	Mitigation strategies
Technology and clinical workflow	Complex workflow that did not match use case Turnaround time and throughput mismatch	The number of steps should be decreased (fewer than three steps are needed for a CLIA-waived test). The number of tests per hour should be specified for single test/run devices in moderate complexity laboratories.
Use case	Reference laboratory test with low throughput High complexity for POC device	A pivot should be made toward a higher throughput reference laboratory test or a POC CLIA-waived test.
Market strategy	Misunderstanding of unmet need Need for refrigerated or frozen reagents	A pivot should be made toward a POC CLIA-waived or OTC test. Lyophilized reagents are needed for these designations.
Clinical studies	Poor understanding of participant inclusion, exclusion, and intended use (symptomatic versus asymptomatic screening)	The highest burden of infection is during the early symptomatic period (the first five days), which may require a more limited use case to achieve the desired sensitivity.
Biosafety contamination	No sample inactivation buffer for POC tests Risk of aerosolization or spills	For CLIA-waived POC tests, biosafety and proper disposal is necessary, whereas for OTC tests it is not required.
Sample type and pitfalls	Salivary sample misunderstandings Difficulties understanding the advantages/disadvantages of each sample type (nasal, mid-turbinate, and NP) Complex sample collection systems	Salivary sample types have been problematic with antigen tests and may require heat inactivation for molecular assays.
CLIA classification	Incorrect understanding of workflow complexity for each CLIA classification Vague instructions for use	Accurate pipetting cannot be done for CLIA-waived tests, and the toxicity of the reagents must be assessed for OTC tests in case of inadvertent ingestion.
Internal assay changes and laboratory information systems	Design freeze Problems with public health reporting with POC and reference laboratory devices Inability to integrate into existing hospital laboratory information systems	Keeping an up-to-date and complete design file is necessary. For use in hospitals, being linked to the laboratory information systems is an added advantage.

common formats for nucleic acid amplification tests are PCR-based and LAMP-based assays.

Assays that are PCR-based require multiple steps of temperature cycling. DNA or RNA strands are denatured at one temperature; primer sequences are then attached (or annealed) to the target amplification zone at a second, lower, temperature; and then the temperature is raised again so that added polymerase can reconstruct the complementary strand for each strand template. This process is cycled 40 or more times to amplify the region of interest, and it requires precise temperature control and some sort of intercalating dye or other analytical method to detect the amplified genes. There are many important design considerations for these reactions, including the temperatures required, the time needed for cycles, the type of detection, and the extraction of the genetic material from the sample.

Assays that are LAMP-based provide amplification at a constant temperature by using a different type of polymerase enzyme that has strand displacement activity in addition to replication activity; this removes the need for a denaturation step. Multiple sets of primers for the target gene sequence are added to the sample, along with the polymerase, and then the temperature is raised to that needed for the target reaction. For amplification, loops are formed that can help with further rounds of replication. This amplification can be detected using intercalating dyes or with simple turbidimetry. Design considerations for these types of assays include the optimal temperature for amplification, the selection of primers and polymerase, the time needed for detection at the necessary sensitivity, the type of detection, and the extraction of the genetic material from the sample.

Direct Detection Assays

While amplification-based assays are very sensitive, they often lean toward higher costs and longer times to results. Direct detection assays frequently trade sensitivity for speed and/or cost. There are a number of ways to perform direct detection assays.

The most common approach is the direct detection of specific antigens (antigen assays) using reagents that target specific proteins from the virus. Antibodies are typically used to interact with sites on the N protein, as this protein does not seem to change much with the different variants, in contrast with the S protein of the virus, which changes frequently. Other types of affinity reagents, such as aptamers, can be substituted for antibodies in these types of assays. Aptamers are short, single-stranded oligonucleotides (RNA or DNA) that are generated through computer modeling (such as Systematic Evolution of Ligands by Exponential Enrichment [SELEX]) and then are tested in the laboratory for their strength of binding to the molecule of interest and iteratively enriched for the best candidates. For COVID-19 assays, none using aptamers has succeeded in receiving authorization at the time of writing this chapter. These affinity reagents (antibodies or aptamers) can be tagged with chemical labels (e.g., fluorescent or chemiluminescent tags) or nanoparticles that can be used for detection, or they can be detected with a second antibody tag. Design considerations for these types of assays include epitope selection (the site for binding), the type of detection, the type of affinity reagent, assay format design (e.g., homogeneous versus heterogeneous design), specimen treatment/extraction to make the epitope available for detection, and the determination of whether an instrument is needed.

Direct detection of nucleic acids is also possible using in situ hybridization. In this approach, localized gene expression can be detected by adding labeled complementary nucleic acid probes to a patient sample where they bind directly to the target RNA or DNA sequence. Detection occurs by then using a second reagent to detect the label. This is a technique often used in anatomic pathology to identify cancer genes in tissue, but it can be adapted to also identify the gene expression of microorganisms in cells. Design considerations for this type of assay include the selection of the target sequence, probe design, the detection scheme, and the specimen treatment needed to make the target available.

When Is an Instrument Needed?

Most central laboratory assays require instrumentation for specimen processing and analysis. For many POC testing options, part of the design process is to determine whether an instrument is needed for the performance of the assay.

Hardware Considerations

When an instrument is needed for testing processes, there are many important considerations, including the method of detection, the user interface and usability, and network connectivity for information management.

Whether direct detection or amplification systems are used, the approach to detection has a critical impact on the analytical sensitivity and overall performance of the assay. Fluorescence is often used due to its sensitivity (e.g. fluorescent dyes used in RT-PCR applications). Electrochemical detection is also used due to its simplicity and compatibility with miniaturization (such as whole blood glucose meters). Visual detection may be used for lateral flow-type assays (such as urine pregnancy kits).

The user interface is critical for POC testing systems to ensure the correct operation of the device and for the capture of important information. The user interface can allow guided testing and troubleshooting to make sure quality control samples are run and for patient identification information. The user interface also allows clear reporting of the result and guides the disposal of materials.

Network connectivity is important for reporting positive results to public health authorities and for transmission of the results to the electronic medical record. Network connectivity is distinct from a laboratory information system interface, which is necessary to facilitate information transfer to the electronic medical record.

Assay Controls

Assay control is necessary to ensure that a test or testing device is working properly, and also to make sure that testing regulations are satisfied. Assay control for POC testing is often lot-based and tested using external materials; this ensures that the reagents are still working properly after the manufacturing and delivery processes. Internal controls for single-use tests are used as process controls to make sure that the sample is appropriate, the fluidics are working properly, and the individual test (e.g., lateral flow assay) or device (e.g., portable meter) is working as intended. For molecular testing, one additional control that can be included is a human gene control that ensures that a swab has been properly performed and that amplification has occurred during the testing process.

Assay Optimization

When focusing on assay optimization, there are some key considerations including how quickly a result is available, how the test will be used, the workflow for the preferred use case, and the performance of the test in terms of false positives and false negatives. For each of these parameters, the key concept will be "fit for purpose," which means "Does this device or test work well enough to be used for a particular application?"

Turnaround Time

When considering how fast the result needs to be available (particularly when using a testing device for which parallel testing is not possible), the developer must first consider how the result will be used. For example, in a home-testing setting, a rapid result is not necessary. A testing time of even 45 minutes can be suitable, as the patient may relax in their own environment or find other things to do while waiting for their result. However, when testing many patients or in a time-sensitive environment, a turnaround time of 15–20 minutes would be desirable. Of course, for manual tests such as lateral flow assays that can be operated in parallel at low cost, the turnaround time is less of a concern.

Workflow

The workflow is particularly important when considering human factors for the operation of the device, as well as the disposal of materials. Key considerations of the workflow include the personnel who will be performing the testing, the setting where the testing will be performed, how the result will be used, and to whom the information will be communicated.

The type of personnel performing the testing is important because it must drive the complexity of the test. A clinical laboratory scientist has vastly different capabilities and perspectives from a non-scientist performing at-home testing.

There are several important considerations related to where a test will be performed. For instance, for a test or device that requires the internet for information transfer or analysis, the availability of reliable WiFi connectivity or cellular service must be considered; something that is suitable for an urban environment in the United States may not be suitable for a more rural area or in other places where resources are limited. Another consideration would be the power for the device: Will it require a plug-in source of energy or is it battery-powered? If battery-powered, will it be a single-use device or rechargeable? In addition, for battery-powered devices, one must ultimately consider the disposal of those devices.

The use case or utilization of the result can drive the design of the device; for instance, a test that will be used for screening at a public event will have different performance requirements from a device that will be used to diagnose and determine eligibility for treatment (e.g., nirmatrelvir–ritonavir [Paxlovid] and tixagevimab–cilgavimab [Evusheld]). To whom the result will be communicated will also drive design and optimization. For at-home testing, a very simple design can be used, and the most important factor will be the clarity of the result for the person performing the test so that they can make appropriate personal health-care decisions. If the test will be utilized in a health-care setting, clarity is certainly important, but there are also considerations regarding tracking within the electronic medical record and the regulatory requirements for testing and the recording of the results.

Test Performance (Sensitivity and Specificity)

The ability of the tests to detect true positives or to rule out true negatives is a critical performance parameter, but the optimal targets for each will depend on how the results will be used. In some cases, triage testing is sufficient for large groups. In this case, one would desire a high clinical sensitivity but could sacrifice specificity.

Sample Pooling

An additional approach to screening large populations is pooled testing, which combines a set number of samples into one test. If the whole pool returns a negative result, then all individuals whose samples were in that pool can be given a negative result. This can increase testing throughput and save the cost of testing each individually. If the pool comes back positive, then each individual must be retested to determine who in the pool caused the result to be positive. Without retesting each individual, there is no method to determine who produced the positive result or if there was more than one infected individual. To achieve the best pooled testing results, the correct pool size and prevalence levels must be selected. If the pool is too large or is in a high prevalence area, the majority of the pools will most probably be positive and everyone will need to be tested again. If the pool is too small, there is minimal benefit in terms of time or expense.[31]

The samples are typically pooled together by two common approaches: swab pooling and media pooling:[32]

1. **Swab pooling:** This involves adding swabs from multiple patients into a single volume of transport media on-site at the time of collection. Dry sample swabs may also be combined in a single tube and transported dry to the laboratory for further processing

2. **Sample/media pooling:** Pooling aliquots of transport media, each containing a single patient sample, can take place in the laboratory during the pre-analytic or analytic phase

Both of these methods have been successfully implemented for SARS-CoV-2 laboratory testing. The FDA has granted EUAs to several testing laboratories for pooled testing using their molecular – mostly PCR – assays.

Additionally, some studies have demonstrated the feasibility for pooled testing in POC settings.[33] Settings with semi-contained or fixed populations (e.g., schools and nursing homes) may also present opportunities for further workflow optimization through the use of pooled sample testing. By arranging a population into cohorts that remain in close proximity, such as in classrooms, those individuals can be regularly tested as a single pool. This allows for rapid identification and quarantine of positive cohorts, with follow-up testing to determine positive individuals. See Berke et al. (2021) for an example of this "pooling in a pod" strategy.[33]

Additionally, in a test utilizing pooled samples, the assay's limit of detection must be sufficient to detect a single positive sample among the pool. This will dictate the maximum number of specimens that can be combined into a pooled sample. For example, a laboratory-based PCR test may be able to test pooled samples containing many more individual specimens than a POC antigen test.

Concept of Trade-Offs

Consideration will often be given to trade-offs between time, analytical sensitivity, clinical performance, cost, and ease of use. Often, increased analytical sensitivity for the analyte of interest will lead to improved clinical performance; however, it will come at an increased cost. There are simple tests such as lateral flow assays that are widely used, but, in those cases, the ease of use and low cost come at the expense of clinical performance.

Preclinical Testing

Prior to the initiation of clinical studies to establish the performance of a particular assay or device, preclinical testing can establish that an assay will perform in a clinical matrix. For example, if an NP swab is to be used, then using an NP swab spiked with viral RNA can test microfluidics or other sample flow issues that may encounter difficulty with clinical matrices that are mucoid or viscous or inhibit RT-PCR reactions. Developers should be sure to use the swab that will be included with the assay or is recommended for the assay. Gamma-irradiated and heat-inactivated organisms can also be used to spike the clinical matrix. The use of an accepted external standard for determining the limit of detection is also helpful (e.g., the Biodefense and Emerging Infections Research Resources Repository [BEI Resources], which is a central repository that supplies organisms and reagents to the broad community of microbiology and infectious diseases researchers). Once acceptable performance has been shown with a spiked matrix to the expected limit of detection, the testing of clinical specimens (preferably blinded) will give an early indication of performance prior to expensive clinical studies to establish sensitivity and specificity.

How to Select a Comparator Assay

An important aspect of determining the analytical performance of an assay is choosing the comparator assay with which the new device will be compared to determine sensitivity (positive percent agreement) and specificity (negative percent agreement) for a premarket submission to the FDA. The selection of this comparator (predicate device) should be done together with the FDA in a prereview. For SARS-CoV-2, for example, the FDA provided a panel for testing, allowing a limit of detection comparison across assays, which showed a five-log difference in detection. If the new device has a very low limit of detection, selection of a less sensitive predicate device could result in a high false-positive rate, whereas a less sensitive new device – if compared with a predicate device with a low limit of detection – could conversely lead to poor overall sensitivity. (The FDA hosts a stable web page with a complete list of FDA-approved comparators, which can be found through a Google search.)

Samples for Preclinical Testing and Desktop Performance

Frozen samples are often a great place to start when determining the desktop performance of a new device. It is important to keep in mind that the detection of viruses may change when testing frozen specimens compared with fresh specimens. Repeatedly, frozen thawed specimens may show results in nucleic acid degradation, so retesting the same specimen at the time of new device testing is desirable. For assays that require a direct swab, this may be more challenging. For antigen tests, there are data showing that frozen thawed specimens can increase sensitivity, presumably due to the release of additional antigens. Procuring samples can be difficult and expensive. Leveraging existing biorepositories from investigators who have previously done device studies or from those who are doing epidemiological studies are potential sources. Often, getting well-curated specimens is also difficult with regard to information around timing in relation to symptom onset, age, and the original result of the comparator assay.

For clinical performance studies that will be submitted to the FDA, the following must be included: the specific patient inclusion and exclusion criteria (the age range with representative positives across the age strata, symptomatic patients, asymptomatic patients, the specimen types and matrices claimed in the intended use, and a geographically diverse patient population), the number of days from symptom onset, the type and number of specimens, directions for use, and a statistical analysis plan that accounts for variances to prevent data bias.

Changing Landscape across the Pandemic

One unanticipated issue during the first two and a half years of RADx Tech was the constant influx of knowledge, which led to changes in the acceptable parameters of performance. For example, antigen assays had to achieve more stringent sensitivity parameters over time. Other challenging issues were viral variants and an assay's ability to detect the virus. For antigen assays, developers were asked to assess performance as new variants emerged; because the N protein changed little compared with the S protein and the majority of antigen assays target the N protein, only a few assays were removed from the market. For molecular assays, single target assays were increasingly discouraged, as one mutation could compromise sensitivity.

Overall, RADx Tech was an unprecedented program that invested a significant amount of money into COVID-19 diagnostics. Over time, the emphasis moved from tests performed in reference laboratories to POC tests and eventually to OTC tests. Depending on the device, assay, and workflow, it is likely that many of these platforms may have the potential to be used with other infectious disease targets, especially those that are in the same sample matrix (such as influenza and respiratory syncytial virus). Those with multiplex capabilities may allow the detection of multiple treatable pathogens, which is exciting.

Providing developers with important data from the research literature and providing opportunities to meet with clinicians and laboratorians proved invaluable in averting misdirection that would be costly and time-consuming. RADx Tech's CRC helped to decrease the development time and showed that successful commercialization and adoption relies on providing assays that meet unmet needs.

Lessons Learned

The lessons learned through the COVID-19 pandemic by the RADx Tech CRC should be considered and applied in future pandemics.

- A complex workflow can eliminate the test utility from a POC or OTC setting. A CLIA-waived test should have fewer than three steps
- Accurate pipetting cannot be done for CLIA-waived tests
- Many POC CLIA-waived or OTC settings do not have the necessary equipment for cold-chain reagents, and developers should pivot toward lyophilized reagents
- For CLIA-waived POC tests, biosafety and proper disposal are necessary; therefore, the inclusion of a sample inactivation buffer eliminates the need for biohazard disposal
- Salivary sample types have been problematic with antigen tests and may require heat inactivation for molecular assays
- The toxicity of the reagents must be assessed for OTC tests in case of inadvertent ingestion
- For use in hospitals, the results of a test being linked to the laboratory information systems is an added advantage

- In most cases, tests must include both a sample adequacy control and an assay control
- For tests requiring swabs, alternative swab manufacturers should be identified and validated to limit supply chain bottlenecks
- Complicated designs with high manufacturing costs, assembly, and components can lead to a cost of goods that make them unattractive at POC or for OTC home self-tests
- The size of and amount of plastic in consumables should be considered during the initial design to ensure an eco-friendly design

References

1. FDA, Emergency Use Authorizations for medical devices (June 15, 2023). https://tinyurl.com/msdhfu5a.

2. S. Pickering, R. Batra, B. Merrick, et al., Comparative performance of SARS-CoV-2 lateral flow antigen tests and association with detection of infectious virus in clinical specimens: a single-centre laboratory evaluation study. *Lancet Microbe*, **2**, 9 (2021), e461–e471.

3. FDA, CLIA waiver by application (May 2, 2022). https://tinyurl.com/yh65vh39.

4. Code of Federal Regulations, Title 42, Chapter IV, Subchapter G, Part 493 (June 13, 2023). https://tinyurl.com/uhhcaysj.

5. O. T. Ng, A. L. Chow, V. J. Lee, et al., Accuracy and user-acceptability of HIV self-testing using an oral fluid-based HIV rapid test. *PLoS One*, **7**, 9 (2012): e45168.

6. R. Weissleder, H. Lee, J. Ko, and M. J. Pittet, COVID-19 diagnostics in context. *Sci Transl Med*, **12**, 546 (2020): eabc1931.

7. N. N. Y. Tsang, H. C. So, K. Y. Ng, et al., Diagnostic performance of different sampling approaches for SARS-CoV-2 RT-PCR testing: a systematic review and meta-analysis. *Lancet Infect Dis*, **21**, 9 (2021), 1233–1245.

8. E. S. Savela, A. V. Winnett, A. E. Romano, et al., Quantitative SARS-CoV-2 viral-load curves in paired saliva samples and nasal swabs inform appropriate respiratory sampling site and analytical test sensitivity required for earliest viral detection. *J Clin Microbiol*, **60**, 2 (2022): e0178521.

9. National Health Service, How to use an NHS COVID-19 rapid lateral flow test (March 21, 2023). https://tinyurl.com/55a7xj6u.

10. R. Ke, P. P. Martinez, R. L. Smith, et al., Daily longitudinal sampling of SARS-CoV-2 infection reveals substantial heterogeneity in infectiousness. *Nat Microbiol*, **7**, 5 (2022), 640–652.

11. Y. C. Manabe, C. Reuland, T. Yu, et al., Self-collected oral fluid saliva is insensitive compared with nasal-oropharyngeal swabs in the detection of severe acute respiratory syndrome coronavirus 2 in outpatients. *Open Forum Infect Dis*, **8**, 2 (2020): ofaa648.

12. A. L. Wyllie, J. Fournier, A. Casanovas-Massana, et al., Saliva or nasopharyngeal swab specimens for detection of SARS-CoV-2. *New Engl J Med*, **383** (2020), 1283–1286.

13. D. R. E. Ranoa, R. L. Holland, F. G. Alnaji, et al., Mitigation of SARS-CoV-2 transmission at a large public university. *Nat Commun*, **13**, 1 (2022), 3207.

14. R. Ke, P. P. Martinez, R. L. Smith, et al., Longitudinal analysis of SARS-CoV-2 vaccine breakthrough infections reveals limited infectious virus shedding and restricted tissue distribution. *Open Forum Infect Dis*, **9**, 7 (2022): ofac192.

15. V. Gniazdowski, C. P. Morris, S. Wohl, et al., Repeated coronavirus disease 2019 molecular testing: correlation of severe acute respiratory syndrome coronavirus 2 culture with molecular assays and cycle thresholds. *Clin Infect Dis*, **73**, 4 (2021), e860–e869.

16. R. Liu, S. Yi, J. Zhang, et al., Viral load dynamics in sputum and nasopharyngeal swab in patients with COVID-19. *J Dent Res*, **99**, 11 (2020), 1239–1244.

17. R. Wölfel, V. M. Corman, W. Guggemos, et al., Virological assessment of hospitalized patients with COVID-2019. *Nature*, **581** (2020), 465–469.

18. J. J. A. van Kampen, D. van de Vijver, P. L. A. Fraaij, et al., Duration and key determinants of infectious virus shedding in hospitalized patients with coronavirus disease-2019 (COVID-19). *Nat Commun*, **12**, 1 (2021), 267.

19. J. Bullard, K. Dust, D. Funk, et al., Predicting infectious severe acute respiratory syndrome coronavirus 2 from diagnostic samples. *Clin Infect Dis*, **71**, 10 (2020), 2663–2666.

20. B. Killingley, A. J. Mann, M. Kalinova, et al., Safety, tolerability and viral kinetics during SARS-CoV-2 human challenge in young adults. *Nat Med*, **28**, 5 (2022), 1031–1041.

21. A. A. R. Antar, T. Yu, N. Pisanic, et al., Delayed rise of oral fluid antibodies, elevated BMI, and absence of early fever correlate with longer time to SARS-CoV-2 RNA clearance in a longitudinally sampled cohort of COVID-19 outpatients. *medRxiv* (2021), https://doi.org/10.1101/2021.03.02.21252420.

22. M. M. Arons, K. M. Hatfield, S. C. Reddy, et al., Presymptomatic SARS-CoV-2 infections and transmission in a skilled nursing facility. *New Engl J Med*, **382**, 22 (2020), 2081–2090.

23. N. W. Furukawa, J. T. Brooks, and J. Sobel, Evidence supporting transmission of severe acute respiratory syndrome coronavirus 2 while presymptomatic or asymptomatic. *Emerg Infect Dis*, **26**, 7 (2020), e201595.

24. S. Hoehl, H. Rabenau, A. Berger, et al., Evidence of SARS-CoV-2 infection in returning travelers from Wuhan, China. *New Engl J Med*, **382**, 13 (2020), 1278–1280.

25. A. Pekosz, V. Parvu, M. Li, et al., Antigen-based testing but not real-time polymerase chain reaction correlates with severe acute respiratory syndrome coronavirus 2 viral culture. *Clin Infect Dis*, **73**, 9 (2021), e2861–e2866.

26. H. K. Siddiqi and M. R. Mehra, COVID-19 illness in native and immunosuppressed states: a clinical–therapeutic staging proposal. *J Heart Lung Transplant*, **39**, 5 (2020), 405–407.

27. N. Sethuraman, S. S. Jeremiah, and A. Ryo, Interpreting diagnostic tests for SARS-CoV-2. *JAMA*, **323**, 22 (2020), 2249–2251.

28. R. L. Smith, L. L. Gibson, P. P. Martinez, et al., Longitudinal assessment of diagnostic test performance over the course of acute SARS-CoV-2 infection. *J Infect Dis*, **224**, 6 (2021), 976–982.

29. M. L. Robinson, A. Mirza, N. Gallagher, et al., Limitations of molecular and antigen test performance for SARS-CoV-2 in symptomatic and asymptomatic COVID-19 contacts. *J Clin Microbiol*, **60**, 7 (2022), e0018722.

30. M. Robinson, C. Gaydos, B. Van der Pol, et al., The Clinical Review Committee: impact of the development of in vitro diagnostic tests for SARS-CoV-2 within RADx Tech. *IEEE Open J Eng Med Biol*, **2** (2021), 138–141.

31. M. G. Aspinall and C. Yamashiro, Pooling test samples: how and when it works, *College of Health Solutions* (November 13, 2020). https://tinyurl.com/mr2fvacc.

32. When to Test, Lab pool testing operational playbook (2022). https://whentotest.org/pooling-playbook.

33. E. M. Berke, L. M. Newman, S. Jemsby, et al., Pooling in a pod: a Strategy for COVID-19 testing to facilitate a safe return to school. *Public Health Rep*, **136** (2021), 663–670.

Chapter 8

Laboratory Verification and Clinical Validation of COVID-19 Diagnostic Assays

Anuradha Rao, Leda Bassit, Julie Sullivan, Wilbur Lam, and Jennifer K. Frediani

Introduction

The first human cases of COVID-19, the disease caused by the severe acute respiratory syndrome coronavirus 2 (SARS-CoV-2) virus, were reported in the news in December 2019. By the end of January 2020, the World Health Organization (WHO) had declared COVID-19 a global health emergency, followed in February 2020 by the declaration of a public health emergency in the United States. On March 11, 2020, the WHO declared the COVID-19 outbreak a global pandemic as cases rose around the world.[1]

To prevent the rapid spread of this infectious airborne disease and to accurately diagnose, treat, and quarantine infected individuals, there was an urgent need for user-friendly, accurate, rapid, and widely available testing for SARS-CoV-2. To meet this challenge, the National Institutes of Health (NIH) launched Rapid Acceleration of Diagnostics (RADx®), a public–private initiative tasked with expanding the development, commercialization, and implementation of COVID-19 testing technologies. This influx of funding and research support led to the development of "first-generation" diagnostic tests that required laboratory verification and clinical validation studies before they could be widely distributed.

In this chapter, we describe the SARS-CoV-2 verification and validation processes that occurred in the laboratory, clinic, and community. A majority of the current successful and widely used SARS-CoV-2 tests developed as part of RADx were evaluated at the Atlanta Center for Microsystems Engineered Point-of-Care Technologies (ACME POCT), based at Emory University, the Georgia Institute of Technology (Georgia Tech), and Children's Healthcare of Atlanta. The combined expertise in microsystems-based technologies at Georgia Tech, the priorities of clinical translation within the biomedical engineering departments at Emory University and Georgia Tech, the renowned clinical acumen at Emory University School of Medicine, and access to large patient populations at Emory University and Children's Healthcare of Atlanta made ACME POCT an ideal location for test verification and clinical validation.

The ACME POCT verification and validation core, headed by Drs. Wilbur Lam, Greg Martin, and Oliver Brand were part of a larger network of clinicians, faculty, clinical coordinators, and virologists who came together to successfully "test the tests."

In the first part of this chapter, we describe laboratory verification and clinical validation studies conducted on first-generation diagnostic tests for SARS-CoV-2, using both live viruses (capable of causing COVID-19) and inactivated viruses (incapable of causing COVID-19). (Note that inactivated viruses cannot be as well detected as live viruses). This is followed by a description of cross-reactivity and specificity studies, in which we evaluated whether tests detected only SARS-CoV-2 and no other coronaviruses. We then discuss the

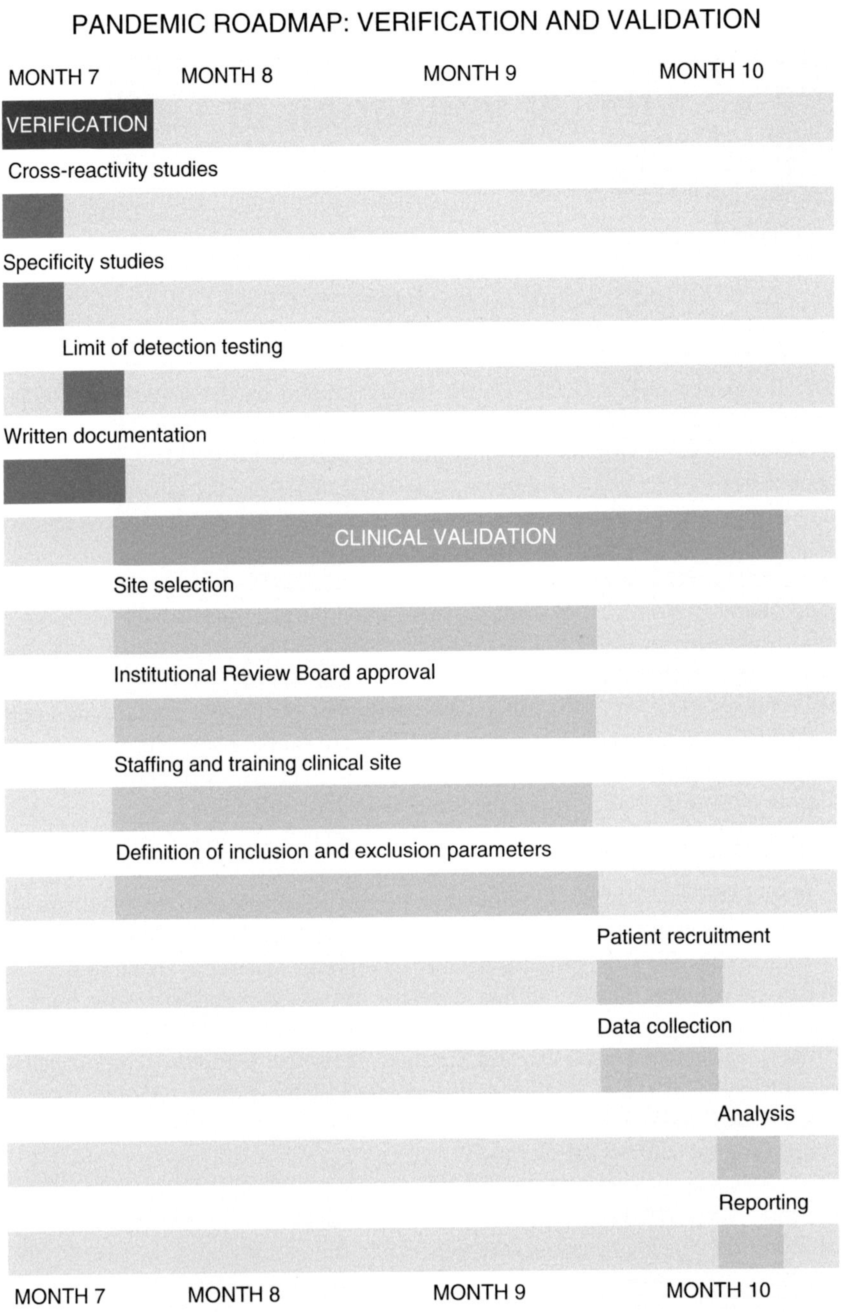

PANDEMIC ROADMAP: VERIFICATION AND VALIDATION

Figure 8.1 This roadmap depicts the vital activities, their chronology, and an estimated time frame in months. In the case of the SARS-CoV-2 pandemic, month 1 was December 2019, the month in which the virus was isolated, sequenced, identified, and published.

The tasks repeat with each new RADx Tech project.

appearance of variants and the establishment of the Variant Task Force (VTF) to evaluate the effectiveness of tests against emerging variants. Next, we describe sensitivity studies using genetically sequenced SARS-CoV-2 remnant clinical samples to determine whether tests could detect low amounts of variants and conclude by describing how test results were documented.

The second part of this chapter describes how clinical validation was done outside the laboratory, in the field. Validation samples were from individuals who suspected they were infected with SARS-CoV-2 and presented to testing centers. We expand on how reaching our goals required the establishment of new partnerships between academic and health-care institutions, staffing and training the large numbers of people needed for this work, and processes that are involved in large-scale data collection, the storage of samples, the documentation of data, and establishing a biorepository. Finally, we describe the lessons learned from clinical testing and how we can prepare for the next pandemic.

Laboratory Verification and Clinical Validation Studies

Outlined in this section are the steps for test verification carried out in the laboratory. In the subsections that follow, we will expand on each step and describe how these RADx-generated protocols may help with accelerated test verification and validation for the next pandemic.

- Limit of detection (LOD) testing using:

  o laboratory-propagated, live (wild-type [WT]) SARS-CoV-2 in a biosafety level (BSL) 3 laboratory. This step is critical because when the tests are deployed to patients, they will be required to detect live virus

  o heat-inactivated (HI) or gamma irradiation-inactivated (GIV) SARS-CoV-2 in a BSL2 laboratory

- Cross-reactivity and specificity studies
- Sensitivity studies using:

  o genetically sequenced SARS-CoV-2 remnant clinical samples containing specific variants

  o the establishment of a biorepository of SARS-CoV-2 variants

- Utilization of LOD and sensitivity studies under the Independent Test Assessment Program (ITAP)
- Documentation and reporting of laboratory testing

Figure 8.2 presents a brief schematic of the events, timeline, and workflow described in our laboratory verification studies.

LOD Testing Using Laboratory-Propagated, Live WT SARS-CoV-2 in a BSL3 Laboratory

Emory University was one of the first places to begin initial SARS-CoV-2 LOD testing protocols. LOD testing is a laboratory technique used to determine the lowest amount of

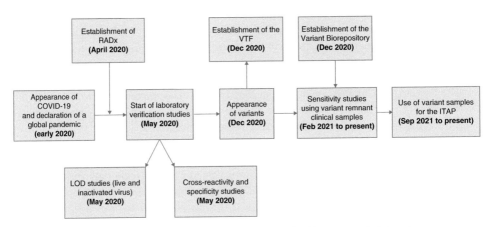

Figure 8.2 Schematic representing the timeline and steps involved in laboratory analytical testing.

a substance (in this case, SARS-CoV-2) that can be detected by a particular test. Emory University has a long history of antiviral drug discovery and is led by Dr. Raymond Schinazi, Director of the Laboratory of Biochemical Pharmacology. Dr. Schinazi's research group had previously developed novel small molecule inhibitors for the treatment of human viral infections such as HIV, herpesviruses, chikungunya, and hepatitis B and C. Importantly, the Laboratory of Biochemical Pharmacology houses a certified BSL3 facility that required only minor modifications to work with SARS-CoV-2. By the time COVID-19 was declared a pandemic, the Schinazi laboratory had already procured the reference strain of SARS-CoV-2 (NR-52281: USA-WA/2020) from the Biodefense and Emerging Infections Research Resources Repository (BEI Resources) and propagated WT virus in monkey kidney Vero cells in its BSL3 facility.

The availability of a BSL3 laboratory approved for use with SARS-CoV-2 ensured that the virology team could propagate and reproducibly quantify the amount of SARS-CoV-2. These quantifications were measured in median tissue culture infectious dose (TCID50/ml), a metric used to quantify and assess the infectivity of a virus in cells. Additionally, the availability of a BSL3 laboratory allowed the preparation of aliquots of live virus for future investigations. An important distinction to note here is the differences between BSL2 and BSL3 laboratories. Table 8.1 breaks down the differences between BSL2 and BSL3 laboratories, but, in summary, BSL3 laboratories have more safety requirements and training.

When the first tests for SARS-CoV-2 that were developed as part of RADx arrived at Emory University, the BSL3 laboratory was well positioned to begin testing with WT SARS-CoV-2. Most of the SARS-CoV-2 tests evaluated during this initial phase were antigen-based lateral flow assays (LFAs) involving an antigen–antibody interaction that produced a colored test line. In such tests, antibodies against a SARS-CoV-2 protein, usually the nucleocapsid (N) protein, are adhered to a nitrocellulose strip. When a test sample containing the N protein (the SARS-CoV-2 antigen) is added to the test strip, it binds to the adhered antibody, causing a colored test line to appear. A limited number of nucleic acid amplification test (NAAT)-based assays that detected viral ribonucleic acid (RNA) instead of protein were also evaluated.

Table 8.1 Differences between BLS2 and BLS3 laboratories. Source: https://researchsafety.gwu.edu/

BSL criteria	BSL2	BSL3
Special practice addressing biological safety cabinet use	A biological safety cabinet (or other containment device) is required for procedures likely to generate aerosols.	A biological safety cabinet (or other physical containment device) is required for all procedures involving manipulation of infectious materials.
Safety equipment addressing protective clothing	Protective laboratory coats, gowns, smocks, or uniforms designated for laboratory use must be worn while working with hazardous materials; protective clothing is not to be worn outside the laboratory and must not be taken home for laundering.	Workers in the laboratory must wear protective clothing with a solid front, such as tie-back or wraparound gowns, scrub suits, or coveralls; protective equipment must not be worn outside the laboratory; protective clothing must be decontaminated before laundering.
Safety equipment addressing glove limitations	Gloves need to be changed when contaminated, when integrity is compromised, or when otherwise necessary.	The same glove-changing verbiage is used as for BSL2, except an additional statement is included advising that two pairs of gloves be worn when appropriate.
Safety equipment addressing eye, face, and respiratory protection	These devices should be used in rooms where infected animals are present based on risk assessment.	These devices must be used in such rooms.

The WT SARS-CoV-2 virus propagated in the Emory University BSL3 laboratory was selected as the virus source for initial test evaluation for two reasons:

1. This was early in the pandemic and, even though SARS-CoV-2-positive individuals were being identified by polymerase chain reaction (PCR) at this time, there was a lack of established protocols to transfer positive clinical samples from a hospital to a laboratory for use in assessing the tests

2. Evaluating prototype tests using non-standardized positive samples without a more complete understanding of virus stability, proper sample storage conditions, or knowing the viral load was problematic. If a test failed, we would not have been able to differentiate between a problem with the test and a problem with the quality of the sample. In contrast, testing using WT virus propagated in the BSL3 facility represented an agile, idealized alternative. Testing in the BSL3 laboratory would be done using live, concentrated, and well-characterized SARS-CoV-2 reconstituted in a compatible test matrix with minimal interfering substances. If tests failed in this ideal scenario, RADx companies would quickly learn that their test performed poorly,

thereby allowing the companies to identify problems early ("fail fast") and redesign their tests

This choice to evaluate tests in the Emory University BSL3 laboratory proved to be an important first step in deciding whether early versions of tests demonstrated sufficient sensitivity and specificity to progress to field studies or whether the tests needed to return to the companies for further development.

For LOD testing, experienced scientists trained in handling live infectious virus and working in a BSL3 laboratory would thaw one vial containing WT virus with a known TCID50/ml. This stock was then used to prepare dilutions of the virus using a test compatible matrix (diluent/buffer) suggested by the device manufacturing company. The matrix was often a nasal wash or nasal rinse obtained from SARS-CoV-2-negative individuals and confirmed by PCR at ACME POCT to be free of the virus. Each dilution was tested three or five times. The lowest virus concentration that produced a positive result (i.e. the highest dilution of virus solution that was positive in three out of three or five out of five replicates) was defined as the LOD for that test. Some tests failed to detect the virus at even the highest concentrations or gave positive results when tested with the matrix alone; such tests were recommended for redesign. Other tests detected the virus at lower amounts and were amenable to field testing after minor modifications.

The use of laboratory-propagated SARS-CoV-2 in a BSL3 facility was a critical bridging step that provided rapid feedback for tests still in the preliminary stages of development. Throughout 2020 and into the beginning of 2021, evaluating the performance of tests using LOD testing in the BSL3 laboratory was done as part of the verification process at ACME POCT. Feedback for tests that failed testing was transmitted quickly to the companies, after which the tests were redesigned and were returned improved for reevaluation or termination. BSL3 testing using live virus and an ideal matrix was an effective way to identify tests that made the cut. Testing in the BSL3 laboratory continued until the appearance of the SARS-CoV-2 alpha variant and the later SARS-CoV-2 variants. In addition to live virus testing in the BSL3 facility, tests were also evaluated using inactivated virus, which we will briefly describe in the next section.

LOD Testing Using HI or GIV Virus in BSL2 Laboratories

Concurrent with live WT testing in the BSL3 facility, we also used inactivated virus to determine LODs in BSL2 laboratories. The major advantage of using inactivated virus over live virus is that testing can be done outside the physical requirements of a BSL3 laboratory. Viruses can be inactivated in two ways:

1. HI: Live virus that has been propagated in a BSL3 laboratory and has a known TCID50/ml is used as starting material. A portion of this stock virus is heated to 65 °C for 30 minutes in a dry heating block. The HI virus is then added to cultured Vero-2 cells, and the cells are observed every day for two weeks for cytopathic effects (changes in cellular morphology) caused by infection. If inactivation is successful, no cytopathic effects are observed. Once the virus stock is confirmed to be inactivated, it can be safely moved out of the BSL3 facility and into a BSL2 laboratory using established transfer protocols. HI is an easier method than GIV because minimal equipment is needed

2. GIV: During GIV, live virus is exposed to gamma radiation, which disrupts the viral RNA genome and renders the virus incapable of replicating. GIV has the advantage over

HI in that GIV preserves viral protein structure, whereas HI can cause changes in protein folding that may affect the binding of viral proteins to test antibodies and the test's apparent sensitivity, thereby affecting the sensitivity of the test

A BSL2 laboratory with a certified laminar flow hood and the use of eye protection, double gloves, a mask, and a laboratory coat are sufficient for use of HI or GIV samples, and the testing protocol follows the same dilution and testing scheme described for live virus. The use of BSL2 facilities significantly increases testing capacity, turnaround, and output, as the number of such available facilities is many times more than that of BSL3 facilities. As mentioned earlier, the training required to work with inactivated virus in a BSL2 environment is considerably less than that needed for a BSL3 environment, meaning that more personnel have access to these materials.

Cross-Reactivity and Specificity Studies

At ACME POCT, early versions of tests produced through RADx were evaluated for specificity (tests should detect only SARS-CoV-2) and cross-reactivity (tests should not give a positive result with other viruses or viral proteins). For these types of studies, we evaluated if the tests indicated a positive result with other members of the coronavirus family, such as SARS-CoV-1, Middle East respiratory syndrome coronavirus (MERS-CoV), and human coronavirus OC43(HCoV-OC43). Inactivated virus samples (HI and GIV) of SARS-CoV-1, MERS-CoV, and HCoV-OC43 were obtained from BEI Resources at known TCID50/ml concentrations. The virus samples were then diluted in saline and tested in a blinded fashion, with GIV SARS-CoV-2 samples mixed in the sample set. After testing was complete, the results were unblinded. A test "passed" when positive results were obtained only in samples containing SARS-CoV-2.

A few early tests were analyzed using a matrix containing a dye called phenol red, which is used to indicate changes in pH. We noticed that just the presence of the dye gave false-positive results in some tests, and such tests were either terminated or redesigned.

Tests analyzed at ACME POCT did not cross-react with the other coronaviruses previously listed. Although we were fortunate that most tests did not cross-react with other coronaviruses, a potential caveat was that the testing for cross-reactivity used inactivated samples. It is possible that potential cross-reactivity could be missed due to the lowered ability of tests to detect inactive virus because, in general, inactivated viruses are not detected as well as live viruses.

Sensitivity Studies

With the first appearance of the alpha variant in December 2020 and the subsequent rapid appearance of beta, gamma, delta, and other variants (termed variants of concern/variants of interest), there was increasing recognition that SARS-CoV-2 was capable of mutating rapidly. This led to two questions relevant to our testing strategy:

1. Could current tests work against new variants?
2. How sensitive were the tests against new variants (i.e. could they detect a new variant with the same sensitivity as the original strain)?

Many aspects of testing could not keep up with the rapid appearance of variants, including the pace needed for isolation of the virus from a clinical sample, laboratory propagation, TCID50/ml calculation, sequencing to ensure that new mutations were not introduced

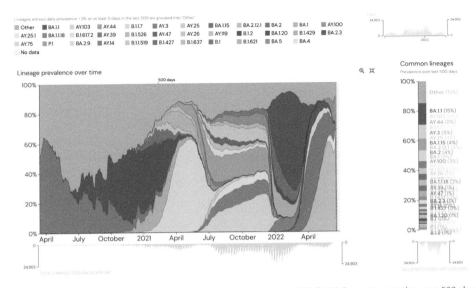

Figure 8.3 Graphical representation of the prevalence of various SARS-CoV-2 lineages over the past 500 days. Screenshot taken from https://outbreak.info/ on July 1, 2022.

during laboratory propagation, and testing every test with each new live variant. This is illustrated in Figure 8.3.

The recognition that SARS-CoV-2 was mutating and would continue to do so led us to search for alternatives to the use of laboratory-propagated samples in testing. Continuous ongoing testing of the tests was required and, as mentioned previously, most of this testing uses N protein-specific antibodies for virus detection. The continual mutation of SARS-CoV-2 always carries the possibility that the gene that produces the N protein of a current variant could mutate and generate an N protein that is sufficiently modified that it escapes detection by current tests. Such a situation would be problematic, as tests could miss positive cases and yield false-negative results. This could cause some people with active SARS-CoV-2 infections to not quarantine or get treatment and contribute to spread of the disease and its downstream consequences. With the appearance of the alpha variant in December 2020, it was decided that we would pivot our testing strategy toward the use of clinical samples for testing in addition to ongoing testing with live virus when needed.

In December 2020, the NIH established the VTF to address this new "variant phase" of the pandemic. The VTF comprises experts from a variety of areas and includes virologists and scientists from academic institutions, former executives with experience in device manufacturing and diagnostics, and staff from federal regulatory and health agencies. The two major goals of the VTF were to:

1. procure live and HI clinical samples for testing and establish a variant biorepository
2. develop protocols to use live and HI variant clinical samples in device testing

As regards the first goal, in consultation with large commercial diagnostic and university-based laboratories, the VTF established protocols and procedures for procuring leftover clinical samples that were positive for SARS-CoV-2 for use by ACME POCT. These laboratories were participants in the Centers for Disease Control and Prevention (CDC) genomic surveillance program, so a portion of all PCR-positive samples was sequenced, and this sequence information was made publicly available. This enabled ACME POCT to start building a biorepository of all currently circulating SARS-CoV-2 variants, with complete sequence information. The VTF met with several companies and universities to ensure that, in addition to them being willing to provide clinical samples to the RADx initiative, these institutions' samples met the quality end points required for the testing protocol. These quality end-point requirements included that:

- the diagnostic companies/university-based laboratories collected the swab (nasal, nasopharyngeal, or mid-turbinate) in at least 1–2 ml of buffer (saline or viral transport media) so that, after testing and sequencing were complete, there was at least 0.5 ml of sample remaining for transfer to ACME POCT
- samples were collected in buffers that preserved the antigen; for example, the collection medium Longhorn PrimeStore molecular transport media was acceptable for NAAT-based assays but not for antigen-based assays. We made this a requirement because we wanted to avoid building separate biorepositories for use with antigen-based versus NAAT-based assays
- companies had the capacity to store samples at –80 °C after testing and to ship the samples to ACME POCT on dry ice in a timely manner

After contacting numerous laboratories, three laboratories met all of these requirements. Material transfer agreements and other formalities were completed, and a variant biorepository was established at Emory University in December 2020. As of the writing of this chapter, whenever a new variant is discovered, we have an established protocol to obtain the samples needed for device testing.

In addition to the three laboratories based in the United States, we have procured SARS-CoV-2-positive samples from Brazil. It is important to establish procedures for international collaboration, as new variants that appear in the United States may have originated in other countries. Our long-term goal is to establish collaborations with laboratories worldwide so that we can build an international biorepository of clinical samples to evaluate the sensitivity of tests against emerging variants and new viruses.

As regards the second goal – to develop protocols to use live and HI variant clinical samples in device testing – after some trial and error, we devised the protocol outlined in Figure 8.4 for the use of variant samples in testing.

As shown in Figure 8.4, we first needed to make a sample pool using clinical samples comprising a specific variant. The creation of such a pool would enable us to have a stock of substrate that could be used for several tests. As the genome sequences of samples were known, we first analyzed sequences using the software Phylogenetic Assignments of Named Global Outbreak Lineages (PANGOLIN) to find samples that were identical in sequence for the N gene, because most tests are designed to recognize N2 (gene or protein) of SARS-CoV-2. Additionally, the cycle threshold (Ct) values of all samples were known. Ct is an indirect measurement of viral load. Real-time reverse transcription PCR is used to measure the amount of viral RNA in a sample, which is then used as a surrogate for the total amount of virus, assuming that the amounts of RNA and protein follow a linear relationship. In general, Ct values ≤ 24 are considered to be reflective of high viral loads, values of 25 to 30 are considered to be intermediate, and Ct values ≥ 30 are considered to be low viral load.

From the set of sequence-matched samples, we picked anywhere from 3 to 50 samples that had an N gene Ct value of < 24 (high viral load) and that had positive test results in one

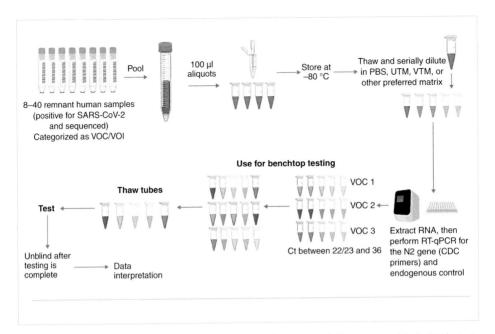

Figure 8.4 Pathway from remnant clinical samples to a blinded variant panel. All panels were blinded to the tester. Data were unblinded and interpreted after testing was complete.

Ct, cycle threshold; PBS, phosphate buffered saline; RT-qPCR, reverse transcription quantitative PCR; UTM, universal transport medium; VOC, variant of concern; VOI, variant of interest; VTM, viral transport medium.

or two Emergency Use Authorization (EUA) antigen tests, to obtain a sample pool of 5 to 20 ml. This pool, made up of low-Ct-value clinical samples, became our variant stock solution, of which we made 100 μl aliquots that were stored at –80 °C. When needed, one aliquot of stock was diluted (two-, five-, or 10-fold) in a pooled nasal wash (Lee Biosolutions) or test specific matrix that was first confirmed to produce a negative test result by ACME POCT internal quality control using N2 primers with the same sequences as those used by the CDC (CDC primers). This dilution series resulted in a panel of tubes, with each dilution differing from the previous by a Ct value of 1 (twofold dilution), 2 (fivefold dilution), or 3 (10-fold dilution).

Early in 2021, we were assessing the tests against anywhere from 9 to 11 variants at a time to ensure all circulating variants were equally detected. For antigen-based assays, we would make five tubes of each variant at fivefold dilutions with Ct values ranging from ~ 18 to ~ 30 for a total of 50 to 60 tubes comprising all circulating variants, including negative controls. A similar panel was created for NAAT-based assays but using 10-fold dilutions. All testing was done in a blinded manner, and results were decoded at the end of the experiment. Whenever possible, testing was done at ACME POCT. However, in the case of more complex assays for which specialized equipment was needed and unavailable on-site, blinded panels of samples for testing were shipped to the company that manufactured the assay.

The comparator at this stage was SARS-CoV-2 B.1.2, which had the closest sequence match to the original Wuhan strain. During sensitivity testing, every 3-Ct change represented a 10-fold difference, a 6-Ct change represented a 100-fold difference, and a 9-Ct change a 1 000-fold difference. If a test detected a variant within 3 Ct values of B.1.2, it was deemed to recognize the variant equivalently and was coded green. A Ct difference of > 3 to ≤ 6 was coded yellow, and a > 6-Ct difference was coded red. All variants that were coded yellow and red were tested further to eliminate any potential effects of pooling and dilutions. For further testing, we used individual patient samples whose Ct values were reassessed by our internal quality control to account for any viral load loss during storage, transport, and re-thawing. Therefore, every test got a "second chance" to pass variant testing. All testing was done in a blinded manner, and results were decoded at the end of the experiment. In Figure 8.5, we illustrate results from a test (Figure 8.5(a)) where all variants tested green and a test (Figure 8.5(b)) that had yellow and red results that were then tested further as described above.

Variant prevalence in the population was closely tracked. Testing at Emory University evolved to deal with the assault of variants during the pandemic. For example, when variants such as alpha, beta, and delta disappeared from circulation, we stopped assessing the tests against these variants. When new variants (BA.1, BA.2, BA.4, BA.5, etc.) arose, we began testing using these samples.

We started testing for only one variant at a time (e.g. delta, BA.1, BA.4, or BA.5 alone) when that variant became the dominant variant after outcompeting others, and then we refined our panel by using twofold dilutions of the low-Ct stock pool. This enabled us to get a better idea of test sensitivity. A twofold dilution series is what is currently being used, such that the panel starts at ~ 19 Ct and goes up to ~ 30 Ct. Table 8.2 shows a dilution series for the BA.1 variant and the results for seven antigen-based tests tested using the same dilution panel. Results from seven LFAs in which the same dilution series was used are also shown. Three vials of virus-negative nasal wash (1, 2, and 3) were included in the testing panel as blinded negative controls.

All testing was done in a blinded manner and, for every test, the direct swab method was used. In this method, 50 μL – or less if specified in the test's instructions for use – was spiked onto a swab and the instructions for use were followed. The use of a standardized test amount allowed us to compare between tests, which was especially important following the establishment of the ITAP, which was created to address the imminent need for high-quality LFAs in the USA. We were testing a vast number of LFAs at the same time and wanted to ensure that only high-quality LFAs were brought into the United States. The testing protocols in our laboratory were done in tandem with clinical field testing, so the question of how the test did in real users' hands was also answered simultaneously.

Lessons Learned from Variant and Sensitivity Studies and the Procurement of Remnant Clinical Samples

Several valuable lessons were learned from the previously discussed studies that involved both the approach to obtaining samples and the actual protocol for using those samples.

- It took a significant amount of time (two months in 2021) to procure the first lot of remnant clinical samples, with another two sources established a few months later. As these contacts are currently in place, it is crucial to not only maintain these relationships but also add new contacts moving forward so that, in the next pandemic, we can procure samples more quickly
- We are working to establish relationships with international laboratories, as we cannot predict where the next pandemic will begin

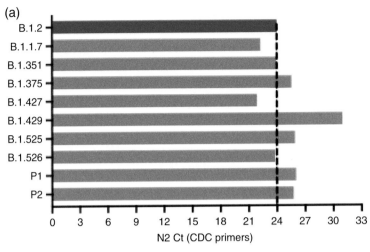

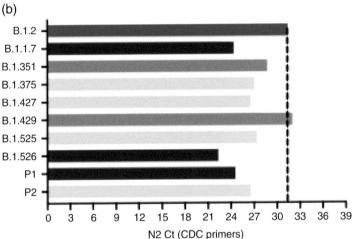

Figure 8.5 (a) Graphical representation of an antigen-based test that detected all variants to within 3 Ct values of B.1.2. (b) Graphical representation of an antigen-based test in which some variants were not detected within 3 Ct values of B.1.2. yellow (> 3 to ≤ 6-Ct difference) and red (> 6-Ct difference) results led to further analysis using individual patient samples of the variant.

- There would be significant public health benefits from an ongoing population surveillance effort to provide clinical samples from patients who present with upper respiratory illnesses across the country. These representative samples can be analyzed against the vast database of viruses currently on hand using sequencing and analysis software developed during this pandemic. Ongoing monitoring will help hospitals and health-care personnel potentially discover a new infection early and act before it becomes a pandemic. Constant vigilance is important
- A plan should be in place to sequence a higher percentage of positive samples from the beginning of the next pandemic and simultaneously study viral evolution. The spike protein gene dropout testing identified the alpha variant but raised the question of

Table 8.2 One-step Ct panel for testing the BA.1 variant: LFA, Ct, and negative nasal wash

BA.1 pool dilutions	Average N2 Ct (n = 9)	Standard deviation of N2 Ct (n = 9)	Percent positive at n = 5						
			LFA 1	LFA 2	LFA 3	LFA 4	LFA 5	LFA 6	LFA 7
Dilution 1	19.8	0.13	100	100	100	100	100	100	100
Dilution 2	20.8	0.13	100	100	100	100	100	100	100
Dilution 3	21.5	0.22	100	100	100	100	100	100	100
Dilution 4	22.7	0.07	100	100	100	100	100	100	100
Dilution 5	23.6	0.12	0	100	100	100	100	100	100
Dilution 6	24.0	0.23	0	60	100	100	100	100	100
Dilution 7	24.8	0.17	0	0	0	100	100	100	100
Dilution 8	25.8	0.07	0	0	0	0	0	0	100
Dilution 9	27.4	0.24	0	0	0	0	0	0	0
Dilution 10	28.1	0.20	0	0	0	0	0	0	0
Dilution 11	29.1	0.14	0	0	0	0	0	0	0
Negative nasal wash 1	0		0	0	0	0	0	0	0
Negative nasal wash 2	0		0	0	0	0	0	0	0
Negative nasal wash 3	0		0	0	0	0	0	0	0

whether we missed positive samples simply because we did not sequence them, and diagnostic PCR testing generated a false-negative result

- It is important to preserve the capacity to culture the virus from remnant clinical samples as we have done. This will enable specialized laboratories to have access to emerging viruses that may be relevant for the development of tests and new therapeutics

In addition to the need to rapidly procure new variant samples, there were additional reasons for using clinical samples instead of relying exclusively on live or inactivated laboratory-propagated virus.

- Several tests were already being sold in pharmacies and used at point-of-care locations. Testing technology had matured, and these tests had already been shown to readily detect SARS-CoV-2 in laboratory and clinical samples. The focus was shifting from evaluating the basic performance of these tests to quickly extending their use to encompass rapidly emerging variants
- Working with live, laboratory-propagated virus meant testing would be restricted to facilities with BSL3 laboratories. This was acceptable during the early development of tests; however, evaluation of the performance of mature test technology with rapidly emerging variants could be achieved more rapidly using clinical samples that could be safely handled in BSL2 laboratories using appropriate personal protective equipment (PPE)

Laboratory protocols are now well established to culture a virus from remnant clinical samples, to make viral stocks for LOD measurements, to make low-Ct pools using remnant clinical samples, and to use dilutions of these pools in a standard matrix for standardized methods of testing (the direct swab method, five replicates). All of these protocols will be published, and it is best to use these as a starting point in the event of the next pandemic.

A pipeline was also established to procure sequenced clinical samples from diagnostic laboratories for use in the verification of tests. The knowledge gained during this phase, the establishment of protocols and procedures to obtain biobanked clinical samples, and the ability to culture new SARS-CoV-2 variants circulating in the population proved to be essential for assessing the tests that came through due to the launch of the ITAP, which is described in the next section.

Use of SARS-CoV-2 Variant Samples for ITAP

By October 2021, the COVID-19 pandemic had already spanned 20 months, and the performance of tests for SARS-CoV-2 detection had improved significantly. However, tests were still not readily available or were expensive in the United States, making people hesitant to test regularly or at the first sign of symptoms. Particularly frustrating was the testing disparity versus other developed countries, where COVID-19 rapid tests were more widely available and either free or purchased at low cost.

To address this need, the RADx Tech initiative established ITAP, in which ACME POCT and contract research organizations would test over-the-counter tests (antigen-based LFAs) already available in overseas markets or under development in the United States. ACME POCT evaluated these tests and determined their LOD for SARS-CoV-2 variants to ensure that the tests met the US Food and Drug Administration (FDA) performance standards needed to be sold and/or distributed in the United States. These tests ultimately became part of the 1 billion COVID-19 tests bought by the United States government for distribution to every household.

An important component of ITAP was assessing the ability of tests to detect new variants of SARS-CoV-2 that were rapidly overtaking previously established variants. At Emory University, Dr. Ann Chahroudi's laboratory had established techniques to culture live SARS-CoV-2 from remnant clinical samples and used that approach to isolate the delta and the BA.1 and BA.2 omicron variants. These variants were propagated in Vero cells, sequenced, and used to generate aliquots with a known quantity of the virus (TCID50/ml). To enable testing in a BSL2 facility, aliquots of SARS-CoV-2 variants were heat inactivated and tested to confirm the loss of infectious virus but the detectable presence of viral RNA and protein. Inactivated virus was diluted to values of TCID50/ml of 10 000, 5 000, 400, 80, 16, and 3.2 and aliquoted into labeled, blinded tubes along with blinded control samples. These panels were then used for range-finding LOD studies, where these dilutions were tested using replicates of five to answer the following two questions.

How Do the Tests Perform against the Delta Variant When Compared with HI WT Virus?

Here we expected tests to perform at least as well as or within one to two TCID50/ml levels for the delta variant when compared with WT virus. For most of the tests that were tested as part of ITAP, WT virus and the delta variant performed similarly or within an acceptable range. Figure 8.6 is a graphical representation of an experiment comparing the LOD of HI WT virus against that of HI delta variant.

As ITAP continued, the delta variant disappeared and was replaced by the BA.1 omicron variant in the US population. We stopped comparing tests with the WT, as the WT (the original Wuhan SARS-CoV-2 variant) had essentially disappeared from most of the world's populations, and moved to testing ITAP LFAs with the delta variant only. As of the writing of this chapter, we are testing with laboratory-propagated BA.4, but we would be able to rapidly pivot toward testing new variants that emerge using "live" remnant clinical samples propagated in the laboratory.

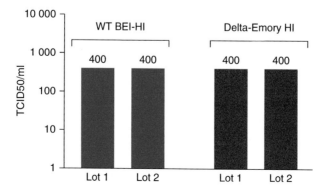

Figure 8.6 Comparison of HI WT from BEI Resources against HI delta variant with three common amino acid changes in the N protein (D63G, R203M, and D377Y).

Do the Tests Exhibit Significant Lot-to-Lot Variability?

Here we tested two different lots for each LFA analyzed in ITAP and found that most tests exhibited very little lot-to-lot variability. For those tests that did show lot-to-lot variability, the differences were within one TCID50/ml level. These results were reassuring, as millions of tests were being distributed, and a lot-to-lot variation would have been problematic.

Along with the use of non-inactivated, live remnant clinical samples, the use of laboratory-propagated virus had two advantages:

1. The use of laboratory-propagated virus ensured that we had a sufficient amount of the virus for a theoretically unlimited number of tests. After evaluating the performance of the initial 25 to 50 tests, additional HI virus pools for panels could be readily prepared from our viral stocks

2. We are constantly monitoring the Global Initiative on Sharing All Influenza Data (GISAID) for new SARS-CoV-2 sequence changes and we could use our banked remnant clinical samples to propagate new variants of interest to ensure that the most "relevant" mutations are being tested in the laboratory. Figure 8.6 illustrates how a specific strain of the delta variant was used in LOD range-finding studies. Since then, we have propagated BA.1 and other variants, which can be used for similar LOD range-finding studies

Documentation and Reporting of Laboratory Testing

A full written document with the following sections is given to each company that provides diagnostic tests for variant testing:

- **Background:** The background section includes a brief description of the current state of the pandemic, the current variant being analyzed, and its prevalence in the United States
- **Purpose of the study:** Each study must meet two goals. Goal (a): determine if the test can detect the variant being tested. Goal (b): determine the relative analytical sensitivity of the test for detecting the variant
- **Materials and methods**
  - **Creation of variant pool:** This section describes how the sample pool was created. The GSAID accession numbers for the samples that went into the pool are made available, as is an analysis of viral genetic sequences of each individual sample used for the pool. Fast-all (FASTA) files uploaded on the Nextclade software (https://clades.nextstrain.org/) and a pictorial representation of N gene mutations in the pool being analyzed are also provided. An aliquot of the pool is serially diluted in Lee Biosolutions negative nasal wash (catalog No. 991-26-P) to obtain a dilution series with a ~ 1 Ct step-wise change encompassing Ct values from ~ 18 to 30. $N2$ Ct values of final pool dilutions to be used for antigen assays, along with line data, are also provided. If genomic equivalent per ml is measured by droplet digital PCR, then that will be provided in the report as well
  - **Test method:** The protocol outlining the initial use/application of the samples has been standardized and follows the "direct swab" process described and accepted by the FDA for analytical testing of spiked/remnant samples. For swab-based assays, testing will follow the direct swab method where, using a graduated pipette, 50 µl is removed from the tube containing the sample solution and applied onto the swab

supplied with the kit, and then the sample swab is processed following the assay-specific instructions for use

- **Results:** A results table (Table 8.3) showing the Ct to which a test gave positive results at n = 5 will be provided, along with how the test's LFA did against two widely used LFAs. These two assays, denoted as assay 1 and assay 2 in Table 8.3, are used as "bookends." For an LFA to be deemed acceptable, it should fall within the bookends, meaning it should do at least as well as assay 1. Results are expressed as the percent positive, and the highest dilution of 100% positive (five out of five) is established as the test sensitivity for that specific pool. Results from bookend assay 1 (bookend test LFA 1) and assay 2 (bookend test LFA 2) are also shown in the table. Three vials of virus-negative nasal wash (1, 2, and 3) are included in the testing panel as blinded negative controls.

The ACME POCT verification core has implemented standardized methods of LOD testing and obtaining remnant clinical samples, established protocols to use these samples in assay development and testing, and established protocols to culture live virus from these samples. The development of these detailed protocols will accelerate laboratory testing in the next pandemic.

Table 8.3 Results from testing an LFA that yielded acceptable results using the FDA-approved direct swab method

Omicron (BA.2) live pool 1	Average N2 Ct	Percent positive		
		Bookend test LFA 1 (n = 5)	Bookend test LFA 2 (n = 5)	Test LFA (n = 5)
BA.2 dilution 1	19.4	100	100	100
BA.2 dilution 2	20.6	100	100	100
BA.2 dilution 3	21.6	100	100	100
BA.2 dilution 4	22.4	100	100	100
BA.2 dilution 5	23.3	100	100	100
BA.2 dilution 6	24.5	0	100	0
BA.2 dilution 7	25.6	0	100	0
BA.2 dilution 8	26.5	0	0	0
BA.2 dilution 9	27.7	0	0	0
BA.2 dilution 10	28.5	0	0	0
BA.2 dilution 11	29.4	0	0	0
BA.2 dilution 12	30.3	0	0	0
Negative nasal wash 1	0	0	0	0
Negative nasal wash 2	0	0	0	0
Negative nasal wash 3	0	0	0	0

Clinical Validation Core

The Clinical Validation Core of ACME POCT was tasked with collecting fresh SARS-CoV-2 samples for the devices we were evaluating. For over-the-counter device testing, we were able to enroll participants who self-collected and performed the test themselves when required. Clinical testing often came after laboratory verification was complete.

Academic and Health-Care Partnerships

When choosing to use an academic health center as a research site, conversations between academic institution leaders and health-care administrators are critical to setting up a Clinical Validation Core quickly and smoothly. In many situations, these are often separate entities (businesses) that will need to support and work together for the success of a Clinical Validation Core. Information sharing is the biggest hurdle. Participant recruitment from a health-care setting can be useful if the laboratory assay is compatible and the researchers are able to obtain laboratory results efficiently. One perk in this partnership is that the health-care entity will likely set up a testing site regardless of the need for research evaluation, will provide easy access to potential research participants, and can expedite the process and prevent duplication of effort. High-level involvement on both sides, including the participation of senior faculty, was found to bridge any gaps between academic and health-care partners and was valuable for expediting study progress. Regulatory protocols were streamlined, including Institutional Review Board (IRB) approvals. We had direct contact with the IRB and could modify our protocol or consents and receive approval quickly and on a designated schedule to prevent interruption in recruitment instead of having to wait sometimes weeks as is the case in typical clinical research projects.

Staffing and Training Clinical Sites

Securing recruitment sites will be integral to a successful future validation program. A semipermanent clinical site for testing will provide stability for staff and community completion of validation tests. There are various options, from hospital settings, inpatient units, and emergency departments to urgent care clinics and drive-through settings in the community. The list that follows summarizes these options and describes the patient profiles typical of each setting and the supplies and staffing requirements we found useful during the COVID-19 pandemic. Hospital and clinic settings may be faster to set up and require less equipment. Community settings will yield the highest recruitment, yet require the most infrastructure, staff, and set-up time.

The following are issues that should be considered when selecting validation sites:

- a connection to the electronic medical record (e.g. special network connections and internal approvals)
- the site's ability to accept symptomatic patients (e.g. proper PPE and barriers if needed)
- security and traffic control in drive-through settings
- electricity needs (e.g. label printing and refrigeration)
- workflow protocols for PPE, sample collection, labeling, storage, and transport
- a portable method of collecting participant data (e.g. tablets with Wi-Fi access)
- a secure, FDA-compliant research database
- supply storage (homebase versus satellite locations)
- one primary laboratory and a back-up laboratory for increased volume
- large drive-through tents with electricity for community settings

- a body of staff that includes a combination of research coordinators and research nurses for both adult and pediatric participants

Plan for Staff Burnout/Turnover

RADx Tech was continuously adapting to the evolving pandemic and required pivots and long hours that put a strain on our staff. This effort called for patience and understanding while being willing to learn and adapt on the job. We were all driven by the noble mission of helping the country. Despite this passion and dedication, we experienced staff turnover and burnout at all levels and constant recruitment was done to meet the ever-changing needs of the pandemic and to make sure that no time was lost onboarding specialized talent – an element that was so crucial for smooth operations. We made sure that we had talented and experienced personnel who were able to address key scientific and clinical challenges that arose as the pandemic continued to sweep through the country. Our organizational chart changed frequently throughout the project, but, in general, we had a chief operating officer who oversaw both laboratory and clinical activities, research faculty for various research questions and operations, program directors to handle the bigger pictures of managing couriers and handling issues that came up with laboratory results or participant complaints, and manager-level staff who handled onboarding and day-to-day staffing activities. We had administrative staff to order supplies, organize events, and handle purchasing and delivering.

Travel Outside the Atlanta Metropolitan Area

During times between surges, we scrambled for positive samples. We created a mobile unit of both staff and supplies that was able to travel outside the Atlanta, Georgia, metropolitan area. Securing locations in areas with high positivity was critical to our mission. This included staff positions, recreational vehicles and other forms of transportation, hotel stays and food for staff, and a faculty lead. This unit was activated when positivity rates dropped below ~ 4%. We combed data from surrounding counties and contacted health departments, churches, and other companies with testing sites and traveled to those communities to not only recruit for research samples but also to help, as these areas were often low on supplies and staff and were overwhelmed. Our most successful trip was in a small town two hours north of Atlanta where, within 10 days, we had set up a large testing site in an outdoor farmers market in the county seat. We tested ~ 600 people in five days. We learned a lot from this trip and were able to plan smarter, but this was only possible because we had the forethought to plan for these situations.

Defining Inclusion and Exclusion Parameters for Devices

Inclusion and exclusion parameters were largely decided based on the device requiring testing. Any person aged 2 years or older was eligible, and we banked specimens for both asymptomatic and symptomatic participants to start. Saliva-based testing or banked saliva samples were completed on those aged 8 years or older to ensure an adequate sample. In general, those participants with symptoms were included for biobanking within 14 days of symptom onset. For most devices, this was shortened to five to seven days depending on device preferences. The symptoms included were based on the current CDC guidelines at the time.

Data Collection and Reporting

Clinical Samples

Specimen types ranged from nasopharyngeal samples to buccal swabs and blood spots. By design, our IRB-approved protocol included every possible specimen type to prevent additional modifications requiring further IRB approval. The biobanking procedure (when a device was not currently being tested) included the comparator (most of the time this was a nasopharyngeal swab, but we did switch to a mid-turbinate swab once this was accepted by the FDA), anterior nares, mid-turbinate, oropharyngeal, and saliva. At times, buccal swabs, breath samples, blood spots, and plasma samples were also collected for various studies or devices. The need for symptomatic versus asymptomatic participants varied throughout the term of the study and was adjusted accordingly. Most of the biobanked samples went to companies requesting frozen samples for preliminary testing and for our own research questions, driven largely by the FDA. A pooling study was also conducted in the pediatric population, in which children were asked to self-swab and samples were pooled to determine the most efficient method of testing in schools and day care settings.

Clinical sample collection was standardized following current CDC guidelines for the specimen type in question. All biobanked samples were logged in a laboratory information management system and frozen at −80 °C. A Tableau dashboard was created to link the laboratory information management system and the REDCap system data together for data queries.

Database Organization

The database chosen for data collection should be compliant with Title 21 of the Code of Federal Regulations, Part 11, for all data that will be sent to the FDA. REDCap has this capability. Data collection should include all of the data required for FDA EUA applications. The RADx database went through many iterations as the pandemic unfolded. At the time of writing of this chapter, the database included the following forms and associated variables:

- **Inclusion/exclusion form:** This form included the participant's age group (pediatric versus adult), medical record number (if from a health-care setting), name, email address, date of birth, age range (to determine if there was a need for consent versus assent), date of screening, and enrollment location. The inclusion criteria questions were as follows: (1) Are you undergoing a COVID-19 test for clinical reasons OR have you previously tested for COVID-19 in the past seven days OR are you willing to undergo COVID-19 testing for research purposes? (2) Is the authorized individual willing to verbally consent? The exclusion criteria were as follows: (1) participation was not feasible due to the participant's medical status and (2) participation in another research study was felt to conflict with this study by the investigators. The form also included the name of the study staff conducting the interview and the language of consent (English or Spanish)
- **Study consent forms:** Assent and consent could both be given in English or Spanish. Once completed, the form triggered an automatic email to the participant that contained a PDF of the consent form signed.
- **Demographics and clinical characteristics:** This form included date of consent, sex at birth, race, ethnicity, city of residence, zip code, phone number, number of people living

in the household, symptoms in the last 14 days (checking all that apply per CDC guidelines), date of earliest symptom onset, whether or not they were currently symptomatic, the symptoms being experienced that day (checking all that apply from the same symptom list), medical conditions (checking all that apply – these ranged from hypertension to asthma and included other and none options), current smoking status, if they drank alcohol in general, if they used products that contain alcohol (e.g. mouthwash – this was for any breath or saliva collection), reason for testing, if they had tested positive previously (if yes, how many times, date of previous test, and type of COVID-19 test), and previous vaccines (if any) with dates

- **Sample collection and results:** This form included the date of visit, sample collected that day (checking all that apply), and if they had eaten or drunk anything within the last 15 minutes. Each specimen type selected had the following elements: date and time of collection, number of swabs collected, device name (if applicable), whether the participant was a known positive or naive, device serial number and lot number (if applicable), device result, date and time of result, and a free text comment section for each specimen collection and/or device

- **Experimental research results:** RADx had separate forms for results that were given to the participant (if they required a standard-of-care test from RADx) and those that were never given back to the participant. These included PCR results and Ct values for any specimen type other than a standard-of-care test, additional antigen testing, and virus sequencing data

- **Standard-of-care test:** RADx Tech implemented a two-part quality check system. The first form included the specimen type, the result, and a question about whether the participant needed PCR results. This question then triggered an additional form to be filled out by the clinical research coordinator (CRC), which then triggered an automatic email sent to two designated CRCs/nurses tasked with double-checking data entry. This follow-up form, once complete, then sent an automatic email to the participant tailored to a positive, a negative, or an indeterminate result with appropriate follow-up information. Located after this question was the laboratory location, assay system, date and time of comparator result, and Ct values. REDCap survey capabilities were used for this process

- **Protocol deviations and adverse events:** Each of these forms included the date and time of the event along with text boxes for descriptions and a drop-down section for whom the event was reported to and who reported it

- **Subject status:** This form was used to create a variable that could then be used to filter out those that had withdrawn or participants that may have started a record and decided not to finish the visit. Various reports were created for each device and each additional research question; a missing data report for quality checks prevented unenrolled participants from being included

- **Gift card distribution:** Each participant was entitled to reimbursement for their time. This form was filled out by an administrative assistant assigned to be the controller of gift card ordering and distribution. This form included the participant's name, email address, date of birth, phone number, and visit date, as well as the type of gift card, whether it was electronic or physical, the gift card number or URL, the compensation amount, the date sent, and a signature of the staff member. Once completed, this form triggered another email to the participant that thanked them for their service and/or included the electronic gift card link. Physical gift cards were rarely used because of tracking purposes, but, in some cases where the participant did not have an email address, the CRC gave a physical card and recorded the necessary information in REDCap

- **Additional forms:** There were a variety of additional forms that RADx at Emory University was responsible for managing. For example, some of the devices tested required usability questions to determine the subjective interpretation of instructions or usage of various devices either by the participant themselves or the CRCs
- **Server back-up procedure:** Emory University's REDCap system administrators have standardized procedures for regular backups of all of the research studies on the server. However, to ensure that study-specific backups were made on a regular basis for RADx, study database administrators adopted a policy whereby a full backup of the study would be made just prior to when any programming or structural changes were made to the database, or weekly if changes were not made

This process is done following the procedures detailed in the document entitled *SYS4 REDCap Database Backup as part of the Standard Operating Procedures for Clinical Trials* developed by the Biostatistics department in the Rollins School of Public Health at Emory University. These procedures require multiple methods of exporting various elements of the data and structure of the RADx database and saving the exported files to a secure and restricted department research drive maintained by the information technologies department at Rollins School of Public Health. Only RADx database administrators have access to the folder on the shared drive where these files are stored. The comprehensive nature of this backup methodology would enable re-creation of the study in any REDCap environment. While Part 11 compliance is recommended, RADx did not have this in place at the start. The backup procedures did not change between REDCap instances.

Lessons Learned

- Having a source of clinical patient-derived samples containing live virus would enable more effective testing for cross-reactivity during a future pandemic
- It is important to establish procedures for international collaboration, as new variants that appear in the United States may have originated in other countries
- Alleviating financial barriers with dedicated funding for hard-to-purchase items is important for the protection of staff and to prevent burnout and turnover – traditionally, federal grants have not allowed certain purchases, such as food/water and wearable items for staff; however, in the case of the pandemic, staff were working outside in extreme heat/cold for 8–10 hours a day, so these items were needed/justified but we were still not allowed to purchase these
- Operations should be simplified – a new site should be created only if absolutely necessary; instead, existing sites should be used
- Staff should be kept as happy as possible, but they should be prepared in advance for an ever-changing and learning environment
- Good relationships are required with those enterprises testing in your area; working partnerships will save time and money and yield high recruitment
- Temperature extremes at outdoor mobile sites should be considered. Refrigeration is needed for all sample types, and some devices may require ambient temperatures
- Although live virus testing has its limitations due to the requirements for a BSL3 facility and highly trained personnel, the maintenance of operational BSL3 facilities is key to

handling a future pandemic. Going forward, institutions (e.g. academic research laboratories) with operational BSL3 facilities should sustain and expand these facilities. This will ensure sufficient viral culture capabilities and facilitate the rapid pivot needed to counter any new emerging viral threats during the next pandemic

- As BSL2 laboratories are readily available and maintained in most academic institutions, it is imperative that these facilities are available for immediate use in the case of a new pandemic
- Established BSL3 laboratories should be maintained and the number of such laboratories should be expanded. Personnel should also be trained to work with infectious agents in these facilities
- Current relationships with diagnostic laboratories (commercial and academic) should be maintained so that samples can be obtained for clinical testing
- Ongoing genomic and global surveillance should be maintained to identify potential emerging infectious diseases
- A list of the key people who established protocols and testing during the current pandemic should be maintained, and a network among them encouraged, so that they can be called on in the future
- Despite several advantages, LOD testing in a laboratory setting is only one part of testing, and it is important to evaluate the performance of tests in clinical and hospital settings as well
- Ideally, testing in the laboratory and the ability to use both live and inactivated virus should be paired with coordination to safely collect and transport samples from the field, enabling a comprehensive approach
- A test may perform well and have an excellent LOD under ideal laboratory conditions but may fail as an in-clinic or at-home test. A test may also only perform moderately well in a BSL3 laboratory setting, and this information can be crucial for the manufacturer to redevelop the assay to ultimately yield a successful test. It should be noted that, in our experience, a test that completely fails BSL3 testing (failed to detect the virus or gave positive results with the matrix alone) is not able to successfully move forward in obtaining an FDA EUA

References

1. WHO, Listings of WHO's response to COVID-19 (June 29, 2020). www.who.int/news/item/29-06-2020-covidtimeline (accessed August 24, 2022).

Importance of Timely Sequencing, Tracking, and Surveillance of Emergent Variants

Jessica Lin, Morgan Greenleaf, Yang Lu, Leda Bassit, Cassandra Wesselman, and Anne Piantadosi

Introduction

Severe acute respiratory syndrome coronavirus 2 (SARS-CoV-2) variants were not a concern during the initial months of the pandemic, as virus evolution at that time was slow. However, in late 2020, the alpha and beta variants emerged (Figure 9.1; see also Table 9.1) and drew attention not only because they were genetically different from the original virus, but also because they were associated with higher transmission and more severe disease, respectively. Their emergence set into motion a massive expansion of SARS-CoV-2 genomic surveillance in the United States, allowing us to be better prepared for subsequent variant evolution. This chapter focuses on understanding the public health consequences of and the response to SARS-CoV-2 variants, but this requires a brief review of a few essential concepts. First, we review virus mutations and evolution to explain how variants arise. Then, we review viral genome sequencing and analysis to explain how variants are discovered and classified.

SARS-CoV-2 Genome Surveillance

Since its emergence, SARS-CoV-2 has been evolving, and scientists have been tracking its evolution for just as long. The evolution of SARS-CoV-2 has repeatedly given rise to new variants (viruses with different sets of mutations), which has presented challenges as regards testing, treatment, and mitigation throughout the pandemic (Figure 9.2). In this chapter, we introduce SARS-CoV-2 variants, describe the unprecedented accomplishments in viral genome sequencing that have allowed us to monitor variants, and discuss the role that the Rapid Acceleration of Diagnostics (RADx®) Variant Task Force (VTF) played in rapidly evaluating diagnostic tests for variants. We use the term "variants" to refer to the World Health Organization (WHO) definitions of variants of concern (VOCs) and variants of interest (VOIs).[1]

In Figure 9.2, the x-axis shows time. The y-axis shows the number of samples sequenced (below the axis) and the prevalence of each variant (above the axis).[1-7] Table 9.1 shows a summary of the VOCs that emerged from January 2020 to December 2022.

SARS-CoV-2 Mutation, Natural Selection, and Evolution

Mutations are a natural by-product of virus replication. As a ribonucleic acid (RNA) virus, SARS-CoV-2 makes copies of its RNA genome using a specific enzyme: RNA-dependent RNA polymerase (RDRP). Viral RDRPs are prone to making errors when copying the viral genome, such as incorporating the incorrect nucleotide (A, C, G, or U). This results in a type of mutation known as a single nucleotide polymorphism (SNP). Other types of mutations

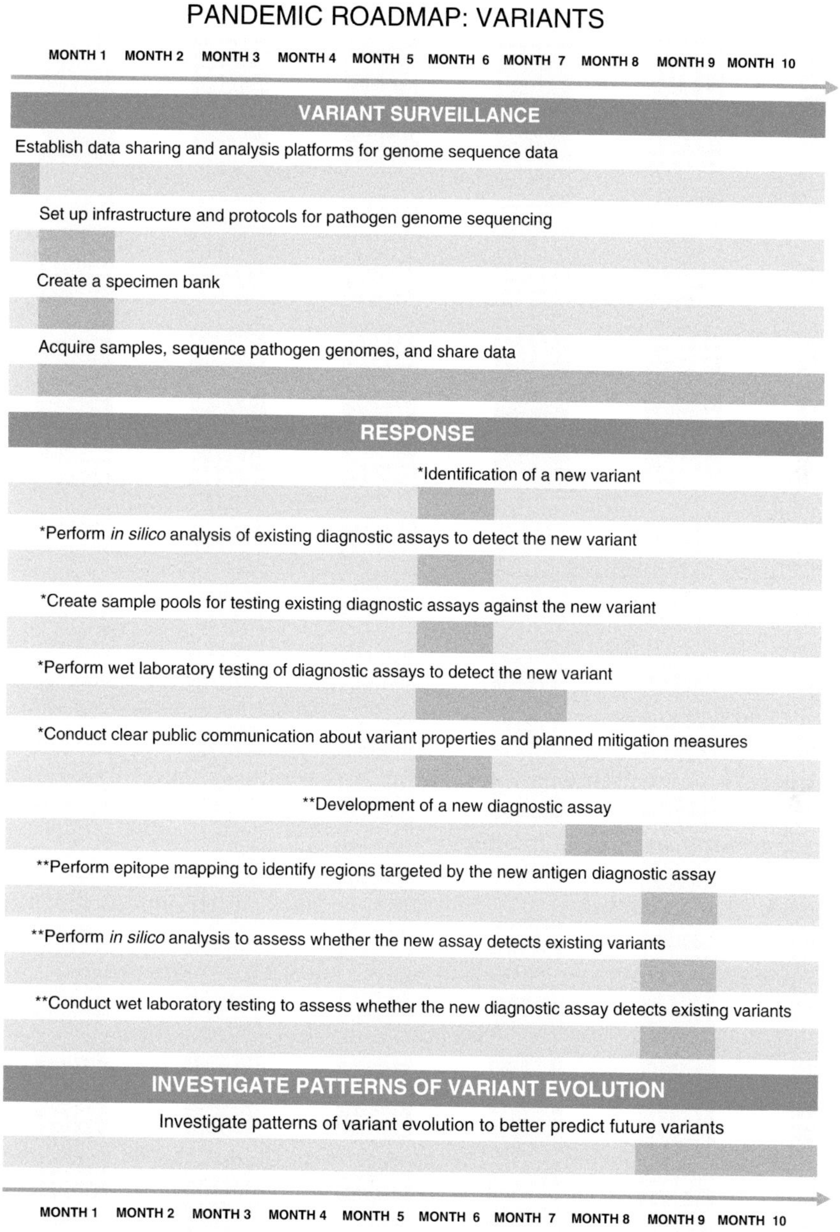

Figure 9.1 This roadmap depicts the vital activities, their chronology, and an estimated time frame in months. In the case of the SARS-CoV-2 pandemic, month 1 was December 2019, the month in which the virus was isolated, sequenced, identified, and published.

This roadmap accounts for two events that are expected to happen repeatedly throughout a pandemic but with uncertain timing: * the emergence of a new variant and ** the development of a new diagnostic assay.

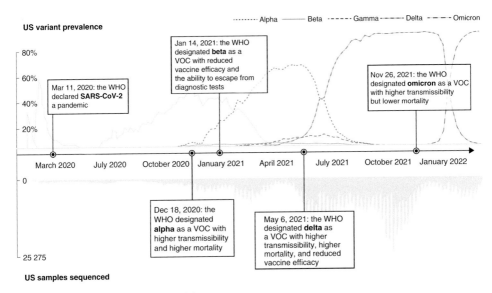

Figure 9.2 Emergence of SARS-CoV-2 VOCs.

can also occur, including (1) deletions, in which part of the parent RNA genome is "skipped," and (2) insertions, in which extra RNA is added. In experimental studies, the SARS-CoV-2 genome accumulates one SNP approximately every 10 replication cycles, which is similar to other coronaviruses, but up to 1 000 times slower than some other RNA viruses.[8] Nevertheless, because of the high rate of virus replication, many mutations may occur over the course of an infection.

The process of evolution requires both mutation and natural selection. Some mutations may impede virus survival and replication; these are called deleterious mutations and are eliminated by natural selection. Other mutations can be neutral; they may or may not persist based on chance in a process known as genetic drift. Relatively few mutations are beneficial to the survival of the virus; these mutations can increase in an infected individual and/or population due to positive selection. When SARS-CoV-2 evolution is monitored by sequencing samples from infected people, we observe the results of a complex interplay between mutation, selection, and drift. All of these processes together result in the accumulation of one SARS-CoV-2 mutation approximately every two weeks at population level.[9] Although technically there is no definition of the number of mutations that is required to call something a new variant, most variants have dozens of mutations compared with the original SARS-CoV-2 virus that emerged in 2019.

Laboratory and Analysis Methods for SARS-CoV-2 Genome Sequencing

One of the key early developments in the pandemic was the quick sequencing and publication of the entire SARS-CoV-2 genome. On January 11, 2020, barely a month after the first patients were reported, researchers from China published the SARS-CoV-2 genome on an open-access website (https://virological.org/).[10–12] This initial sequence allowed scientists to

Table 9.1 Summary of SARS-CoV-2 variants: January 2020 to December 2022

WHO designation	Pango* nomenclature	Month when first identified	Nucleocapsid protein mutations
N/A (original virus)	B.1.2	December 2021	D377Y, P67S, P199L
Alpha	B.1.1.7	December 2020	R203 K, G204 R, D3X, S235F
Gamma	P.1	December 2020	R203 K, G204 R
Zeta	P.2	April 2020	R203 K, G204 R, M231I, A119S
Beta	P.1.351	January 2021	T205I
	B.1.375	September 2020	T205I, L139F
Epsilon	B.1.427	June 2020	T205I
	B.1.429	June 2020	T205I, M234I
Eta	B.1.525	November 2020	T205I, A12G, S2Y, D3del
Iota	B.1.526	November 2020	M1X, M234I, P199L
Lambda	C.36	June 2021	P13L, R203 K, G204 R, G214C, T366I
Mu	B.1.621	December 2020	T205I
Delta	B.1.617.2	December 2020	D63G, R203 M, G215C, D377Y
Omicron	BA.1	November 2021	P13L, E21del, R32del, S33del, R203 K, G204 R, D343G
	BA.2	November 2021	P13L, E21del, R32del, S33del, R203 K, G204 R, S413 R
	BA.4	January 2022	P13L, G30G, E21del, R32del, S33del, S413 R, P151S
	BA.5	February 2022	P13L, G30G, E21del, R32del, S33del, S413 R
	BQ.1	July 2022	P13L, R203 K, E136D, G204 R, del31/33 S413 R

* Pango: Phylogenetic Assignment of Named Global Outbreak Lineages.

quickly develop polymerase chain reaction (PCR)-based diagnostic tests, track disease spread and evolution, and start to develop SARS-CoV-2 vaccines.

Detection of mutations and variants relies on sequencing SARS-CoV-2 from clinical samples. In the laboratory, RNA is extracted and turned into sequencing libraries (Figure 9.3), which are strands of nucleic acid that can be read by a sequencing machine. Sequencing libraries are usually made by converting RNA into complementary DNA (cDNA), which is broken into fragments before amplifying and adding specific adapters to the fragmented cDNA for reading by the sequencing machine. Sequencing machines provide output in the form of reads, which are strings of nucleotides (A, T, C, and G) corresponding to the genetic sequences of the input libraries. The time required for SARS-CoV-2 sequencing

Process patient samples for molecular tests

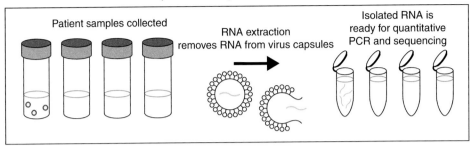

RT-PCR for COVID-19 diagnosis

Sequence positive samples

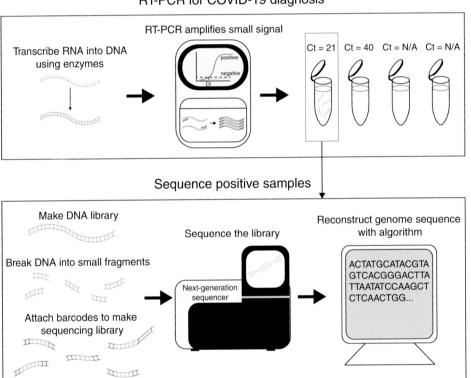

Figure 9.3 Patient sample processing for molecular diagnostic tests and genomic sequencing.
Ct, cycle threshold; RT-PCR, reverse transcription PCR.

can range from one to three days, and the cost is less than $100 per sample (not including personnel and overhead costs).[13]

Most SARS-CoV-2 genome sequencing is performed with techniques that generate short reads (150–500 base pairs), but some techniques can generate long reads (up to 10 000 base pairs). Sequencing can be performed using a targeted approach, which uses specific primers to sequence the virus of interest, or an unbiased approach (also called metagenomic or "shotgun" sequencing), which sequences all of the nucleic acids present in a sample and can be useful in identifying and sequencing new viruses.

Sequencing reads are grouped by sample, checked for quality, and assembled into a complete genome sequence. The consensus sequence of a sample reflects the most common nucleotide at each position, and this is used for most reporting and analysis.

Because of the high mutation rate of RNA viruses, a sample from one individual may contain many viruses, some of which are slightly different from the others. If needed, deep sequencing and analysis of minor variants can be used to investigate within-sample variation.

Analysis of SARS-CoV-2 Sequences

Consensus sequences from different samples can be compared with one another through alignment, in which each position in the genome is represented along a common x-axis, allowing direct comparison of the nucleotides and/or amino acids in each sample. A common reference, the initial Wuhan-Hu-1 strain in the case of SARS-CoV-2, allows all samples to be compared with the same initial sequence.[14]

Alignment allows for easy identification of SNPs, deletions, and insertions. It is also frequently used to determine in which gene a mutation occurs and whether an SNP is non-synonymous (resulting in an amino acid change) or synonymous (not changing the amino acid or protein). Sequences are compared to observe the accumulation of mutations and to discover new variants.

In addition to examining specific mutations, it can be informative to study the evolutionary history of a group of sequences using a phylogenetic tree. When reading a phylogenetic tree, the horizontal distance between sequences (x-axis) reflects how closely related the sequences are. Closely related sequences form a cluster on the tree, and the ancestor of a cluster contains the set of mutations shared by sequences in that cluster. For SARS-CoV-2, large clusters are defined as lineages, and lineages with important biological properties may be defined as VOCs. Figure 9.4 shows a phylogenetic tree representing the evolutionary history of SARS-CoV-2 variants.

SARS-CoV-2 Variants

Databases and Initiatives for SARS-CoV-2 Genomic Surveillance

When researchers sequenced the initial SARS-CoV-2 genome in January 2020, they were able to immediately upload the sequence to several existing, publicly available, databases, including GenBank and the GISAID database.

These databases were crucial for the surveillance and tracking of virus evolution in real time. The National Institutes of Health (NIH) National Center for Biotechnology Information (NCBI) maintains several resources that allow researchers to submit and access data freely. For example, GenBank is a database of publicly available genome sequences that are frequently annotated and linked with metadata.[16, 17] The Sequence Read Archive is a repository for raw sequence data, which is important in monitoring data quality and integrity. The NCBI developed modules specific to SARS-CoV-2, facilitating rapid data deposition and retrieval.[18]

Launched in 2008 along with its EpiFlu™ database, GISAID is an independent, nonprofit organization to facilitate the transparent and timely sharing of data – including sequence

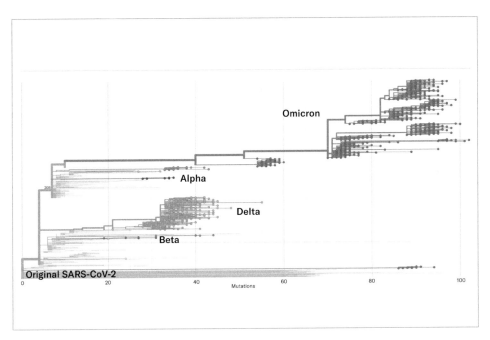

Figure 9.4 Phylogenetic tree of SARS-CoV-2 variants. SARS-CoV-2 variants were visualized using the Nextstrain dashboard and data from the Global Initiative on Sharing All Influenza Data (GISAID).[15]

data and clinical and epidemiological data – to monitor and guide responses to disease outbreaks.[19] Because of GISAID's previous experience with influenza data sharing, it was able to quickly respond to the new viral pandemic, creating a new SARS-CoV-2 database: EpiCoV.

As the virus spread to different countries, many institutions began to sequence SARS-CoV-2 from patient samples and upload the sequences to these databases. In the United Kingdom, various academic and public health institutions came together in April 2020 to form the COVID-19 Genomics UK (COG-UK) Consortium, which aimed to sequence SARS-CoV-2 viral genomes for monitoring disease outbreaks and variants.[20] By April 2021, a year after the establishment of COG-UK, the United Kingdom had shared over 379 000 sequences; by 2022, that number was over 2 million.[21, 22] In May 2020, the US Centers for Disease Control and Prevention (CDC) established the SARS-CoV-2 Sequencing for Public Health Emergency Response, Epidemiology, and Surveillance (SPHERES) consortium to expand and coordinate SARS-CoV-2 genomic surveillance.[23, 24] SPHERES grew from the CDC's Advanced Molecular Detection program, which had previously been established to build genomics capacity in public health laboratories throughout the United States. Through SPHERES, the CDC brought together public health laboratories, academic groups, and biotechnology companies that were performing large-scale SARS-CoV-2 testing and thus were well positioned to begin sequencing. The CDC's genomic surveillance response included funding mechanisms, communication and discussion around best practices, and an online COVID Data Tracker.[25] In other parts of the world, regional coalitions were created for the same purposes, such as the Network for Genomic Surveillance in South Africa and the COVID-19 Genomic Surveillance Regional Network established by the Pan American Health Organization for sharing sequence data in Latin American and Caribbean countries.[26–28]

In addition to collecting SARS-CoV-2 data, these organizations also provided support to researchers and clinicians in standardizing sequencing protocols, accessing sequencing facilities, and analyzing the sequence data they obtained. The GISAID data sharing agreement, which gives appropriate credit to those who upload data, also encouraged many researchers, particularly those from less developed countries, to upload data without fear of having their data used without credit.

Thanks to these efforts, by the end of the first pandemic year, over 1.2 million SARS-CoV-2 genomes had been sequenced worldwide.[22] In comparison, the EpiFlu database accumulated just over 170 000 influenza sequences in the eight years between its launch in 2008 and 2016.[29] This enormous quantity of SARS-CoV-2 sequence data allowed virus evolution to be tracked in real time at a scale not seen before.

Because of this unprecedented quantity of data, advances in computational and bioinformatics tools were necessary to categorize and analyze the sequences. One major platform that provides bioinformatic tools to help visualize genetic differences of viral sequences is Nextstrain, an open-source platform that provides code, data curation, and an interactive visualization dashboard (see Figure 9.4).[15] Early in the pandemic, Nextstrain quickly developed a bioinformatics pipeline to analyze SARS-CoV-2 genome data from databases such as GenBank and that of GISAID. Its visualization tools and accessibility allowed researchers and clinicians without extensive bioinformatics experience to analyze and visualize the large quantity of sequencing data being generated and to make decisions based on the analyses.

As another example, https://outbreak.info/ from Scripps Research offers a suite of reports and tools based on SARS-CoV-2 genomic data from GISAID.[30] The lineage and mutation trackers on https://outbreak.info/ provide customizable reports of frequency over time and by location for specific lineages and mutations. The lineage comparison tool allows the comparison of mutation frequencies between lineages. Searches for specific mutations and lineages are linked with relevant publications to facilitate the exploration of genotype–phenotype correlations.

Pre-variant Context

In the initial stages of the pandemic, the possibility of new variants was not a major concern, in part because of the slow mutation rate of coronaviruses generally, which is attributable to an enzyme they carry to "proofread" their genome as it is replicated.[8, 31] Other issues were prioritized during the early pandemic, such as the supply of N95 masks, disposable gowns, gloves, respirators, and other personal protective equipment for hospitals, health-care staff, and patients. There was an urgent need for real-time PCR machines in hospitals, for Clinical Laboratory Improvement Amendments (CLIA)-certified laboratories, and for reagents for molecular COVID-19 diagnostic testing. In addition, the disease severity and mode(s) of transmission of COVID-19 were not well understood and drew most of the research focus.

Initially, genetic drift – that is, small random mutations in the SARS-CoV-2 genome – were used primarily for molecular or genomic epidemiology, namely the practice of using genomic data to understand disease transmission dynamics. This allowed researchers and public health officials to trace the mechanisms of COVID-19 spread, both locally and globally.[32–35]

The first variant of SARS-CoV-2 that showed evidence of having effects on virus transmission was detected as early as February 2020, when the D614G mutation was found in patient samples in Europe and the Americas. This mutation, in which an aspartic acid is replaced by glycine in the SARS-CoV-2 spike protein, was associated with higher viral loads and increased transmission of the virus, although it did not appear to increase disease severity.[36–39] Because of this increased transmission, by May 2020, the D614G variant comprised the majority of global cases. Despite these properties and the initial concern, the D614G variant was ultimately a minor player in the variant narrative, as it would soon be overshadowed by additional variants.

Growing Public Awareness of Variants

The first variants to enter wider public awareness were detected in the United Kingdom (B.1.1.7) and South Africa (B.1.351) in late 2020, later named the alpha and beta variants, respectively. The alpha variant, which first emerged in the United Kingdom around September 2020, had 17 mutations, 8 of which were present on the spike protein. This variant showed evidence of increased infectivity (a 43–90% increase in transmission) compared with previous variants and outcompeted other variants to become the dominant strain in the United Kingdom by January 2021.[40, 41] Around the same time, the beta variant and the gamma variant (P.1), with the latter first detected in Brazil, also showed increased transmissibility and some evidence of immune escape.[42–45] The alpha, beta, and gamma variants brought the topic of variants into the public eye and sparked debate about the potential effects of variants on therapeutic, diagnostic, and preventive measures.

All of the variants contained mutations in the spike protein, which was the main target for many of the approved vaccines that were just beginning to roll out. In addition, all of these variants showed some ability to avoid the immune response against the original SARS-CoV-2 virus and, in some cases, against vaccine-elicited immunity.[41–46] Researchers and the public alike feared that vaccines developed against the original Wuhan strain might not be effective against these new variants.

Diagnostic tests, which were largely based on the original Wuhan sequence of the virus, were also affected by the mutations. The US Food and Drug Administration (FDA) identified tests that would potentially have a reduced performance due to mutations, including the Meridian Bioscience Revogene SARS-CoV-2 assay, the Applied DNA Science Linea COVID-19 Assay Kit, the Tide Laboratories DTPM COVID-19 Reverse Transcription (RT)-PCR Test, the Accula SARS-CoV-2 Test, TaqPath COVID-19 Combo Kit, and the Xpert Xpress SARS-CoV-2 test.[47] Some of these manufacturers have since modified their products and they no longer exhibit mutation deficiencies. The alpha variant could be differentiated from previous variants using some reverse transcription (RT)-PCR tests, as it caused PCR markers of the nucleocapsid (N) gene and spike (S) gene to drop out or lose signal.[48, 49] This raised concerns about the detectability of potential future variants with even more mutations.

Another fear – increased disease severity – was realized by a VOC that gained traction in May 2021. The delta variant, first detected in India, quickly took hold to become the dominant variant globally. In addition to even higher transmissibility and immune evasion, which drove a wave of COVID-19 cases in the USA and worldwide, the delta variant also showed signs of causing more severe disease and increased hospitalization compared with previous variants.[50–52] This contradicted a common public opinion that the virus would evolve to be less virulent.

The rollout of vaccines and increasing immunity from prior infections created additional selective pressure for the virus, and later variants showed a marked increase in immune escape. The omicron variant, which was first reported in South Africa in November 2021, was declared a VOC by the WHO due to the highest number of mutations (approximately 55) from the original strain, including more than 30 mutations in the S protein.[53, 54] The omicron variant showed a slightly higher increase in transmissibility than the delta variant, but a decrease in disease severity.[55–57] The most marked change was in omicron's ability to evade immunity from both previous infections and vaccines. Omicron showed resistance to neutralization by the sera of vaccinated and previously infected patients, as well as by many of the monoclonal antibodies developed as therapeutics against COVID-19.[54, 58, 59] This immune evasion led to a surge of reinfections and prompted vaccine updates.[60–62]

The emergence of variants has been rapid, with several VOCs emerging and disappearing in merely two years, each with distinct genetic and phenotypic characteristics. Real-time detection and characterization of these variants have been crucial to shaping the public health response and will likely continue to play a large role in the response to this pandemic and future pandemics.

Variant Names and Nomenclature

With the rapidly increasing number of SARS-CoV-2 genomes available in public databases, researchers needed a way to discuss the different variants. Thus, in the initial months of the pandemic, three major naming conventions were established:[63]

1. The GISAID naming convention groups genomes into high-level phylogenetic clades based on mutations but does not take into consideration the biological significance of the mutations.[64] Thus, despite the prominence of the GISAID database, this naming convention is rarely used
2. Nextstrain proposed a nomenclature based on global prevalence and phylogenetic characteristics that assigns each major clade an alphanumeric code based on the year and order in which the clades appeared. Additional updates to the naming criteria allowed researchers to account for regional differences in variant prevalence, public health designations, and the rise of less genetically distinct subvariants[65–67]
3. The Pango nomenclature groups virus genomes into lineages, which are given alphanumeric codes consisting of a letter followed by up to three numbers (such as B.1.1.529 for the omicron variant).[68] Lineages are designated based on periodic assessment of circulating variants, a feature that allows for prioritization and discussion of the most significant variants at any given time[69]

Although these nomenclature systems facilitated scientific discussion of the virus, the increase in public awareness of variants meant that members of the public and the media were paying close attention to the research. By early 2021, it became clear that the existence of multiple naming conventions, as well as the complex alphanumeric codes used in each, were confusing to the public. Many news sources began referring to the dominant variants by names based on the location where they were first discovered, such as "the UK variant" and "the South Africa variant." This led to stigma and sometimes political retaliation against the countries in the form of travel bans.

To remedy this, the WHO announced a new naming convention. In February 2021, although the WHO had previously provided working definitions of VOCs and VOIs based on phenotype and public health significance, it had not given any official names to the existing variants.[70, 71] After consultation with experts, at the end of March 2021, the WHO announced that it would assign names based on the Greek alphabet to the various VOCs and VOIs. Under this naming convention, the B.1.1.7 variant identified in the United Kingdom was designated the alpha variant and the B.1.351 variant discovered in South Africa was designated the beta variant.[72]

Because of the global nature of the pandemic, there were differences in local variant prevalence, and many countries had their own criteria for designating VOCs and VOIs. In the USA, the government established the SARS-CoV-2 Interagency Group, which meets regularly and classifies variants as VOCs, VOIs, or variants being monitored (VBMs) based on their transmissibility, severity, immune escape, and prevalence in the USA.[73] The FDA has also set a threshold for closer monitoring of emerging variants, namely those variants that are present in more than 5% of samples sequenced.[74]

Impact of Variants on Molecular Diagnostic Tests

As SARS-CoV-2 continues to accumulate mutations compared with the original sequence, molecular diagnostic tests based on the original SARS-CoV-2 sequence are more likely to miss new variants. This can lead to an increase in false-negative tests and can potentially interfere with efforts to control the spread of COVID-19.

Most of the available molecular diagnostic tests are based on RT-PCR technology, which uses specific primers to amplify one or more regions of the SARS-CoV-2 genome. Targets for RT-PCR diagnostic tests can be located across different genes, and many tests include two or three targets, usually genes that encode important structural proteins of SARS-CoV-2. When mutations arise in a specific target region, a test may give false-negative results or partially false-negative results if mutations affect only one of multiple targets. A prominent example of this is S gene target failure (SGTF), in which a six-nucleotide deletion leads to the loss of the S gene PCR signal but not the N gene or ORF1ab signals for widely used assays such as the TaqPath COVID-19 PCR (ThermoFisher). This six-nucleotide deletion was first present in the alpha variant, and monitoring SGTF proved to be an accurate mechanism for monitoring the emergence of this variant.[48, 49, 75] The delta variant did not contain the six-nucleotide deletion and thus did not exhibit SGTF, although there was some decrease in signal for the N gene target.[76] The omicron variant also contained the six-nucleotide deletion leading to SGTF, again allowing a mechanism to monitor the rise of the omicron variant without decreasing the diagnostic power of the tests.[75]

In February 2021, the FDA published guidelines for evaluating molecular diagnostic tests against emerging variants, listing several recommendations to mitigate the impact of variants on molecular diagnostic tests.[74] Molecular diagnostic tests with multiple targets are more robust than single-target tests and are less likely to fail with new variants. In addition, choosing targets in more highly conserved areas of the genome may decrease the chance of false negatives for new variants. There is also a need for continuous monitoring of circulating variants and routine updates of tests if new mutations begin to cause issues, particularly with the rapid mutation of the virus.

Although issues with molecular tests are easy to predict from variant genome sequences, the impact of new variants on antigen diagnostic tests is more difficult to foresee, and evaluation methods are discussed in the next section.

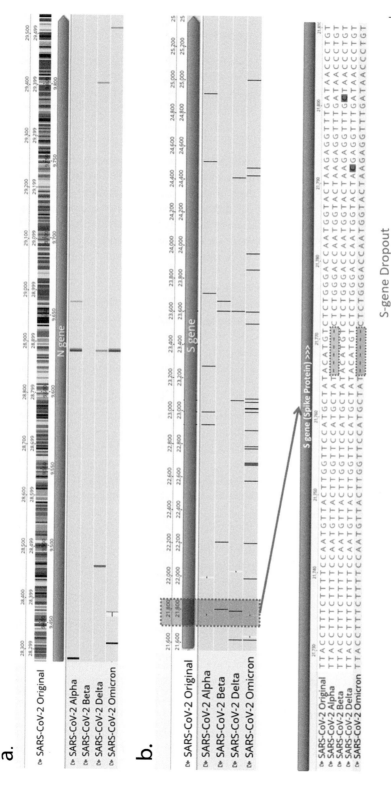

Figure 9.5 Alignment of the SARS-CoV-2 N protein and part of the S gene. Panel (a) shows amino acid mutations and deletions in the N protein compared with Wuhan-Hu-1. Panel (b) shows nucleotide changes in the S gene and a close-up of SGTF.

Impact of Variants on Antigen Diagnostic Tests

To date, one antigen test has suffered performance degradation from a specific variant mutation. The Quidel Sofia SARS Antigen FIA test was unable to detect variants with the N: D399N mutation found in a small percentage of B.1.429 variants.[77] This "miss" was confirmed by the RADx Tech VTF with laboratory methods described in the "RADx VTF" section.

Subvariants

Throughout 2022, the omicron variant remained dominant. Several subvariants of omicron – BA.2, BA.3, BA.4, and BA.5 – surfaced during the summer and fall of 2022 and carried additional mutations that differentiated them from the original omicron strain (BA.1).[78] These subvariants did not have enough genetic differences to be classified as a separate variant, yet they showed clear phenotypical differences in their higher transmission rates (BA.2) and immune evasion (BA.4 and BA.5).[79–81] The immune escape for BA.4 and BA.5 is much greater than for previous variants, and these two strains show the ability to escape from immunity elicited by BA.1 and BA.2.[82]

In response to the decreased efficacy of vaccines to prevent COVID-19 infection, the FDA announced a planned update to messenger RNA (mRNA) COVID-19 vaccines to protect against BA.4 and BA.5.[61] However, even as the public health response tried to keep up, the virus continued to evolve. In the fall of 2022, two additional variants, BQ.1 and BQ.1.1, began to circulate widely and threatened to cause another wave of COVID-19 in the United States.[83] These variants show resistance to neutralizing antibodies, increased transmissibility, and potential immune escape.[84–86]

Fortunately, bivalent vaccine boosters that contain mRNA to protect against both the original SARS-CoV-2 strain and the BA.5 omicron variant have shown improved efficacy against these newly emerged omicron variants compared with the original formula.[87–89] However, the threat of continued evolution and immune escape of SARS-CoV-2 remains.

Only time can tell where the next major variant will originate, what properties it will have, and if we will be able to predict it and rapidly respond. The emergence of variants has highlighted the importance of global collaboration in the real-time genomic tracking of pandemics, but the story is far from over.

RADx VTF

The RADx VTF is focused on assessing the effectiveness of RADx technologies against variants. It is an interdisciplinary group comprising federal agencies, diagnostic device manufacturers, private and public bioinformatics companies and organizations, large laboratory organizations, and academic institutions (Figure 9.6).

This group was initially started and led by Richard Creager, Ph.D., and Eric Lai, Ph.D., with three goals:

1. testing assays of concern as identified by the FDA
2. providing go/no-go decision points for RADx-supported assays requesting clinical trial support
3. testing all RADx companies against known VOCs

At its core, the RADx VTF was charged with ensuring that diagnostic assays supported by RADx could reliably and effectively detect SARS-CoV-2 variants and mutations in a quickly changing virus. It is worth reemphasizing that the creation of the RADx VTF would not have

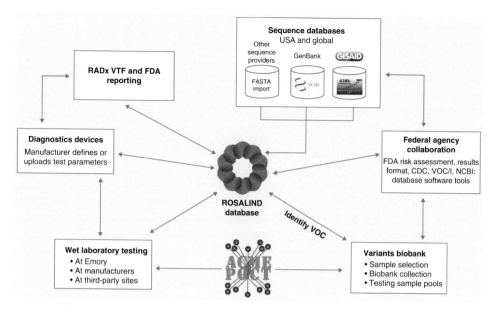

Figure 9.6 RADx VTF organization and collaboration.

been possible without rapid and flexible funding for surveillance and the collection of variant samples, the execution of testing, the reporting of results, and administration of the program.

In February 2021, the FDA issued the *Policy for Evaluating Impact of Viral Mutations on COVID-19 Tests: Guidance for Test Developers and Food and Drug Administration Staff.*[74] Since mutations in the viral genome can affect the hybridization of test reagents with SARS-CoV-2, this report recommended evaluating hybridization changes using an *in silico* analysis to identify a mutation expected to result in a mismatch (or mismatches) within the target primer/probe binding site(s) of the SARS-CoV-2 diagnostic test.

The report suggested that investigations of the impact of hybridization should be done in three stages, each providing a more accurate evaluation of test performance than the last:

1. *in silico* calculation
2. wet testing of genomic material
3. wet testing of virus isolates with a mutation

This guidance was applicable to nucleic acid amplification tests (NAATs), antigen tests that detect SARS-CoV-2, and serology tests that detect antibodies to SARS-CoV-2.

ROSALIND Diagnostic Monitoring System

In collaboration with ROSALIND (www.rosalind.bio), the RADx VTF developed a comprehensive platform, the ROSALIND Diagnostic Monitoring System (DxM), that integrates bioinformatic *in silico* modeling with clinical in vitro laboratory testing to assess the impact of SARS-CoV-2 mutations on both NAATs and antigen assays. This work was supported in part by the National Institute of Biomedical Imaging and Bioengineering of the NIH under award numbers 75N92019P00328, U54EB015408, and U54EB027690 as part of the RADx initiative.

The ROSALIND DxM automatically imports sequences from US and global databases through a data connectivity agreement with GISAID for complete, daily, worldwide downloads from the GISAID EpiCoV database.[29] Sequences not tagged with "is complete" and sequences with an "n_content" of more than 0.05 are excluded before pairwise whole-genome alignments of all sequences are performed using LASTZ v1.04.02 to align each GISAID sequence to the Wuhan-Hu-1 strain (Wuhan/WIV04/2019).[14, 90] Since January 2020, ROSALIND DxM has compiled, searched, and analyzed 12 936 617 sequences (as of 21 September 2022) from GISAID.

The ROSALIND software uses the basic local alignment search tool to find the position of primers and probes on the same Wuhan strain.[14] The Bioconductor package for genetic variants, VariantAnnotation v1.20.2, is then used for the translation of nucleotide mutations into amino acids in R v3.3.2, and the identification of amino acid substitutions or frameshifts is used to determine a unique mutation incident.[91]

Incidents are defined as unique combinations of mutations that span the region of the genome or proteome being assayed with the molecular test. For example, a typical PCR diagnostic test will consist of several reactions, each reaction containing a forward and reverse primer and usually a probe sequence used for the actual detection. Typically, these molecular tools are designed with high precision to provide both high sensitivity and high specificity to a particular pathogen (in this case, the RNA sequence of the SARS-CoV-2 virus). However, dropout can occur if any of the primers or probes fail to bind to the target sequence. ROSALIND's scoring system assesses the predicted severity of an incident to identify which emerging mutations may be likely to drop out.

The scoring system returns a score between 0 and 5, with a score of 0 meaning that the mutation incident is very unlikely to affect the test and 5 meaning that urgent laboratory testing is required. The combination of incidents and severity scores is used to assess the overall potential impact on the performance of the assay.[92] For a PCR assay, an SNP in the middle of the primer is unlikely to cause an issue, but the same SNP toward the 3' end could prevent the amplification needed to start or be as efficient as without the SNP. Multiple adjacent SNPs, as well as indels (insertions or deletions of one or more nucleotides in a DNA sequence), can also affect the assays.

Antigen mutations may also affect the performance of a diagnostic test, but predicting this effect is difficult due to the complex three-dimensional structure and dynamic behavior of proteins in solution. This is further complicated by the fact that the location of the epitopes of most diagnostic probes is unknown. The ROSALIND DxM software identifies amino acid changes and deletions and uses this information to generate its risk scores. A simple scoring system was implemented that considers two factors: (1) the severity of the amino acid change and (2) the surface accessibility of the mutated residue. The severity of an amino acid change is based on general exchangeability scores derived from experimentally evaluated effects of mutations on protein function.[93] Surface accessibility scores are determined using published structures of S and N proteins and calculations of the solvent-accessible surface area for each residue.[94] For the S protein, both the open and the closed conformations of the SARS-CoV-2 S protein receptor binding domain are considered. Missing residues, such as unresolved regions in the S protein or regions predicted to be intrinsically disordered in the N protein, are considered solvent accessible.

Table 9.2 NAAT severity score calculation

Nucleotide Change	PCR	LAMP	FISH	CRISPR
One SNP	+0	+0	+1	+1
Two SNPs	+1	+1	+2	+2
Three SNPs	+2	+2	+3	+3
More than three SNPs	+4	+4	+4	+4
Adjacent SNPs	+2	+2	+2	+2
One base indel	+1	+1	+2	+2
Indel of two or more bases	+3	+3	+3	+3
SNP or indel location				
SNP in ultimate or penultimate base of 3' end of primer	+3 (per SNP)	+3 (per SNP)*	N/A	N/A
SNP in ultimate or penultimate base of 5' end of primer	N/A	+3 (per SNP)**	N/A	N/A
SNP in third, fourth, and fifth base from 5' end of primer	N/A	+3 (per SNP)**	N/A	N/A
SNP in third, fourth, and fifth base from 3' end of primer	+2 (per SNP)	+2 (per SNP)*	N/A	N/A
SNP in probe	+2 (per SNP)	N/A	N/A	N/A
Indel in final 5 bases from 3' end of primer	+2	+2 (per SNP)*	N/A	N/A
Indel in final 5 bases from 5' end of primer	N/A	+2 (per SNP)**	N/A	N/A
Indel in probe	+2	N/A	N/A	N/A
Delta temperature of melting (°C)				
≥ 5 and < 8	+2	+2	+2	+2
≥ 8	+4	+4	+4	+4

LAMP, loop-mediated isothermal amplification; FISH, fluorescence in situ hybridization; CRISPR, clustered regularly interspaced short palindromic repeats.
* For forward 2 primer (F2), back 2 primer (B2), forward 3 primer (F3), back 3 primer (B3), forward loop primer (FL), and back loop primer (BL).
** For forward 1 primer complementary (F1c) and back 1 primer complementary (B1c).

Developers of NAATs upload primer and probe sequences into the ROSALIND DxM, and antigen test developers upload target epitope regions. The ROSALIND DxM automatically assesses each test design against all available sequences and assigns a severity score (NAATs) or risk score (antigen tests) based on the potential impact of emerging SARS-CoV-2 variants on diagnostic performance. In addition to incident scoring, the ROSALIND DxM also computes the incident prevalence, that is, the percent of samples with that unique set of mutations. Combining the risk score and the incident prevalence is key when ordering the results of *in silico* analysis so that test manufacturers can identify the most important incidents. An incident with a score of 3 and a prevalence of 10% is more urgent to investigate than an incident with a score of 5 but a prevalence of 0.1%.

The ROSALIND DxM currently supports PCR, LAMP, FISH, CRISPR, and antigen molecular assays for performing these different assessments. The ROSALIND DxM also offers a system to track the verification and notes associated with the incident investigation so that the platform keeps in one place the full history of the potential issue and the associated testing.

Together, these analyses complete the first stage of the FDA policy for evaluating the impact of viral mutations on testing assays. Based on these results, continued in vitro testing takes place with the RADx VTF, and results are fed back into the ROSALIND DxM to improve scoring algorithms. These results are then reported to the NAAT or antigen companies.

Sample Banking

To accomplish the second and third stages of the FDA policy for evaluating the impact of viral mutations, wet laboratory testing was performed using an extensive biobank of samples created at Emory University. This biobank, which comprises thousands of remnant clinical samples (RCSs), allowed the team to rapidly test and screen diagnostic assays for rare or common mutations. First, the RADx VTF established contractual relationships with large laboratories that were performing testing commercially or on behalf of the CDC. These laboratories included Helix, LabCorp, and the University of Washington. These laboratories provided fully sequenced RCSs that were both live and heat-inactivated, as well as the corresponding metadata, including sequence information. Next, the RADx VTF used bioinformatic tools, such as Pangolin, Nextclade, and the ROSALIND platform, to identify variants and mutations of interest within the samples, and these samples were sent to Emory University for future use.

Samples were stored at –80 °C at the Children's Clinical and Translational Discovery Core, and the corresponding metadata and sequence files were stored within the ROSALIND platform. Once stored, the samples allowed the RADx VTF to select and test assays against specific variants and mutations. The biobank eventually contained more than 10 000 unique sequenced samples.

Laboratory Methods to Assess Test Performance

Over the first two years of the pandemic, tremendous progress was made in developing and improving both molecular and antigen diagnostic tests for SARS-CoV-2 and its variants. This progress was in part due to the efforts of clinical and research laboratories at Emory University. In 2020, Emory University built a system of clinical and high biosafety level (BSL) laboratories to rapidly and efficiently evaluate the sensitivity and specificity of new diagnostic tests through the NIH/RADx initiative, as discussed in Chapter 4.

This system involved using live, highly concentrated SARS-CoV-2 (WA1/2020 Wuhan-Hu-1 wild-type [WT] strain) cultured and propagated in a BSL3 facility, which had been certified for containing and working with live, infectious material. Fortunately, the BSL3 facility at Emory University was already working with the WT SARS-CoV-2 virus for drug discovery purposes, which facilitated the use of cultured live viruses to evaluate the performance of the NIH/RADx diagnostic tests. The WT virus was ordered from the Biodefense and Emerging Infections Research Resources Repository (BEI Resources), an NIH-run repository for infectious disease researchers, and passaged twice in Vero E6 cells for propagation of large volumes of the SARS-CoV-2 provirus. An aliquot of each passage was re-sequenced by next-generation sequencing as a quality control to verify the integrity of the virus and the absence of additional mutations grown in culture (only viruses without extra relevant mutations in any gene were used). The WT virus was then subcultured twice and titrated for foci-forming units, half-maximal tissue culture infectious dose (TCID50), and the determination of cycle threshold (Ct) values by quantitative RT-PCR methods. After the highly concentrated WT virus stock was made and aliquoted (200 μl or ~ 200 cryotubes), it was stored at –80 °C until further use.[95, 96]

In the first year of the pandemic, we used well-characterized, live WT viruses to evaluate the limit of detection (LoD) of the NIH/RADx diagnostic tests in the BSL3 laboratory. First, an aliquot of the WT virus was thawed and serially diluted in an appropriate matrix (saline, phosphate-buffered saline, viral transport medium, universal transport medium, commercially available saliva or nasal wash, etc.). Next, the serial dilutions were spiked onto the swab or test device of a diagnostic test, and the test's instructions for use were followed. A laboratory result report with photographs of the antigen or molecular-based assay was generated two to three days after receiving the tests and evaluated in an NIH-like study session. Finally, the company would receive a report, together with the results generated with clinical or inactivated WT viruses by other Emory University laboratories.[97]

In the BSL3 laboratories, we tested approximately 28 rapid tests using WT strains. After propagation of the viral stocks (passage 2), the stocks were sequenced to check that no significant mutations were present in the viral genome, including in the S and N genes. To check the levels of infectivity of the viral stocks, a focus-forming assay was performed with live propagated viruses in the BSL3 laboratory. An example of an infectivity assay in Vero E6 cells with the WT viral stock used to determine the LoD of the rapid tests is shown in Figure 9.7.

Serially diluted SARS-CoV-2 WA-1/2020 frozen stock was incubated with cells in an assay to determine the presence of the virus. The presence of dots indicates infection and the expression of SARS-CoV-2 S protein receptor binding domain antigens.

For each test evaluated in the BSL3 laboratories, an algorithm was used that collected the following information:

- device number
- company name
- device name
- sample type (nasopharyngeal swab, anterior nasal swab, saliva, etc.)
- target

  o protein (S or N protein)

  o gene (S, N, ORF1a/b, envelope [E], etc.)

- test type

  o antigen (LFA)

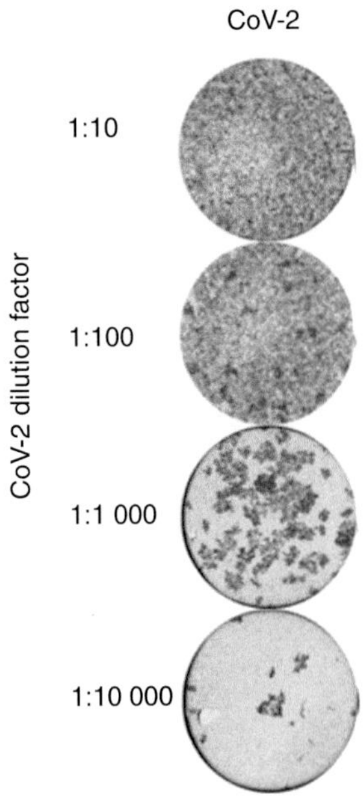

CoV-2

Figure 9.7 Focus-forming infectivity assay of WT SARS-CoV-2.

o molecular (PCR, LAMP, CRISPR, etc.)

- LoD TCID50/ml
- copies of genome-equivalent droplet digital PCR or real-time quantitative PCR
- notes

As the virus began to mutate – a fact that was becoming evident with the rise of the D614G variant as early as April 2020 – we needed to adopt a new strategy to reevaluate the LoD of rapid tests for their ability to detect new and future mutations or variants of SARS-CoV-2, as the RADx rapid tests were developed based on the genome sequence (nucleotides and amino acids) of the WT (Wuhan-Hu-1) unmutated virus. The first diagnostic tests for COVID-19 targeted only one gene, the S protein, further raising fears of false negatives.

To work with emerging variants from December 2020 onward (see Table 9.1 for an evaluation of variants over time), the RADx VTF procured RCS variants that had been confirmed to be positive by ultra-deep sequencing and from different vendors (i.e. Helix, LabCorp, and the University of Washington). We created the most extensive biobank of emerging SARS-CoV-2 variants in the USA. Using samples from our biobank, we developed panels of RCSs by making pools for each variant that appeared with a frequency of ≥ 5% in the USA or in a state or for a VOC/VOI that had a fast growth rate, namely doubling every 14 days nationally or regionally (for a more detailed explanation of how panels and pools are created for in vitro laboratory testing with VOCs and VOIs, see Chapter 8). As of the writing of this chapter, we have created 17 RADx VTF pools with different VOCs/VOIs or VBMs to monitor their impact on RADx diagnostic tests, with several mutations in the N gene.[98, 99]

How to Pick Vendor(s) of RCSs to Build a Powerful Biobank of All Known VOCs/VOIs in the USA

Initially, we requested that each vendor send several frozen RCS variants (at least three different variants that were prevalent during the period of testing) with low Ct values or high viral loads, together with sequences and all available Ct values. The RCS variants must be frozen and sent to our laboratories in a minimum volume of 0.5 ml of specified matrix, preferably saline. If the vendor inactivated the RCS, the process of inactivation must be provided. Samples are received, thawed, and tested using two to three antigen-based assays and at least one molecular-based assay. Once the results are evaluated by the RADx VTF, they are sent to the vendor. Approvals of which vendors to pick are based on RCS quality and sequences and whether the samples are feasible for molecular and antigen-based tests. An international biobank is also being procured with other countries, including Brazil, to expand our biobank with emerging VOCs/VOIs or mutations not found in the USA but detected abroad.

How to Pick RCS Variants from a Vendor

Vendor(s) must send a list of sequences and Ct values of all frozen RCSs weekly. The RADx VTF constantly checks for VOCs/VOIs or mutations of interest and low Ct (high viral load) selections. A list of samples of interest is sent to the vendor, and the vendor ships the samples to the Emory University laboratory weekly. FASTA files of all samples are uploaded into the ROSALIND DxM system, which also imports sequences from GISAID and GenBank, among others. The RADx VTF consistently uses the platform to pick the desired RCSs from vendors.

At the beginning of the RADx VTF, we used Excel spreadsheets (macro-system) of all of the mutations to choose the desired group of samples that had the same profile. Several days were spent searching and picking samples in this way. Then, the sequences of approximately 30 to 50 samples were uploaded into Nextclade to be analyzed in phylogenetic trees and matrices. We then picked the most similar sequences of a specific variant to use when creating the pooled panels. The ROSALIND DxM uses LASTZ to align each sequence to the Wuhan-Hu-1 WT strain. A single mutation of interest is easily selected among thousands of RCSs. Several samples containing the desired mutation can easily be used to test against a specific diagnostic antigen or molecular assay.

Epitope Mapping

The RADx VTF also evaluated the impact of a mutation on diagnostic antigen tests by using a new epitope mapping assay. Epitope mapping is the process of predicting how a viral protein's structure will change based on changes in its amino acid sequence and how changes in protein structure will affect antibody binding. This is an important technique for predicting how antigen tests, most of which are antibody-based, will perform against new variants with known genetic mutations. Traditional methods for epitope mapping include site-directed mutagenesis, peptide arrays, and mass spectrometry to locate and infer the effects of amino acid substitutions on antibody binding. However, many of these methods do not directly measure the binding of antibodies and rely on predictions of epitope shape change that may be inaccurate.

A new method, developed by researchers at Emory University, uses rapid screening of direct antibody binding to almost all potential single amino acid mutations of a viral protein, which allows for preemptive detection of mutations that might affect antibody binding. This method uses a lentivirus-mediated mammalian surface-display platform for the SARS-CoV-2 N protein, the most abundant SARS-CoV-2 protein and the target of most rapid antigen-based tests.[100] The new system predicts the performance of rapid antigen tests against past, current, and possible future variants of SARS-CoV-2 and can identify mutations with the potential to cause available rapid COVID-19 antigen tests to fail.

Future of SARS-CoV-2 Evolution

Anticipating virus evolution is a key part of controlling endemic viruses, as well as preventing future pandemics. Thus, much effort has been put into attempting to predict how future variants of SARS-CoV-2 might look. To predict future variants, we can attempt to determine the origins of existing variants and look toward the evolution of similar respiratory viruses.

Despite the incredible amount of collaboration and effort put into sequencing and analyzing sequences, we have yet to find an established pattern in the way that SARS-CoV-2 variants emerge. Although many expected a stepwise evolution, in which new variants are direct descendants of previous ones, genomic analysis shows that many of the VOCs that emerged in 2021 arose from unrelated lineages of SARS-CoV-2. Most notably, the omicron variant is more closely related to the alpha variant than to the delta variant (the latter having preceded it chronologically), and it did not evolve directly from either.

One theory for this unusual pattern of evolution is that the virus evolved in immuno-compromised individuals with persistent COVID-19 infections. Researchers have detected several of the mutations found in the S protein in immunocompromised people who were infected with COVID-19 before the emergence of the omicron variant.[101–103] A second theory for the origin of omicron is that it evolved in an animal host and jumped back into humans with many additional mutations. This theory is supported by the detection of SARS-CoV-2 in many animal species such as white-tailed deer, minks, and cats, several of which can also transmit the virus back to humans.[104–107]

Another way to predict how SARS-CoV-2 variants may evolve is to look at the evolution of other endemic viruses. Globally, there are seasonal coronaviruses causing mild disease that have been circulating among the population for years. A study of these coronaviruses shows that, rather than increasing transmission, the viruses tend to evolve toward increasing immune escape.[108, 109] Influenza virus, one of the most prominent seasonal viruses, also manages to remain in circulation by continuously evolving toward immune evasion, which necessitates annual flu vaccines.[110]

The SARS-CoV-2 variants have begun to show a trend of increased immune evasion over increased severity. As of the end of 2022, the newest highly circulating variants were all from the omicron lineage and were closely related to previous dominant variants, such as BA.1.

We have yet to determine whether SARS-CoV-2 evolution will continue this trend or if additional unrelated variants will come from unexpected places. Regardless of how the virus evolves, we must continue to monitor it through sampling and genomic sequencing to update prevention, diagnostic, and treatment efforts.

Lessons Learned

The challenges presented by the emerging variants of COVID-19 taught us important lessons that should be deployed, when necessary, in the future.

- Established sequence databases and the early release of the first SARS-CoV-2 genome sequence allowed researchers to begin tracking changes in the SARS-CoV-2 genome immediately
- Data sharing and open sequence sharing are crucial for coordinated global monitoring of variants
- Variant nomenclature should be established early and uniformly to prevent confusion among the public and to mitigate reactionary policy decisions
- Target selection for both vaccines and diagnostics should be varied and not concentrated on a single portion of the genome
- Early determination of the transmissibility and severity of new variants can greatly help the public health response
- RCSs should be obtained early. If possible, clinical laboratories should be asked to store all positive samples at −80 °C from the very beginning
- A repository of RCSs for variants with an increased prevalence of ≥ 5% should be built and samples should be selected with Ct values ≤ 20
- Continued collaboration between clinical and research organizations will be critically important for selecting and storing crucial samples early and facilitating the efficient and responsive testing of new diagnostic tests during pandemics
- A robust bioinformatics platform like the ROSALIND DxM is fundamental to speeding up the selection of suitable variant samples for testing and assessing the risk of decreased test sensitivity with new variants
- Having a large, reliable number of samples from a large geographic area enabled the RADx VTF to identify, order, and test rare variants before they became prevalent in the population
- A combination of government-supported and private software organizations enabled the rapid analysis of samples for mutations and sequence quality

References

1. WHO, Classification of omicron (B.1.1.529): SARS-CoV-2 variant of concern (November 26, 2021). https://tinyurl.com/yc57rbme (accessed December 19, 2021).

2. F. Campbell, B. Archer, H. Laurenson-Schafer, et al., Increased transmissibility and global spread of SARS-CoV-2 variants of concern as of June 2021. *Euro Surveill*, **26**, 24 (2021), 2100509.

3. T. Nyberg, K. A. Twohig, R. J. Harris, et al., Risk of hospital admission for patients with SARS-CoV-2 variant B.1.1.7: cohort analysis. *BMJ*, **373** (2021), n1412.

4. WHO, Weekly epidemiological update on COVID-19 – 20 July 2021 (2021). https://tinyurl.com/bdd6f82t (accessed August 15, 2022).

5. Public Health England, Risk assessment for SARS-CoV-2 variant Delta (2021). https://tinyurl.com/yckpacmk (accessed July 25, 2021).

6. Public Health England, SARS-CoV-2 variants of concern and variants under investigation (2021). https://tinyurl

.com/4jbzmt3h (accessed January 4, 2023).

7. T. Nyberg, N. M. Ferguson, S. G. Nash, et al., Comparative analysis of the risks of hospitalisation and death associated with SARS-CoV-2 Omicron (B.1.1.529) and Delta (B.1.617.2) variants in England: a cohort study. *Lancet* **399**, 10332 (2022), 1303–1312.

8. M. Amicone, V. Borges, M. J. Alves, et al., Mutation rate of SARS-CoV-2 and emergence of mutators during experimental evolution. *Evol Med Public Health*, **10**, 1 (2022), 142–155.

9. S. Duchene, L. Featherstone, M. Haritopoulou-Sinanidou, et al., Temporal signal and the phylodynamic threshold of SARS-CoV-2. *Virus Evol*, **6**, 2 (2020): veaa061.

10. WHO, Listings of WHO's response to COVID-19 (2020). www.who.int/news/item/29-06-2020-covidtimeline/ (accessed June 21, 2022).

11. J. Cohen, Chinese researchers reveal draft genome of virus implicated in Wuhan pneumonia outbreak (January 11, 2020). https://tinyurl.com/4sjfhy76 (accessed June 21, 2022).

12. E. Holmes, Novel 2019 coronavirus genome – SARS-CoV-2 coronavirus (2020). https://virological.org/t/novel-2019-coronavirus-genome/319 (accessed June 21, 2022).

13. C. R. Paden, Y. Tao, K. Queen, et al., Rapid, sensitive, full-genome sequencing of severe acute respiratory syndrome coronavirus 2. *Emerg Infect Dis*, **26**, 10 (2020), 2401–2405.

14. F. Wu, S. Zhao, B. Yu, et al., A new coronavirus associated with human respiratory disease in China. *Nature*, **579**, 7798 (2020): 265–269.

15. J. Hadfield, C. Megill, S. M. Bell, et al., Nextstrain: real-time tracking of pathogen evolution. *Bioinformatics*, **34**, 23 (2018): 4121–4123.

16. D. A. Benson, M. Cavanaugh, K. Clark, et al., GenBank. *Nucleic Acids Res*, **41**, D1 (2013), D36–42.

17. NCBI, GenBank overview. www.ncbi.nlm.nih.gov/genbank/ (accessed July 6, 2022).

18. NCBI, NCBI SARS-CoV-2 resources. www.ncbi.nlm.nih.gov/sars-cov-2/ (accessed September 12, 2022).

19. Y. Shu and J. McCauley, GISAID: Global initiative on sharing all influenza data – from vision to reality. *Euro Surveill*, **22**, 13 (2017), 30494.

20. COG-UK, History of COG-UK (2021). www.cogconsortium.uk/about/about-us/history-of-cog-uk/ (accessed July 5, 2022).

21. UK Health Security Agency, UK completes over 2 million SARS-CoV-2 whole genome sequences (February 10, 2022). https://tinyurl.com/yky7u7u9 (accessed July 7, 2022).

22. A. Maxmen, One million coronavirus sequences: popular genome site hits mega milestone. *Nature*, **593**, 7857 (2021), 21.

23. CDC, CDC launches national viral genomics consortium to better map SARS-CoV-2 transmission (May 1, 2020). https://tinyurl.com/yxpj93vw (accessed July 7, 2022).

24. CDC, SPHERES (April 9, 2021). www.cdc.gov/coronavirus/2019-ncov/variants/spheres.html (accessed June 21, 2023).

25. CDC, COVID Data Tracker (2020). https://covid.cdc.gov/covid-data-tracker (accessed September 12, 2022).

26. N. Msomi, K. Mlisana, and T. de Oliveira, A genomics network established to respond rapidly to public health threats in South Africa. *Lancet Microbe*, **1**, 6 (2020), e229–230.

27. J. A. Leite, A. Vicari, E. Perez, et al., Implementation of a COVID-19 Genomic Surveillance Regional Network for Latin America and Caribbean region. *PLoS One*, **17**, 3 (2022): e0252526.

28. Pan American Health Organization, COVID-19 Genomic Surveillance Regional Network (2022). https://tinyurl.com/yc8akdnr (accessed July 7, 2022).

29. S. Elbe and G. Buckland-Merrett, Data, disease and diplomacy: GISAID's innovative contribution to global health. *Glob Chall*, **1**, 1 (2017), 33–46.

30. K. Gangavarapu, A. A. Latif, J. L. Mullen, et al., Outbreak.info genomic reports: scalable and dynamic surveillance of SARS-CoV-2 variants and mutations. *medRxiv* (2022). https://doi.org/10.1101/2022.01.27.22269965 (accessed September 12, 2022).

31. L. van Dorp, M. Acman, D. Richard, et al., Emergence of genomic diversity and recurrent mutations in SARS-CoV-2. *Infect Genet Evol*, **83** (2020), 104351.

32. O. Pybus, A. Rambaut, L. du Plessis, et al., Preliminary analysis of SARS-CoV-2 importation & establishment of UK transmission lineages (2020). https://tinyurl.com/4fhex3vn (accessed June 6, 2022).

33. M. M. Arons, K. M. Hatfield, S. C. Reddy, et al., Presymptomatic SARS-CoV-2 infections and transmission in a skilled nursing facility. *N Engl J Med*, **382**, 22 (2020), 2081–2090.

34. N. F. Müller, C. Wagner, C. D. Frazar, et al., Viral genomes reveal patterns of the SARS-CoV-2 outbreak in Washington State (2021). https://github.com/blab/ncov-wa-d614g (accessed July 1, 2022).

35. D. S. Candido, I. M. Claro, J. G. de Jesus, et al., Evolution and epidemic spread of SARS-CoV-2 in Brazil. *Science*, **369**, 6508 (2020), 1255–1260.

36. B. Korber, W. M. Fischer, S. Gnanakaran, et al., Tracking changes in SARS-CoV-2 spike: evidence that D614G increases infectivity of the COVID-19 virus. *Cell*, **182**, 4 (2020): 812–827.

37. E. B. Hodcroft, M. Zuber, S. Nadeau, et al., Emergence and spread of a SARS-CoV-2 variant through Europe in the summer of 2020. medRxiv (2021) https://doi.org/10.1101/2020.10.25.20219063.

38. E. Volz, V. Hill, J. T. McCrone, et al., Evaluating the effects of SARS-CoV-2 spike mutation D614G on transmissibility and pathogenicity. *Cell*, **184**, 1 (2021), 64–75.

39. L. Zhang, C. B. Jackson, H. Mou, et al., SARS-CoV-2 spike-protein D614G mutation increases virion spike density and infectivity. *Nat Commun*, **11**, 1 (2020), 6013.

40. N. G. Davies, S. Abbott, R. C. Barnard, et al., Estimated transmissibility and impact of SARS-CoV-2 lineage B.1.1.7 in England. *Science*, **372**, 6538 (2021): eabg3055.

41. P. Supasa, D. Zhou, W. Dejnirattisai, et al., Reduced neutralization of SARS-CoV-2 B.1.1.7 variant by convalescent and vaccine sera. *Cell*, **184**, 8 (2021), 2201–2211.

42. C. K. Wibmer, F. Ayres, T. Hermanus, et al., SARS-CoV-2 501Y.V2 escapes neutralization by South African COVID-19 donor plasma. *Nat Med*, **27**, 4 (2021), 622–625.

43. Q. Li, J. Nie, J. Wu, et al., SARS-CoV-2 501Y.V2 variants lack higher infectivity but do have immune escape. *Cell*, **184**, 9 (2021), 2362–2371.

44. P. Wang, R. G. Casner, M. S. Nair, et al., Increased resistance of SARS-CoV-2 variant P.1 to antibody neutralization. *Cell Host Microbe*, **29**, 5 (2021), 747–751.

45. D. Planas, T. Bruel, L. Grzelak, et al., Sensitivity of infectious SARS-CoV-2 B.1.1.7 and B.1.351 variants to neutralizing antibodies. *Nat Med*, **27**, 5 (2021), 917–924.

46. D. A. Collier, A. De Marco, I. A. T. M. Ferreira, et al., Sensitivity of SARS-CoV-2 B.1.1.7 to mRNA vaccine-elicited antibodies. *Nature*, **593**, 7857 (2021), 136–141.

47. FDA, Tests expected to fail to detect the SARS-CoV-2 omicron variant and sub-variants (2022). https://tinyurl.com/mrya77nm (accessed January 4, 2023).

48. N. L. Washington, S. White, K. M. S. Barrett, et al., S gene dropout patterns in SARS-CoV-2 tests suggest spread of the H69del/V70del mutation in the US. *medRxiv* (2020). https://doi.org/10.1101/2020.12.24.20248814 (accessed July 19, 2022).

49. P. Wollschläger, D. Todt, N. Gerlitz, et al., SARS-CoV-2 N gene dropout and N gene Ct value shift as indicator for the presence of B.1.1.7 lineage in a commercial multiplex PCR assay. *Clin Microbiol Infect*, **27**, 9 (2021), 1353.e1–1353.e5.

50. R. Earnest, R. Uddin, N. Matluk, et al., Comparative transmissibility of SARS-CoV-2 variants Delta and Alpha in New England, USA. *Cell Rep Med*, **3**, 4 (2022), 100583.

51. A. Sheikh, J. McMenamin, B. Taylor, and C. Robertson, SARS-CoV-2 Delta VOC in Scotland: demographics, risk of hospital admission, and vaccine effectiveness. *Lancet*, **397**, 10293 (2021), 2461–2462.

52. S. W. X. Ong, C. J. Chiew, L. W. Ang, et al., Clinical and virological features of severe acute respiratory syndrome coronavirus 2 (SARS-CoV-2) variants of concern: a retrospective cohort study comparing B.1.1.7 (Alpha), B.1.351 (Beta), and B.1.617.2 (Delta). *Clin Infect Dis*, **75**, 1 (2022), e1128–1136.

53. C. Jung, D. Kmiec, L. Koepke, et al., Omicron: what makes the latest SARS-CoV-2 variant of concern so concerning? *J Virol*, **96**, 6 (2022), e02077–21.

54. J. Hu, P. Peng, X. Cao, et al., Increased immune escape of the new SARS-CoV-2 variant of concern Omicron. *Cell Mol Immunol*, **19**, 2 (2022): 293–295.

55. K. P. Y. Hui, J. C. W. Ho, M. Cheung, et al., SARS-CoV-2 Omicron variant replication in human bronchus and lung ex vivo. *Nature*, **603**, 7902 (2022), 715–720.

56. WHO, Severity of disease associated with Omicron variant as compared with Delta variant in hospitalized patients with suspected or confirmed SARS-CoV-2 infection (June 7, 2022). www.who.int/pub lications-detail-redirect/9789240051829 (accessed July 21, 2022).

57. F. Abdullah, J. Myers, D. Basu, et al., Decreased severity of disease during the first global Omicron variant covid-19 outbreak in a large hospital in Tshwane, South Africa. *Int J Infect Dis*, **116** (2022), 38–42.

58. L. Liu, S. Iketani, Y. Guo, et al., Striking antibody evasion manifested by the Omicron variant of SARS-CoV-2. *Nature*, **602**, 7898 (2022), 676–681.

59. D. Planas, N. Saunders, P. Maes, et al., Considerable escape of SARS-CoV-2 Omicron to antibody neutralization. *Nature*, **602**, 7898 (2022), 671–675.

60. J. R. C. Pulliam, C. van Schalkwyk, N. Govender, et al., Increased risk of SARS-CoV-2 reinfection associated with emergence of Omicron in South Africa. *Science*, **376**, 6593 (2022): eabn4947.

61. P. Marks, Coronavirus (COVID-19) update: FDA recommends inclusion of omicron BA.4/5 component for COVID-19 vaccine booster doses, *FDA* (June 30, 2022). https://tinyurl.com/2p7tnf7f (accessed July 21, 2022).

62. Pfizer, Pfizer and BioNTech announce omicron-adapted COVID-19 vaccine candidates demonstrate high immune response against omicron (June 25, 2022). https://tinyurl.com/muc8ftjp (accessed July 21, 2022).

63. F. Konings, M. D. Perkins, J. H. Kuhn, et al., SARS-CoV-2 Variants of Interest and Concern naming scheme conducive for global discourse. *Nat Microbiol*, **6**, 7 (2021), 821–823.

64. GISAID, Clade and lineage nomenclature aids in genomic epidemiology studies of active hCoV-19 viruses (March 2, 2021). https://tinyurl.com/yhya9y3x (accessed June 28, 2022).

65. E. B. Hodcroft, J. Hadfield, R. A. Neher, and T. Bedford, Year-letter genetic clade naming for SARS-CoV-2 on Nextstrain.org (June 2, 2020). https://tinyurl.com/cnmw s8f5 (accessed June 28, 2022).

66. T. Bedford, E. B. Hodcroft, and R. A. Neher, Updated Nextstrain SARS-CoV-2 clade naming strategy (January 6, 2021). https://tinyurl.com/53aeyjsu (accessed June 28, 2022).

67. C. Roemer, E. B. Hodcroft, R. A. Neher, and T. Bedford, SARS-CoV-2 clade naming strategy for 2022 (April 29, 2022). https://tinyurl.com/4bdkftz8 (accessed July 11, 2022).

68. Pango Network, What are Pango lineages? (2022). https://tinyurl.com/ycytjtbv (accessed June 28, 2022).

69. A. Rambaut, E. C. Holmes, Á. O'Toole, et al., A dynamic nomenclature proposal for SARS-CoV-2 lineages to assist genomic epidemiology. *Nat Microbiol*, **5**, 11 (2020), 1403–1407.

70. WHO, WHO announces simple, easy-to-say labels for SARS-CoV-2 variants of interest and concern (May 31, 2021). https://tinyurl.com/y2umf75f (accessed June 28, 2022).

71. WHO, COVID-19 weekly epidemiological update (February 25, 2021). https://tinyurl.com/55vm2fnk (accessed July 12, 2022).

72. WHO, Tracking SARS-CoV-2 variants (2021). www.who.int/en/activities/tracking-SARS-CoV-2-variants/ (accessed December 27, 2021).

73. CDC, SARS-CoV-2 variant classifications and definitions (2022). https://tinyurl.com/5n6srche (accessed June 6, 2022).

74. FDA, Policy for evaluating impact of viral mutations on COVID-19 tests (2021). https://tinyurl.com/5atty76z (accessed January 4, 2023).

75. FDA, SARS-CoV-2 viral mutations: impact on COVID-19 tests (2022). https://tinyurl.com/2upu8w6s (accessed July 25, 2022).

76. S. C. Holland, A. Bains, L. A. Holland, et al., SARS-CoV-2 Delta variant N gene mutations reduce sensitivity to the TaqPath COVID-19 multiplex molecular diagnostic assay. *Viruses*, **14**, 6 (2022), 1316.

77. L. Bourassa, G. A. Perchetti, Q. Phung, et al., A SARS-CoV-2 nucleocapsid variant that affects antigen test performance. *J Clin Virol*, **141** (2021), 104900.

78. E. Mahase, Covid-19: What do we know about Omicron sublineages? *BMJ*, **376** (2022), o358.

79. J. Wise, Covid-19: Omicron sub variants driving new wave of infections in UK. *BMJ*, **377** (2022), o1506.

80. Q. Wang, Y. Guo, S. Iketani, et al., Antibody evasion by SARS-CoV-2 Omicron subvariants BA.2.12.1, BA.4, & BA.5. *Nature*, **608**, 7923 (2022), 603–608.

81. S. Xia, L. Wang, Y. Zhu, L. Lu, and S. Jiang, Origin, virological features, immune evasion and intervention of SARS-CoV-2 Omicron sublineages. *Signal Transduct Target Ther*, **7**, 1 (2022), 1–7.

82. Y. Cao, A. Yisimayi, F. Jian, et al., BA.2.12.1, BA.4 and BA.5 escape antibodies elicited by Omicron infection. *Nature*, **608**, 7923 (2022), 593–602.

83. WHO, TAG-VE statement on Omicron sublineages BQ.1 and XBB (October 27, 2022). https://tinyurl.com/wz24x74m (accessed December 8, 2022).

84. P. Arora, A. Kempf, I. Nehlmeier, et al., Omicron sublineage BQ.1.1 resistance to monoclonal antibodies. *Lancet Infect Dis*, **23**, 1 (2023), 22–23.

85. D. Planas, T. Bruel, I. Staropoli, et al., Resistance of Omicron subvariants BA.2.75.2, BA.4.6 and BQ.1.1 to neutralizing antibodies, *bioRxiv* (2022). https://doi.org/10.1101/2022.11.17.516888 (accessed December 9, 2022).

86. P. Qu, J. P. Evans, J. Faraone, et al., Distinct neutralizing antibody escape of SARS-CoV-2 omicron subvariants BQ.1, BQ.1.1, BA.4.6, BF.7 and BA.2.75.2, *bioRxiv* (2022). https://doi.org/10.1101/2022.10.19.512891 (accessed December 8, 2022).

87. J. Zou, C. Kurhade, S. Patel, et al., Improved neutralization of Omicron BA.4/5, BA.4.6, BA.2.75.2, BQ.1.1, and XBB.1 with bivalent BA.4/5 vaccine, *bioRxiv* (2022). https://doi.org/10.1101/2022.11.17.516898 (accessed December 9, 2022).

88. Pfizer, Pfizer and BioNTech announce updated clinical data for omicron BA.4/BA.5-adapted bivalent booster demonstrating substantially higher immune response in adults compared to the original COVID-19 vaccine (November 4, 2022). https://tinyurl.com/bdhekpzz (accessed December 9, 2022).

89. R. Link-Gelles, Effectiveness of bivalent mRNA vaccines in preventing symptomatic SARS-CoV-2 infection – increasing community access to testing

program, United States, September–November 2022. *MMWR Morb Mortal Wkly Rep*, **71**, 48 (2022), 1526–1530.

90. R. S. Harris, *Improved Pairwise Alignment of Genomic DNA*, Thesis (2007). www.bx.psu.edu/~rsharris/rsharris_phd_thesis_2007.pdf (accessed September 21, 2022).

91. V. Obenchain, M. Lawrence, V. Carey, et al., VariantAnnotation: a Bioconductor package for exploration and annotation of genetic variants. *Bioinformatics*, **30**, 14 (2014), 2076–2078.

92. S. Lefever, F. Pattyn, J. Hellemans, and J. Vandesompele, Single-nucleotide polymorphisms and other mismatches reduce performance of quantitative PCR assays. *Clin Chem*, **59**, 10 (2013), 1470–1480.

93. L. Y. Yampolsky and A. Stoltzfus, The exchangeability of amino acids in proteins. *Genetics*, **170**, 4 (2005), 1459–1472.

94. R. Fraczkiewicz and W. Braun, Exact and efficient analytical calculation of the accessible surface areas and their gradients for macromolecules. *J Comput Chem*, **19**, 3 (1998), 319–333.

95. E. J. Nehl, S. S. Heilman, D. Ku, et al., The RADx tech test verification core and the ACME POCT in the evaluation of COVID-19 testing devices: a model for progress and change. *IEEE Open J Eng Med Biol*, **2** (2021), 142–151.

96. P. E. George, C. L. Stokes, L. C. Bassit, et al., Covid-19 will not "magically disappear": why access to widespread testing is paramount. *Am J Hematol*, **96**, 2 (2021), 174–178.

97. J. D. Roback, E. A. Tyburski, D. Alter, et al., The need for new test verification and regulatory support for innovative diagnostics. *Nat Biotechnol*, **39**, 9 (2021), 1060–1062.

98. J. K. Frediani, J. M. Levy, A. Rao, et al., Multidisciplinary assessment of the Abbott BinaxNOW SARS-CoV-2 point-of-care antigen test in the context of emerging viral variants and self-administration. *Sci Rep*, **11**, 1 (2021), 14604.

99. A. Rao, L. Bassit, J. Lin, et al., Assessment of the Abbott BinaxNOW SARS-CoV-2 rapid antigen test against viral variants of concern. *iScience*, **25**, 3 (2022), 103968.

100. F. Frank, M. M. Keen, A. Rao, et al., Deep mutational scanning identifies SARS-CoV-2 Nucleocapsid escape mutations of currently available rapid antigen tests. *Cell*, **185**, 19 (2022), 3603–3616.

101. B. Choi, M. C. Choudhary, J. Regan, et al., Persistence and evolution of SARS-CoV-2 in an immunocompromised host. *N Engl J Med*, **383**, 23 (2020), 2291–2293.

102. V. Borges, J. Isidro, M. Cunha, et al., Long-term evolution of SARS-CoV-2 in an immunocompromised patient with non-Hodgkin lymphoma. *mSphere*, **6**, 4 (2021), e00244-21.

103. S. A. Kemp, D. A. Collier, R. P. Datir, et al., SARS-CoV-2 evolution during treatment of chronic infection. *Nature*, **592**, 7853 (2021), 277–282.

104. B. B. Oude Munnink, R. S. Sikkema, D. F. Nieuwenhuijse, et al., Transmission of SARS-CoV-2 on mink farms between humans and mink and back to humans. *Science*, **371**, 6525 (2021), 172–177.

105. T. Sila, J. Sunghan, W. Laochareonsuk, et al., Suspected cat-to-human transmission of SARS-CoV-2, Thailand, July–September 2021. *Emerg Infect Dis*, **28**, 7 (2022), 1485–1488.

106. M. Martins, P. M. Boggiatto, A. Buckley, et al., From deer-to-deer: SARS-CoV-2 is efficiently transmitted and presents broad tissue tropism and replication sites in white-tailed deer. *PLoS Pathog*, **18**, 3 (2022), e1010197.

107. S. V. Kuchipudi, M. Surendran-Nair, R. M. Ruden, et al., Multiple spillovers from humans and onward transmission of SARS-CoV-2 in white-tailed deer. *Proc Natl Acad Sci*, **119**, 6 (2022), e2121644119.

108. R. T. Eguia, K. H. D. Crawford, T. Stevens-Ayers, et al., A human coronavirus evolves antigenically to escape antibody immunity. *PLoS Pathog*, **17**, 4 (2021), e1009453.

109. K. E. Kistler and T. Bedford, Evidence for adaptive evolution in the receptor-binding domain of seasonal coronaviruses OC43 and 229e. *eLife*, **10** (2021), e64509.

110. V. N. Petrova and C. A. Russell, The evolution of seasonal influenza viruses. *Nat Rev Microbiol*, **16**, 1 (2018), 47–60.

Chapter 1

The RADx® Regulatory Core and Its Role in COVID-19 Emergency Use Authorizations

Erika Tyburski and Cathryn Cambria

Introduction

The objective of this chapter is to describe the regulatory landscape during the COVID-19 pandemic in relation to the development of diagnostic tests for severe acute respiratory syndrome coronavirus 2 (SARS-CoV-2) and Emergency Use Authorization (EUA) approval by the US Food and Drug Administration (FDA). This chapter summarizes the genesis of the Rapid Acceleration of Diagnostics (RADx®) Regulatory Core and the validation testing requirements for molecular and antigen EUA submissions. The catalytic role of the Atlanta Center for Microsystems Engineered Point-of-Care Technologies (ACME POCT) as a coordinator and supporter of RADx on the development and clinical validation of tests in record time is discussed in detail. Founded in 2018, the ACME POCT is a team of academic and medical institutions, including Emory University, Georgia Tech, and Children's Healthcare of Atlanta, that works with industry and government to foster collaboration among clinicians, technologists, and entrepreneurs. Our center is one of five in the National Institutes of Health (NIH)-funded Point-of-Care Technology Research Network (POCTRN) and is led by principal investigators Greg Martin, M.D., Oliver Brand, Ph.D., and Wilbur Lam, M.D., Ph.D.

The mission of ACME POCT is to accelerate the innovation and translation of microsystems-engineered technologies, including microfluidic or microsensors-based point-of-care (POC) technologies, many of which are diagnostic or monitoring devices. In early 2020, conversations began around our center's involvement in assisting our nation by supporting test developers to significantly increase the diagnostic testing solutions available for COVID-19.

First, our center was requested to identify the resources that would be required to shepherd the rapid development of tests. We knew these resources would include regulatory and quality support and a direct line to the FDA. We presented the NIH with a condensed timeline for helping teams achieve EUAs in a matter of weeks and months instead of years. When the RADx initiative was officially launched, our stomachs flipped – we were excited and terrified by how much was at stake. Ultimately, over the course of RADx, eight regulatory team members worked with 35 project teams to obtain more than 30 EUAs, ultimately enabling millions of COVID-19 tests to make their way into laboratories, schools, POC settings, and homes.

RADx Regulatory Core

In April 2020, the ACME team met with the POCTRN chief, Steve Schachter, M.D., to share the list of resources and human capital that we felt would be essential to shepherd diagnostic tests for SARS-CoV-2 to market with speed and at scale. Along with the other POCTRN

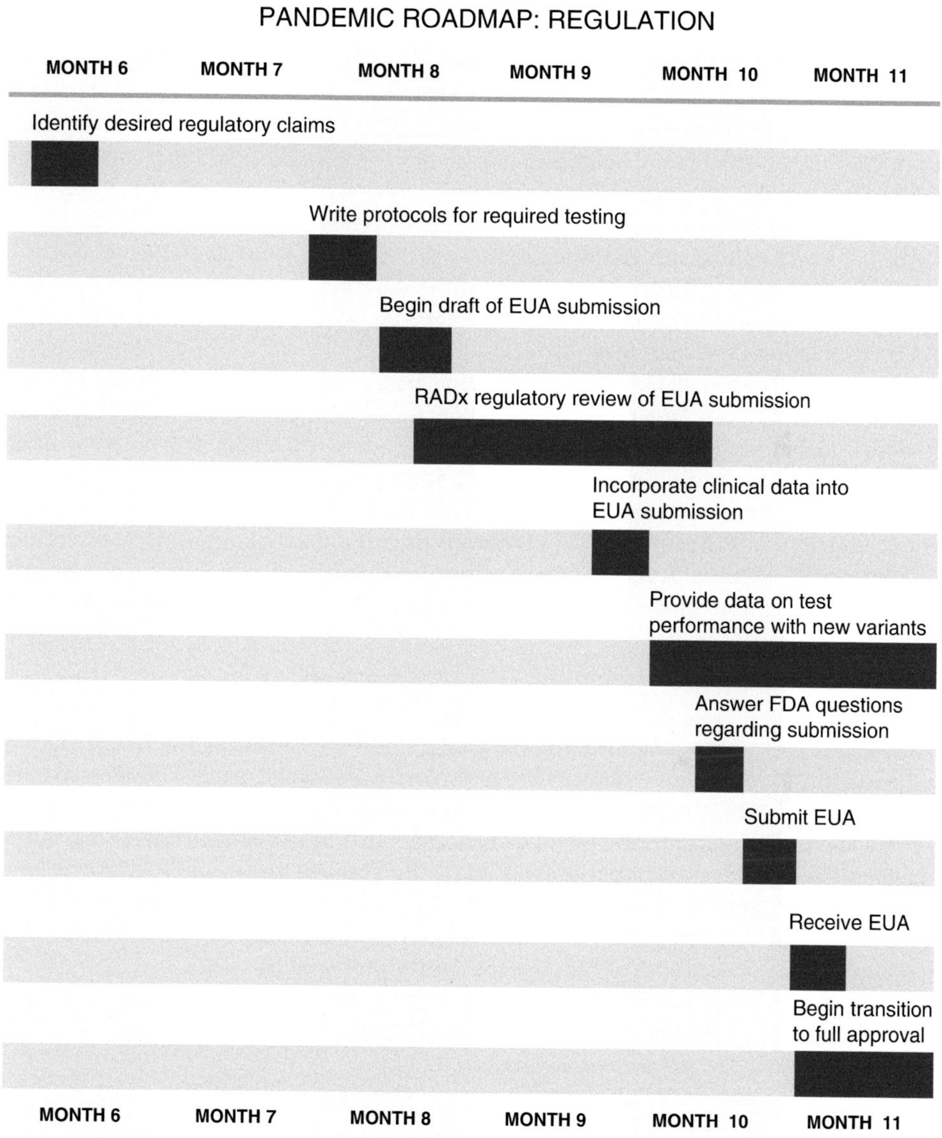

PANDEMIC ROADMAP: REGULATION

Figure 10.1 This roadmap depicts the vital activities, their chronology, and an estimated time frame in months. In the case of the SARS-CoV-2 pandemic, month 1 was December 2019, the month in which the virus was isolated, sequenced, identified, and published.

The tasks repeat with each new RADx Tech project.

centers, we were urged to establish proposals and budgets for verification testing, virology laboratory expertise and laboratory access, and additional operations support. Within 48 hours, we submitted a fully developed budget several times the size of our five-year center budget. We quickly engaged with a regulatory consultant within our Atlanta circle and formed our ACME regulatory team of three.

We knew that a critical factor in the success of this effort would be establishing a direct line with the FDA. Together, NIH and POCTRN worked with the FDA to put a plan in place. Typically – that is, not in a public health emergency – in vitro diagnostic tests are reviewed by the FDA via submissions under Section 510(k) of the Federal Food, Drug and Cosmetic Act and Q-submission meetings (Q-submissions are a way to request feedback from the FDA), which were scheduled 60–75 days in advance. By June 2020, we had established weekly meetings about the RADx pandemic response with the FDA every Wednesday. The calls were moderated by Dr. Nancy Gagliano, and representatives across RADx were welcome to join and listen in as we presented the latest questions on behalf of the RADx Tech teams. We were astonished at how quickly the machine was moving. As the pipeline of RADx teams grew, additional regulatory consultants joined the RADx team. The RADx Regulatory Core was born.

The goal of the Regulatory Core was to offer regulatory and quality consultation and services to RADx Tech project teams to support the de-risking of these technologies and to optimize their chances for deployment. To that end, we continued to interact with the FDA regularly to ask questions, to determine appropriate use cases and use settings for proposed testing technologies (i.e. performed by laboratories with a Clinical Laboratory Improvement Amendments [CLIA] certificate [high/moderate complexity], performed by laboratories with a CLIA certificate of waiver [POC settings], and for use in home self-testing), and to identify the validation testing required for a specific technology to obtain an EUA.

FDA's Role

The FDA is responsible for protecting the public's health by ensuring the safety, efficacy, and security of human and veterinary drugs, biological products, medical devices, cosmetics, products that emit radiation, and our nation's food supply. As it pertains to medical devices and in vitro diagnostics, the FDA typically – that is, not in the context of a public emergency – reviews several types of applications, for example 510(k) applications, de novo applications, and premarket approvals (PMAs). The type of application depends on whether there is a preexisting FDA-cleared product to which the candidate product can establish substantial equivalence (both technically and for the proposed use case), as well as the risk categorization. Differences in risk are assigned different classes; class I devices demonstrate low risk, class II devices demonstrate moderate risk, and class III devices demonstrate high risk, as summarized as follows and in Table 10.1:

- **510(k):** In general, if the risk of the proposed product is similar to that of existing products on the market and there is substantially equivalent technology being used, the path is a 510(k) premarket notification, wherein the sponsor establishes substantial equivalence of the proposed product to a predicate and the FDA "clears" the device for market
- **PMA:** When no such predicate exists and the proposed product has a significant risk profile, the sponsor must pursue "approval" via a PMA path
- **De novo:** For devices that do not have a suitable predicate but have less risk than a PMA product, the FDA created the de novo pathway for device pre-market notification "clearance"

Table 10.1 Typical regulatory paths (in vitro diagnostics)

Class	Risk level	Controls required	Typical premarket path	Examples
Class I	Low	Exempt from premarket notification and/or regulatory controls are applied (e.g. general controls and good manufacturing practices unless specifically exempted)	510(k) or 510(k) exempt	Total cholesterol, triglycerides
Class II	Moderate	General and special controls are applied (informed by guidance documents)	510(k) or de novo application	Blood glucose monitors (i.e. the majority of POC in vitro diagnostics)
Class III	High	General, special, and PMA controls are applied	PMA	Implantable pacemakers

Emergency Use Authorization

The Public Health Service Act, under section 319, allows the Secretary of the Department of Health and Human Services (HHS) to declare a public health emergency. After a 90-day period, a public health emergency is either renewed by the secretary or terminated if the secretary declares that the public health emergency no longer exists. On February 4, 2020, on the basis of a section 319 determination, the HHS Secretary declared a public health emergency due to the emergence of COVID-19. On March 24, 2020, the HHS Secretary justified the authorization of emergency use of in vitro diagnostics for the detection and/or diagnosis of this novel coronavirus (2019-nCoV) pursuant to section 564 of the Federal Food, Drug and Cosmetic Act, subject to the terms of any authorization issued under that section, enabling the EUA regulatory pathway. The pathway enables the FDA to weigh the benefits of new products against the risks to address the public health emergency when no alternatives exist.

The EUA path typically requires a much smaller quantity of data to determine effectiveness than what is required for a 510(k), de novo, or PMA application, and reviewing EUAs is prioritized to ensure products become available in a timely manner. Devices following the 510(k) path are "FDA cleared" through premarket notification, de novo devices are granted marketing authorization under a new classification regulation, PMA devices are "FDA approved," and EUAs are totally separate.

Shortly after the announcement, the FDA released guidelines on how to request an EUA. Three categories of tests were immediately addressed: tests that detect actual virus or ribonucleic acid (RNA) (molecular tests), tests that detect antigen proteins from virus (antigen tests), and tests that detect the presence of antibodies after exposure to the virus (serology tests). For the purposes of COVID-19 detection during active infection, the RADx Tech initiative focused on antigen and molecular tests.

Molecular Tests

Most molecular tests for SARS-CoV-2 rely on a workflow similar to that of real-time reverse transcription polymerase chain reaction (RT-PCR) tests. These assays extract, amplify, and/or multiply the number of viral RNA molecules present in a respiratory sample via chemicals and heat cycling. Using this workflow, RNA is replicated after each heat cycle, whereby each cycle consists of different temperatures held for different amounts of time. The number of heat cycles needed to detect the target is inversely proportional to the amount of virus in the sample, that is, the lower the number of cycles, the higher the viral load. This is where the term cycle threshold (Ct) value comes from: the number of heat cycles a device completes before the virus is detected in the sample. Although Ct is a number, Ct values are not quantitative when it comes to comparing samples between different molecular platforms. This is because the assays work differently and have different heat cycles; thus, cycle thresholds vary across platforms.

Molecular testing with viral extraction and heat cycling is considered the most sensitive category of COVID-19 testing due to its ability to detect even small amounts of virus from a single sample. While RT-PCR is the most traditional method for detecting the COVID-19 virus, it typically requires complex instrumentation run by trained personnel and is a time-consuming method, taking several hours to complete a single test. Other molecular testing methods, such as loop-mediated isothermal amplification (LAMP) tests, can be done with a single constant temperature and do not require thermal cyclers, thus reducing cost and the time to complete a test (typically under one hour).

Antigen Tests

The majority of antigen tests detect the presence of antigen proteins on the surface of a virus. For COVID-19 tests, the most commonly targeted proteins are the spike (S) protein and the nucleocapsid (N) protein. The S protein is located on the surface of the coronavirus, while the N protein is expressed during replication of viral RNA. This means that the N protein is typically more conserved, even as a virus mutates into different variants or strains, making it a common target for antigen assays.

The typical workflow for an antigen test is direct detection of the protein in the sample via an enzyme-linked immunosorbent assay (ELISA), wherein antibodies for the target antigen are bound to a surface, most often a nitrocellulose strip. If the antigen protein is present, it will be collected at the antibody site and exhibit a color. Many antigen tests are lateral flow assays, similar to pregnancy tests, where the antibody–antigen reaction happens in a short time (15 minutes or less) and a line is exhibited that is visible to the naked eye. Antigen tests are usually not as sensitive as molecular tests across stages of infection because there are times when viruses express higher and lower levels of protein. Some may argue that what antigen tests lack in sensitivity they make up for in affordability, rapid time to result, and simple workflows that can be conducted in remote and home settings by lay users. Furthermore, it can be argued that serial testing (i.e. testing of an individual multiple times over a specific duration of hours/days) can drastically improve sensitivity.[1]

With an unprecedented demand for testing that was growing rapidly, the industry quickly realized that testing efficiency needed to be improved. There simply are not enough laboratories, personnel, instrumentation, or supplies to conduct RT-PCR tests on hundreds of millions of US citizens at once.

Diagnostic tests are typically conducted in high- or moderate-complexity laboratories and are categorized as such under CLIA. In addition, there are tests categorized as CLIA waived, which are performed in CLIA-waived laboratories (typically POC environments), while other tests that can be performed via self-testing at home, which are cleared or authorized for home prescription and over-the-counter use and are not regulated under CLIA. Because the EUA path is designed to be fast to market, tests that receive an EUA from the FDA are not formally CLIA categorized, but rather are deemed for use in a specific setting by the FDA, that is, in either high- or moderate-complexity settings and in CLIA-waived settings or in home settings.

Improving test throughput and efficiency meant enabling more testing to be done in simpler settings, outside high- and moderate-complexity laboratories. However, designing tests and workflows for POC and at-home settings poses significant challenges. In CLIA-waived or POC settings, staff are minimally trained and testing methods must be simple enough to preclude requiring outside training or specialized, calibrated, or otherwise maintained equipment, apart from the testing materials provided with a test kit or system. Home testing methods must be as simple as possible and must include internal onboard controls sufficient to communicate to a layperson whether the test is working.

To address shortcomings in COVID-19 test availability, the RADx Tech initiative had two main areas of focus:

1. The improvement in efficiency and throughput of traditional, laboratory-based RT-PCR testing methods
2. The validation of novel testing methods that could be used by untrained personnel in the simplest of environments. For our regulatory team, that meant assessing tests for their compatibility with broader use cases and assisting companies with the validation testing required to achieve an EUA through either of these paths

Anatomy of an EUA Application

The RADx Tech Regulatory Core was involved in the planning and review of countless validation studies that were required to be granted an EUA. All molecular and antigen test EUA submissions required validation data in five areas:

1. limit of detection (LoD) (analytical sensitivity)
2. inclusivity (analytical reactivity)
3. cross-reactivity (analytical specificity) and interference testing
4. stability
5. clinical evaluation results

EUA submissions for CLIA-waived testing sites (POC) and home self-tests also needed to include usability and flex studies. These are described in greater detail in the "Usability Studies" and "Flex Studies" subsections under the "Clinical Evaluation" section that follows.

Note, depending on the specific test methodology, being granted an EUA could require additional testing that is specific to the assay. The list above does not include all elements of an EUA submission and focuses on validation requirements expressed by the FDA via EUA templates.

Limit of Detection (Analytical Sensitivity)

The LoD is defined as the lowest concentration of an analyte in a sample that can be consistently detected with a stated probability (typically at 95% certainty). The LoD is typically evaluated following the Clinical and Laboratory Standards Institutes (CLSI) guidance entitled *CLSI EP17 Evaluation of Detection Capability for Clinical Laboratory Measurement Procedures*. An LoD study should be the first analytical study completed for an EUA and consists of two parts: the preliminary LoD and the confirmed LoD.

For all sample types being pursued, the FDA recommends that the preliminary LoD be determined by testing a two- or threefold dilution series (using a negative matrix and inactivated virus of a currently circulating variant/strain) of three replicates per concentration, which is then confirmed with 20 replicates of the concentration determined to be the preliminary LoD. The preliminary LoD is the lowest concentration that gives positive results 100% of the time, and the final or confirmed LoD is the lowest concentration at which at least 19 of the 20 replicates are positive. The preliminary LoD studies should include at least one concentration that does not yield 100% positive results. When presenting the data in an EUA submission, it is important to show both passing and failing results of LoD testing.

Inclusivity (Analytical Reactivity)

A COVID-19 EUA submission had to address how the sponsor would monitor and assess the impact of new and emerging variants, mutations, and strains of the SARS-CoV-2 virus on the performance of the assay. Mutations (defined as changes in the genomic sequence from the wild type or the original strain, including amino acid insertions, deletions, and substitutions) have been detected in the SARS-CoV-2 genome throughout the pandemic, resulting in many virus variants. Mutations and variants can affect both molecular and antigen test performance. To assess the impact of new variants, molecular test sponsors were encouraged to consult the Global Initiative on Sharing All Influenza Data (GISAID) database of SARS-CoV-2 sequences with regular frequency (e.g. every two weeks or at least monthly) to confirm which sequences were prevalent in at least 5% of the population. For any viral mutations and variants that are identified as prevalent and/or clinically significant, as described above, sponsors needed to assess whether the resulting predicted amino acid change(s) in the viral proteins were critical to the test design.

For molecular assays, this can be accomplished via *in silico* analysis of published SARS-CoV-2 sequences compared with the assay's primers and probes. For antigen assays, an epitope map is a useful tool in assessing the potential effects of emerging mutations and variants. An epitope map is assay-specific and is completed via experimentally identifying the binding site (epitope) of an antibody on its target antigen (typically the S or N protein).

If mutations are found to be critical to the test design, such mutations and variants should be evaluated using clinical (or contrived as available and as appropriate) samples to assess the impact of the mutation or variant on test performance. The aggregate effect of the mutations should not reduce the clinical performance of the test by 5% or more. Therefore, this part of an EUA submission needed to include a plan specific to the assay for monitoring new variants, as well as a plan for assessing if any prevalent variants affected assay performance.

Cross-Reactivity (Analytical Specificity) and Interference Testing

Cross-reactivity studies are performed to demonstrate that the test does not react with related pathogens, high-prevalence disease agents, or normal or pathogenic flora that are reasonably likely to be encountered in the clinical sample or matrix. The FDA recommended that specific species be tested for respiratory and saliva samples according to Tables 10.2 and 10.3.

The sponsor must first have completed cross-reactivity testing, which tests for the chances of false-positive results when a species is present in a negative matrix. Then, if species are not cross-reactive, they also needed to be tested for microbial interference, wherein species are tested in combination with inactivated SARS-CoV-2 at two or three times the LoD of the assay to assess for the potential of false negatives. Testing is recommended to be in triplicate for each condition and at concentrations of 10^6 colony-forming units (CFU)/ml (or higher for bacteria) and 10^5 plaque-forming units (PFU)/ml or median tissue culture infective dose (TCID50)/ml (or higher for viruses) as shown in Tables 10.2 and 10.3.

Note, FDA EUA templates for COVID-19 assays should be checked for the most up-to-date list of organisms and agents to be tested. Additionally, when a concentration is not provided in the EUA template, the sponsor should check *CLSI EP07 Interference Testing in Clinical Chemistry*. If a concentration is not available in CLSI EP07, then the sponsor should provide an explanation or justification of the concentration selected.

Interference testing is also required of samples that contain a potential interfering substance with and without inactivated SARS-CoV-2 virus at two or three times the LoD. The list of interfering substances to be tested varies based on the sample type of the assay, as shown in Tables 10.4 and 10.5.

If an assay used a biotin capture system, biotin interference testing was also required. For antigen assays, a high-dose hook effect analysis was also required. The assay must be tested at very high concentrations of SARS-CoV-2 to ensure that the test does not produce false-negative results at very high concentrations of the virus.

Stability

There are several parts of the stability section of an EUA: sample stability, transport/shipping stability, and shelf-life stability.

Sample stability

Sample stability testing is designed to ensure that samples remain viable during collection and during any perceived wait times before testing according to assay instructions for use. For tests designed for POC and home settings, testing is required to be performed for time periods that are at least 10% longer than claimed in the instructions for use to show robustness, even in nonideal conditions. Each sample stability claim is supported by testing at least 30 samples at one or two times the LoD, 10 samples at three to five times the LoD, and 10 samples that are negative. This design may also be used to support the use of frozen samples if the sponsor used frozen or banked samples to support the clinical validation of the assay. In this case, the sponsor would conduct the testing on both fresh and frozen samples to show equivalence in performance.

Table 10.2 Recommended list of organisms to be analyzed *in silico* and by wet testing for all respiratory samples[*]

High-priority pathogens from the same genetic family	High-priority organisms likely present in respiratory samples
Human coronavirus 229E (wet testing)	Adenovirus (e.g. C1 Ad. 71) (wet testing)
Human coronavirus OC43 (wet testing)	Human metapneumovirus (wet testing)
Human coronavirus NL63 (wet testing)	Parainfluenza virus 1–4 (wet testing)
MERS coronavirus (wet testing)	Influenza A and B (wet testing)
SARS coronavirus (wet testing)	Enterovirus (wet testing)
Human coronavirus HKU1 (*in silico* [protein blast] testing)	Respiratory syncytial virus (wet testing)
	Rhinovirus (wet testing)
	Haemophilus influenzae (wet testing)
	Streptococcus pneumoniae (wet testing)
	Streptococcus pyogenes (wet testing)
	Candida albicans (wet testing)
	Pooled human nasal wash – representative of normal respiratory microbial flora (wet testing)
	Bordetella pertussis (wet testing)
	Mycoplasma pneumoniae (wet testing)
	Chlamydia pneumoniae (wet testing)
	Legionella pneumophila (wet testing)
	Staphylococcus aureus (wet testing)
	Staphylococcus epidermidis (wet testing)
	Mycobacterium tuberculosis (*in silico* [protein blast] testing)[**]
	Pneumocystis jirovecii (*in silico* [protein blast] testing)[**]

MERS, Middle East respiratory syndrome; SARS, severe acute respiratory syndrome.
[*] Content of table reproduced directly from FDA template.[2]
[**] *M. tuberculosis* and *P. jirovecii* are applicable to lower respiratory matrices only (e.g. bronchoalveolar lavage and sputum).

Table 10.3 High-priority organisms likely present in saliva samples: recommended list of organisms to be analyzed *in silico* and by wet testing of saliva samples[*, **]

Other high-priority pathogens from the same genetic family	High-priority organisms likely in the circulating area
Human coronavirus 229E (wet testing)	Adenovirus (e.g. C1 Ad. 71) (wet testing)
Human coronavirus OC43 (wet testing)	Human metapneumovirus (wet testing)
Human coronavirus NL63 (wet testing)	Parainfluenza virus 1–4 (wet testing)
MERS coronavirus (wet testing)	Influenza A and B (wet testing)
SARS coronavirus (wet testing)	Rhinovirus (wet testing)
Human coronavirus HKU1 (*in-silico* [protein blast] testing)	Respiratory syncytial virus (wet testing)
	Herpes simplex virus 1 (wet testing)
	Epstein–Barr virus (wet testing)
	Cytomegalovirus (wet testing)
	Moraxella catarrhalis (wet testing)
	Porphyromonas gingivalis (wet testing)
	Bacteroides oralis (wet testing)
	Nocardia species (wet testing)
	Streptococcus mutans (wet testing)
	Streptococcus mitis or other viridans streptococci (wet testing)
	Eikenella species (wet testing)
	Neisseria species (wet testing)
	Candida albicans (wet testing)
	Pseudomonas aeruginosa (wet testing)
	Staphylococcus epidermis (wet testing)
	Streptococcus salivarius (wet testing)

MERS, Middle East respiratory syndrome; SARS, severe acute respiratory syndrome.
* Content of table reproduced directly from FDA template.[2]
** These organisms should be analyzed/tested in addition to the ones included in Table 10.2.

Transport Stability

Transport stability is designed to characterize the potential effects of storage variability on the unopened kit or assay. The most common transport studies include summer and winter cycling and extended thermal exposure studies. Summer cycling includes storage at several

Table 10.4 List of potential interfering substances recommended for testing when the candidate test is indicated for respiratory samples*

Potential interfering substances	Concentration
Whole blood	4%
Mucin	0.5%
Chloraseptic (menthol/benzocaine)	1.5 mg/ml
Naso GEL (NeilMed)	5% v/v
CVS Nasal Drops (phenylephrine)	15% v/v
Afrin (oxymetazoline)	15% v/v
CVS Nasal Spray (cromolyn)	15% v/v
Zicam	5% v/v
Homeopathic (Alkalol)	1:10 dilution
Sore throat phenol spray	15% v/v
Tobramycin	4 µg/ml
Mupirocin	10 mg/ml
Fluticasone propionate	5% v/v
Tamiflu (oseltamivir phosphate)	5 mg/ml

v/v, volume per volume (volume concentration of a solution).
* Content of table reproduced directly from FDA template.[3]

temperatures above room temperature for specified time frames. Winter cycling includes storage at several temperatures below room temperature for specified time frames. The assay is then tested using samples prepared at three to five times the LoD, preferably on at least three lots with five replicates per lot. Open kit stability should also be assessed, when applicable. This is especially important for POC tests, when an operator may be delayed in performing the test steps because of a busy working environment, or in the case of a home self-test, owing to potential distractions in a home setting.

Shelf-Life Testing

Real-time shelf-life testing is required to support the labeling of the assay. During the pandemic, accelerated shelf-life testing data were generally not acceptable to support long shelf-life claims at the time of authorization. Real-time shelf-life studies are ongoing and constantly updated. At the time of granting of an EUA, sponsors were granted six months of stability to enable speed to market. As a condition of authorization, sponsors are required to complete real-time shelf-life testing using a protocol agreed with the FDA and must report to the FDA with each time point of new data.

Table 10.5 List of potential interfering substances recommended for testing when the candidate test is indicated for saliva and oral samples[*]

Substance	Concentration[**]
Cepacol lozenges (benzocaine/menthol)	3 mg/ml
Cough drops (dextromethorphan HBr)	
Robitussin	
Chloroseptic sore throat spray (phenolglycerin)	5% v/v
Emergen-C (zinc, magnesium, riboflavin, vitamin C)	
Crest/Listerine mouthwash (eucalyptol, menthol, methyl salicylate, thymol)	5% v/v
Act dry mouth lozenges (isomalt, xylitol, glycerin)	
Toothpaste (Colgate)	0.5% v/v
Nyquil (acetaminophen, doxylamine succinate, extromethorphan HBr)	
Mucin: bovine submaxillary gland, type I-S	2.5 mg/ml
Human genomic DNA	10 ng/µl
Vaseline (petroleum Jelly)	
Nicotine	0.03 mg/ml
Alcohol (ethanol)	5%
White blood cells/leukocytes	1 to 5×10^6 cells/ml
Whole blood	2.5%

[*] Content of table reproduced directly from FDA template.[3]
[**] For concentrations not specified in the EUA templates, sponsors should propose a reasonable concentration found in physiological levels, as applicable to the candidate assay.

Clinical Evaluation

A clinical evaluation is designed to evaluate the performance of the assay on real clinical samples, by the target end users, and in the desired use setting. The requirement for high-complexity laboratories, moderate-complexity laboratories, and CLIA-waived testing sites (POC settings) is to collect and report data on a minimum of 30 positive and 30 negative samples. In general, tests designed for the home (self-testing) require a minimum of 30 positive and 100 negative samples. Testing must be done on the candidate assay and a high sensitivity molecular comparator (typically an RT-PCR EUA assay with a separate extraction step). Of the positive samples tested, there is also a requirement for at least 25% of the samples to be low positive results according to the Ct value of the comparator for a molecular candidate assay; this figure is 10–20% for an antigen candidate assay. In general, for molecular tests, the positive percent agreement (PPA) between the candidate and comparator assays is expected to be 95% or more. In general, for antigen tests, the PPA is expected to be 80% or more. The negative percent agreement (NPA) is expected to be 98% or more.

Additional studies required for POC tests that are "deemed CLIA-waived" and home (non-laboratory) tests are summarized in the following subsections.

Performance around LoD

Performance around LoD is part of the clinical evaluation for CLIA-waived (POC) assays. This substudy is designed to assess if the untrained operators can perform the test correctly to identify negative samples and positive samples at very low viral load of less than two times the LoD. During the clinical evaluation, contrived samples are incorporated into the POC workflow. Operators are blinded to the status of these samples and process at least three low positive samples and three negative samples as if they were clinical samples. These results are reported separately from the clinical PPA and NPA calculations.

Flex Studies

Flex studies are conducted to support the robustness of the assay during nonideal use by untrained operators for either the POC or home use setting. Flex studies should be informed by a detailed risk analysis conducted by the sponsor that is specific to the assay's technology, use case, and workflow. In general, the FDA recommends testing the following: testing at high heat and humidity, testing after a delay in sample testing or test read time, testing early or after delays and disturbances in test steps, testing with sample volume variability, and testing with buffer volume variability and with test read time variability. Each testing condition should be compared with control (ideal use) results done with at least triplicate negative and triplicate positive samples at two or three times the LoD.

Usability Studies

Usability studies are generally conducted before the clinical evaluation to inform any changes to the workflow or labeling that would improve performance or usability by a lay user. Results are also used to support an assay's ease of use by the target POC operator or home user. In general, the design comparison is similar to the clinical evaluation, but the study participants are observed more closely to determine if they are performing the test accurately. Participants are also surveyed after completion of the test and specifically asked about ease of use.

Protocols, raw data, and summarized results of the studies are provided along with the EUA submission to support the validation of the assay for an EUA. It is important to note that, upon authorization, each sponsor received a post-market commitment letter detailing the requirements of the sponsor that would continue after authorization.

Post-Market Commitments

To enable speed to market, the FDA has the authority to require sponsors to complete certain tasks and ongoing studies as post-market commitments. The commitments are made public on the FDA's website in sponsor letters of authorization upon the granting of an EUA. Such commitments typically include making instructions for use and other labeling documentation publicly available on the FDA's website, post-market clinical evaluations, ongoing shelf-life studies, and notifications to the FDA of any changes to labeling or distributors. Some commitments have timelines associated with them, to which sponsors and FDA reviewers agree prior to the issuance of an EUA.

EUA Process Evolution

The previous sections summarize the typical anatomy of an EUA. Although all EUAs include these parts, the EUA process evolved as the pandemic continued, as summarized in the following subsections.

Ebbs and Flows

There have been a few notable points of flexibility in the pandemic, specifically with respect to the availability of clinical samples. For example, there were some time periods when prevalence plummeted, and it became difficult to obtain the 30 positive samples needed for a complete EUA clinical evaluation. Despite the prevalence dropping, there was still a need to improve testing availability, as many locations began to require screening programs to mitigate disease spread. In this case, the FDA extended flexibility to sponsors, accepting a portion of the clinical sample requirement at the time of authorization and agreeing to review the balance of clinical sample testing results as the evaluation continued after authorization as a post-market commitment. We saw this flexibility wane as prevalence returned and positive clinical samples became available once more. Often, the availability of positive samples would rebound due to the emergence of a new variant. As new variants emerged, the FDA added new recommendations into EUA templates, including the recommendation to complete analytical testing with the most common variants or strains in circulation. Indeed, the first strains detected (Wuhan and Washington) became obsolete after the subsequent variants replaced them (e.g. omicron). This also led to the FDA–RADx initiative for variant analysis called the Variant Task Force for continued assessment of the impact of new variants on EUA tests (see Chapter 9 for more information).

Laboratory-Developed Tests

Another example of the evolving regulatory EUA landscape concerns laboratory-developed tests (LDTs). LDTs are generally deemed low-risk products/tests that are designed, produced, manufactured, and limited to performance within a single CLIA-certified laboratory for clinical use. The FDA has traditionally exercised enforcement discretion over LDTs, and these laboratories independently validate the testing offered under CLIA regulations. During the pandemic, under the FDA's authority for COVID-19 tests, many laboratories created and independently validated their methods and did serve as a testing resource through the agency's EUA review process. However, from August 2020 to November 2021, the FDA's authority over LDTs was revoked. The guidance document entitled *Policy for Coronavirus Disease-2019 Tests During the Public Health Emergency (Revised)* was issued on November 15, 2021, and required LDTs to be reviewed by the FDA to obtain an EUA.

New Right of References

Right of reference (RoR) is a term used to describe a sponsor's ability to reference an external group's work to substantiate a claim. RoRs are important for the entire industry, as they are designed to allow sponsors to leverage previous work and alleviate the burden for future sponsors. The FDA established the device master file system to preserve trade secrets and confidential data of a company. Throughout the pandemic, sponsors leveraged several RoRs for testing. For example, the Centers for Disease Control and Prevention and ThermoFisher issued RoRs to allow the FDA to review their confidential information in the context of the applicant's EUA submission for SARS-CoV-2 detection without allowing the applicant to have direct access to the information. The FDA also collaborated with RADx POCTRN centers and ACME POCT for creating an RoR for pediatric self-swabbing[4] (FDA master file number MAF3543) and with the Center for Advancing Point of Care Technologies (CAPCaT) for establishing the performance of serial testing for antigen home tests.[1] Both RADx RoRs have been used by the FDA to make generalizable conclusions about pediatric self-swabbing and serial testing. The FDA based its recent recommendation for serial testing labeling for all antigen tests on the CAPCaT dataset.

The EUA path is designed to address shortages in traditionally used testing methods to enable more testing throughput. As more and more tests become available on the market via EUA, needs are addressed, and the need for additional EUA tests goes down. This is especially true when prevalence dips and the national demand for testing drops. On the other hand, we have been shown time and time again that we should not become complacent because prevalence can rise just as fast as it falls. Even now, at the time of writing this chapter, we continue to see the FDA's approach to EUAs evolve. Currently (in winter 2022), we are experiencing a season with a high incidence of acute respiratory illnesses that include COVID-19, influenza, and respiratory syncytial virus (RSV), sometimes coexisting with one another. This has created the need for more access to multiplex tests for the identification of a respiratory illness when symptoms are often nonspecific. As such, RADx has started a new initiative for multiplex tests, and the FDA recently granted an EUA for POC assays that differentiate between COVID-19, influenza A, and influenza B.

Regulatory Future for COVID-19 Tests

The RADx Tech Regulatory Core has been a huge success. Having streamlined the process with the FDA and assisted more than 30 RADx Tech teams with their regulatory paths for EUA, we are often faced with lingering questions: How long will the pandemic last? How long will sponsors be able to market COVID-19 tests with an EUA? When will I have to convert my EUA into a 510(k) or de novo application?

Although we cannot answer when a pandemic may be declared "over" or when EUA assays will no longer be marketed, we are making efforts to set sponsors up for success when approaching their full authorizations (510[k] or de novo). We are discussing requirements and working with the FDA to optimize the chances of pooling EUA data with full authorization data. Full authorization will require additional clinical sample testing and reproducibility and repeatability testing, but sponsors should engage with their FDA reviewer to confirm what additional considerations should be made. Additionally, sponsors should consult the *Best Practices for the Design of Accessible COVID-19 Home Tests*[5] created by the RADx Accessibility Group during test design to address text perception, general readability and layout, physical embodiment, graphics, images, symbols, and language to ensure an accessible test. Test accessibility is an ongoing collaborative effort between RADx and the FDA.

Pandemic Response, Over-the-Counter Tests, and POC Tests Forever Changed

The COVID-19 pandemic has been one of the longest lasting public emergencies worldwide. As the virus spread, the USA had to rapidly address testing needs. RADx has been one of the most impactful collaborations between the US government, regulating agencies, and industry in working toward the common goal of making reliable testing available in a more timely manner. Work by the NIH, the POCTRN centers, the FDA, the Centers for Medicare and Medicaid Services, and all of the sponsors we have supported at the time of writing this book has resulted in 50 EUA tests that have been deployed in all settings across the USA – from high-complexity laboratories with automation and robotics to drastically improve testing capacity, through POC settings for rapid testing in local pharmacies and tent drive-throughs, to the home setting, where millions of US citizens have been delivered self-tests right to their front door. This pandemic has truly highlighted the power of streamlining the regulatory approach, which should be preserved to remain prepared for any new health emergency that the USA may face.

Particularly for POC and home tests, RADx Tech assisted the FDA in identifying the sponsors' and testing facilities' questions, which led to appropriate test designs to support highly specific use cases, ranging from high-volume university screening programs to individuals testing themselves at home. As a result, we have been able to witness the power of providing simple yet reliable testing in the hands of the general population to assist in a widespread effort to curb the spread of a deadly virus.

At the start of the pandemic, very few in the general population knew how to collect a nasal or saliva sample. Very few knew what a PCR test was and how it was different from a rapid test. Now, our neighbors, relatives, and colleagues can perform a COVID-19 home test and have even followed up with confirmatory testing after receiving a rapid test result. Many are reporting results to their health-care providers or even reporting on websites and smartphone apps with ease. Furthermore, some families have even mirrored testing requirements for travel for their own family events and requested rapid test results to determine if the group should gather for a holiday. Having experienced this firsthand in the lead author's family, we were able to identify family members who were positive for COVID-19 and prevent them from infecting others. Knowledge of not only how to perform home tests *but also what to do with the results* has unlocked the potential for more POC and home testing. As such, home testing has enabled self-screening and has the potential to lower infections at the community level.

The widespread foundation of knowledge and demand allows for the creation of new POC and home tests, and pathways in between, such as the observed telehealth testing. Indeed, rapid POC and self-tests have become ubiquitous, commonplace, and expected by the public. Even three years after the beginning of the pandemic, there is a strong demand for multiplex tests for other respiratory illnesses alongside COVID-19, such as influenza, RSV, and even strep throat, from both health-care providers and the general population alike – and there are many test developers and manufacturers aiming to fill that demand. Recently, we have seen a few multiplex POC assays receive EUAs, and we look forward to the potential for multiplex tests for home use. We have also seen recent interagency support for increasing domestic manufacturing throughput for testing to prepare for any future public health emergencies.[6] Overall, we expect that rapid, POC, and self-testing will extend to conditions beyond respiratory illnesses as a new standard of test availability and preparedness. We will remember this pandemic and the foundation of knowledge that was built to make long-standing testing availability the new standard for generations to come.

Lessons Learned

Valuable lessons were identified through the implementation and execution of the RADx Tech Regulatory Core, as follows:

- Direct and frequent communication between RADx Tech and the FDA allowed for efficient information sharing as the virus evolved and pandemic needs shifted. Fluid communication helped in the determination of appropriate use cases and use settings for proposed testing technologies
- This pandemic enabled widespread POC and home self-testing. The RADx Tech initiative created important RoRs for test developers, including bridging the gap for pediatric self-swabbing and determining effective testing frequency for serial home testing
- There is a strong continued desire to have multiplex tests for respiratory illness (COVID-19, influenza A, influenza B, and/or RSV, among others) for differentiating respiratory illnesses in both POC and home settings

References

1. A. Soni, C. Herbert, H. Lin, et al., Performance of screening for SARS-CoV-2 using rapid antigen tests to detect incidence of symptomatic and asymptomatic SARS-CoV-2 infection: findings from the Test Us at Home prospective cohort study. *medRxiv* (2022). https://doi.org/10.1101/2022.08.05.22278466.

2. FDA, *Template for Developers of Molecular Diagnostic Tests* (2021). www.fda.gov/media/135900/download.

3. FDA, *Template for Developers of Antigen Tests* (2021). www.fda.gov/media/137907/download.

4. J. J. Waggoner, M. B. Vos, E. A. Tyburski, et al., Concordance of SARS-CoV-2 results in self-collected nasal swabs vs swabs collected by health care workers in children and adolescents. *JAMA*, **328**, 10 (2022), 935–940.

5. US Access Board, *Best Practices for the Design of Accessible COVID-19 Home Tests*. www.access-board.gov/tad/radx.

6. J. S. Eglovitch, Budget law calls for BARDA and FDA to establish "warm base" manufacturing to better prepare for future pandemics. *Regulatory Focus* (January 16, 2023).

Chapter 11

Commercialization and Market Assessment of COVID-19 Assays

Manuel Kingsley, Sunshine Moore, Heath Naquin, Eliseo Velasquez, Emily Kennedy, and Grace Bendinger

Introduction

Commercialization is the process of bringing products and services to market, that is, moving intellectual assets out of theoretical practice and into active use within a commercial environment. Typically, the commercialization process (also known as technology transfer) includes an ideation (or funnel) phase, business setup, beta market testing, stakeholder engagement, and business development.

In the Rapid Acceleration of Diagnostics (RADx®) Tech context of a global pandemic, the National Institutes of Health (NIH) supported a funnel/deep dive phase designed to fund projects developing severe acute respiratory syndrome coronavirus 2 (SARS-CoV-2) assays with the best chance of scientific and technical viability, with less emphasis on commercial viability. Once selected, the individual steps in the commercialization process were engineered to occur simultaneously rather than sequentially. RADx Tech portfolio companies needed to pursue clinical validation and regulatory approval in parallel with developing core business functions, conducting market research and financial modeling, preparing to scale up production and distribution, and engaging potential buyers. To accomplish this, RADx Tech provided projects with extensive support in both their clinical and their commercial operations.

This chapter explores the process of bringing RADx-funded products to market, the core functions of the RADx Tech commercialization team, the go-to-market strategies and testing approaches that worked well, regulatory and policy barriers that hindered broader commercial success, the impact of digital solutions on future diagnostic workflows, and the lessons learned to inform future pandemic preparedness.

Commercialization centers on the intersection between scientific advancement, product development, and market dynamics. For example, an established contract manufacturing firm may be able to produce and distribute millions of tests, but that does not automatically translate to widespread accessibility. Bringing new diagnostics to market takes five to seven years, on average. RADx Tech sought to make fast, cheap, reliable, and user-friendly tests widely accessible in less than eight months. Ultimately, RADx Tech's success is reflected in the number of Emergency Use Authorizations (EUAs) approved in such a short time frame (50 EUAs in under three years) and the sheer volume of tests produced (5 billion as of November 2022). However, some tests were more commercially successful than others.

Core Functions

The RADx commercialization team played a role that was complementary to yet distinct from other RADx segments. Whereas the Deployment Core assisted portfolio companies in scaling up manufacturing, securing raw materials, and contracting with suppliers to ensure they could

211

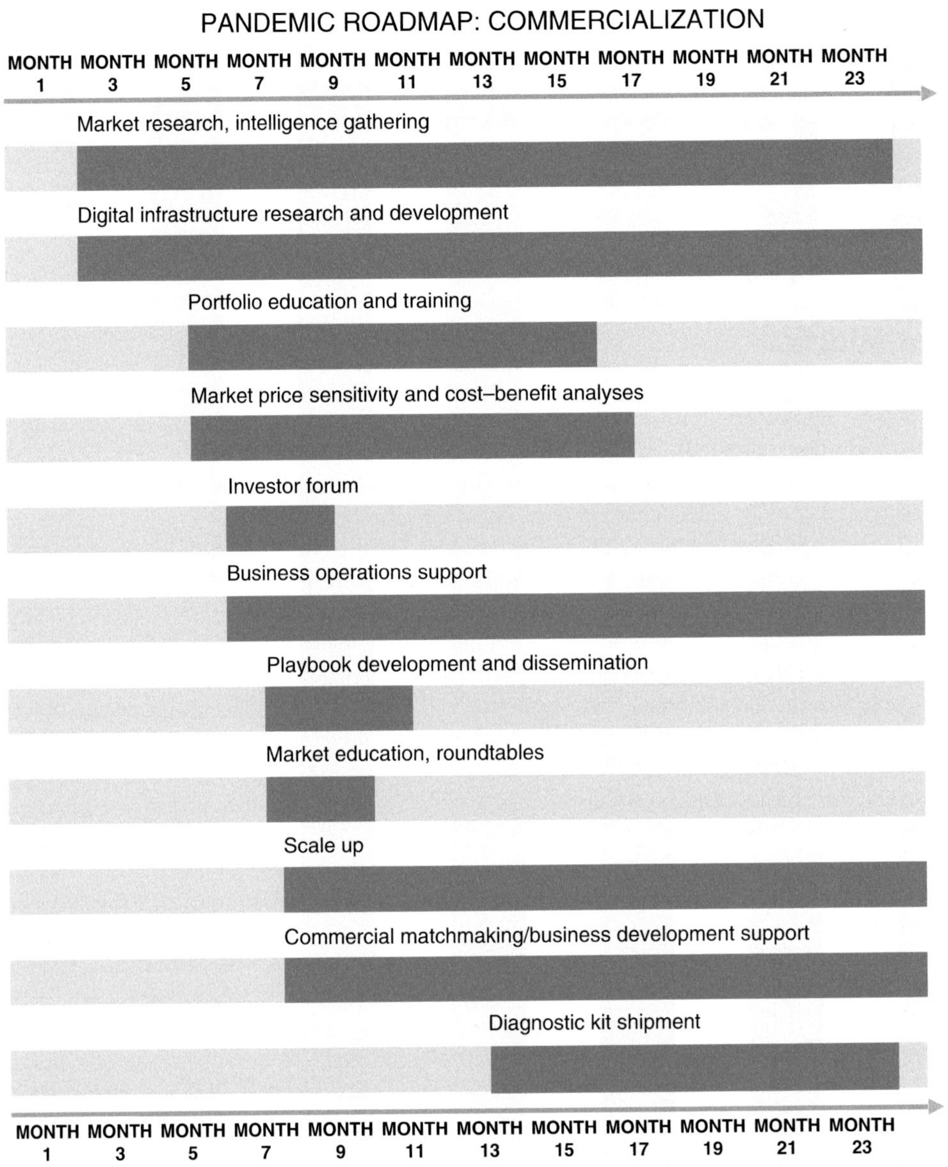

Figure 11.1 This roadmap depicts the vital activities, their chronology, and an estimated time frame in months. In the case of the SARS-CoV-2 pandemic, month 1 was December 2019, the month in which the virus was isolated, sequenced, identified, and published.

produce and deliver the volume of tests needed to fulfill purchase orders, the Commercialization Team assisted portfolio companies in scaling up *business* operations to make their products commercially viable in the market. Likewise, the Regulatory Team assisted portfolio companies with their regulatory submissions to the US Food and Drug Administration (FDA), whereas the Commercialization Team regularly identified

Table 11.1 Typical commercialization process

Phase	Description
Ideation/funnel	Technical product development, market discovery and exploration (current "state of the art"), and understanding of regulatory approval pathways
Business setup	Preparing for scaling up production and distribution, solidifying the business model, and direct market feedback and insights
Beta market testing	Seeking insights from select real-word applications to inform final product development and use cases before mass production
Stakeholder engagement	Formal engagement with potential buyers and strategic partners, and market adoption
Business development	Engagement of marketing, sales, pricing, forecasting, and other core business functions to inform and launch "go-to-market" strategies

Table 11.2 RADx Tech Commercialization Team core functions

Core function	Description
Internal capabilities assessments	Assessment of RADx applications from both a business and a commercial perspective
Market research	Research on the total addressable market, target/ideal customers, the competitive landscape, pricing, purchaser attitudes, and perceived barriers
Education and business support	Ongoing education, coaching, and webinars on government contracting, the competitive landscape, investment preparedness, and other areas identified as gaps
Market intelligence and business development	Investor forums, procurement opportunities, matchmaking introductions, and market updates
Market education	Webinars, online calculators, and implementation guides
Regulatory and policy analysis	Identification of non-FDA-related policy and regulatory barriers that impacted the portfolio's commercial success
Digital solutions and emerging diagnostic workflow	Introductions to technology support vendors and the assessment of real-world use cases and reporting challenges

non-FDA-related regulatory and public policy issues that impacted the success or failure of adopting testing at a broad scale.

Core Function 1: Internal Capabilities Assessments

During the deep dive/funnel process, RADx primarily evaluated applicants on the scientific potential of their diagnostic proposals. To a lesser extent, we evaluated applications on the commercial viability of the applicants' products and the business acumen of their teams. As a result, portfolio companies had a wide range of commercial experience. Most companies in the RADx portfolio fell into one of three categories: accelerators, incubators, and mid-size companies.

- **Accelerators:** These were companies with existing diagnostic products on the market and significant existing operational infrastructure. The Commercialization Team assisted these companies by providing market intelligence, communicating customers' needs, and relaying up-to-date public health guidance
- **Incubators:** These were smaller, less experienced companies that had never brought a diagnostic to market. Many had academic backgrounds but no commercial expertise and needed a broader array of assistance than larger market players. Their scientific approaches were sound, but they did not have the ability to scale up their operations at the pace or scope needed to produce and deliver millions of tests. The Commercialization Team assisted these companies in their go-to-market planning and connected them with commercial partners
- **Mid-size companies:** These companies knew the regulatory landscape, had staffing and manufacturing capabilities, and had already succeeded in commercializing other diagnostic products on a small scale. They had not produced at the scale that the pandemic required, but they had existing infrastructure and core business functions in place. The Commercialization Team assisted these companies with real-time market intelligence, business development, and refining their go-to-market planning

The companies that were most successful were those that presented the highest potential for scientific *and* commercial viability. Future projects should make sure that the portfolio of companies is balanced, namely that diagnostic innovation is balanced with the need to scale. The selection process should also include a stronger emphasis on evaluating each company's business and commercial potential. The following criteria should be added as part of the application process:

1. *Operational readiness reviews* to identify gaps and needs early on. This could be done via a quantitative rubric and should include rigorous due diligence
2. *Capability assessments* to understand the expertise, business acumen, and personalities within the organization and what additional staffing resources may be needed to augment the company's team
3. *Virtual or on-site visits* to calibrate discussions, verify facts, and determine what is reasonably achievable. These visits help reduce funding and execution risk by identifying strengths and weaknesses that might not be evident in an applicant's submission documents or via remote discussions

Finally, each application should be reviewed by dual team leads with complementary expertise (i.e. one with a technology/science background and one with commercial experience) to provide a more comprehensive perspective when evaluating submissions and throughout the RADx Tech process. Dual team leads were employed on a limited basis but proved to have significant advantages.

Core Function 2: Market Research

For COVID-19 diagnostic companies, projecting what the market landscape would look like once they received their EUAs was a prominent challenge. Companies typically spend months or even years analyzing market potential, researching customer needs and attitudes, scoping out the competitive landscape, developing pricing models, securing distribution channels, and on various other topics. However, the pandemic threw every aspect of traditional market research into chaos.

For example, traditional diagnostic customers (governments, laboratories, and medical providers) were not the only purchasers in this market. Use cases continually shifted from traditional health-care settings to mass community sites and drive-throughs, to schools/workplaces, and eventually to homes. In a matter of a few months, community-based organizations, large employers, school districts, pharmacies/retailers, the travel industry, and individual consumers needed access to test kits and supplies. Moreover, demand oscillated throughout various phases of the pandemic, including lockdowns and reopenings, the approval of the first vaccines, and each new surge and variant. Supply, too, was difficult to project, as component and packaging manufacturers suffered from the same supply chain and labor shortages as other parts of the economy. All of these factors, including widespread price volatility and a chaotic competitive landscape, made it difficult for portfolio companies to project the market weeks, let alone months or years, in advance.

RADx Tech projected that the United States would need to be able to produce 6.5 million tests per day or nearly 50 million tests per week, but exactly what type of tests would be needed, who would pay for them, and how and to whom they would be administered was not immediately clear. These answers had significant implications for product design, customer education, distribution, marketing, and sales.

Case Study

An employer in the top 50 of the Fortune 500 seeking 10 000 point-of-care (POC) tests per week was looking for test suppliers. The company anticipated paying $50–100 per test and needed the first shipment within two weeks. At that time, only a few RADx Tech companies had received EUAs for POC rapid antigen tests and were beginning to ramp up production for inventory that had already been prepurchased by government agencies. The soonest a company could commit to providing 10 000 tests per week was 30–45 days. A month later, the employer had already extended its work-from-home policy, no longer felt a sense of urgency to return to in-person operations, and was only willing to pay $5 per test due to the reallocation of their testing budget to support work-from-home equipment, IT support, and other remote operations. This example illustrates the challenges of projecting supply, demand, pricing, and other considerations from both the test purchasers' and the test manufacturers' perspectives.

Quantitative Database

To understand the sheer size of the total addressable market, the RADx Tech Commercialization Team aggregated projections of national daily testing needs from various trusted sources (e.g. Harvard University; Johns Hopkins University; the Rockefeller Foundation; the Massachusetts Institute of Technology (MIT) Institute for Data, Systems, and Society; Health Advances; and AdvaMed) and shared them with portfolio companies. In early summer 2020, we estimated that the USA's testing demand ranged from roughly 1–1.2 million per day for viral mitigation to approximately 4.3 million per day for viral suppression.

Not all tests would be suitable for all types of testing locations and circumstances. Therefore, we conducted quantitative and qualitative market analyses to identify the potential customer base, best use cases, and desirable characteristics for various types of tests that were in development. We built a database using publicly available national data on the number and distribution of individuals across different sectors of the economy. We focused on sectors that typically require in-person interactions (as opposed to office-based employment sectors that could potentially sustain work-from-home policies). Where available, we broke down the data by state, subcategory, the total number of employers/institutions, the total number of locations, and the total number of people to be tested (employees, staff or volunteers, and students/residents) as shown in Table 11.3.

Stakeholder Engagement

We supplemented the quantitative data with surveys and in-person interviews of stakeholders who required testing programs. As listed in Table 11.4, these stakeholders included chambers of commerce executives, cities and counties, education agencies, foundations that work with community-based organizations, representatives from the travel industry, restaurant associations, self-insured employers, medical wholesalers, distributors, and retailers. Interactions took the form of roundtables, webinars, 1:1 conversations, in-person and email surveys, and formal research funded by RADx. With testing needs continually evolving, this level of engagement provided a vital link between test makers and test purchasers/users and should be replicated in the future.

During interviews, we gathered information on purchasers' attitudes, concerns, interests, and perceived challenges to testing. We identified desirable test characteristics and price sensitivities for different use cases and populations and shared them with all portfolio companies. Portfolio companies could use this information to adjust their scientific approaches if needed and inform their go-to-market strategies. Many of our findings are useful for future pandemic preparedness efforts.

The qualitative findings from the RADx market research are as follows:

1. **Developers need to consider the end user.** Our research pointed to a potential disconnect between development and commercial potential. Diagnostic developers generally view their technology from a performance perspective, focusing on specimen and assay type, clinical indications (or contraindications), and accuracy (specificity, sensitivity, false positives, and false negatives). While these performance attributes are critical for regulatory approval, they do not completely align with the end user's perspective. Purchasers are sensitive to price, ease of use, convenience, and turnaround times. They care about accuracy and reliability but are willing to make trade-offs to achieve desired outcomes, such as the ability to test more people more frequently and at lower cost, or the ability to scale operations using more user-friendly, less resource-intensive testing methods, even if they are slightly less accurate.

2. **Different use cases require different kinds of tests.** Purchasers' willingness to trade certain test attributes for others varied by sector, setting, population, and unique needs. For example, urgent care clinics value accuracy over cost, as they need to make clinical decisions based on test results and are not the ultimate payer for tests. By contrast, large employers prioritize price because they are directly incurring the cost for testing their workers.

Table 11.3 RADx commercial testing market database components

Sector	Data distribution	Further detail
Kindergarten to 12th grade (K–12) education	By state, district, campus, and type (public, private, or charter)	Teachers, students, and faculty
Child-care facilities and licensed child-care providers	By state	Staff and children enrolled
Higher education (universities and colleges)	By state, campus, and type (public, for-profit, or not-for-profit)	Staff, students, and athletes
American Indian and Alaska Native population	By state and tribe	Total individuals who identify as American Indian and Alaska Native
Homeless shelters	By state, location, and beds	Staff and residents
Emergency responders	By state, agencies, and type (fire, ambulance/emergency medical services, or law enforcement)	Employees and volunteers
Skilled nursing, long-term care, other health-care facilities	By state and location	Staff and residents
Manufacturing	By state, plants, and type (automotive, etc.)	Employers and employees
Hospitality, travel, leisure	Nationally by type (hotels, restaurants, casinos, fitness, or amusement parks)	Employers and employees
Mining, oil, energy	By state and location	Employers and employees
Retail/customer service (non-sales staff)	Nationally by type (clothing, furniture, gas station, personal/health care, pharmacy, building/gardening, etc.)	Employers and employees
Distribution/transportation	Nationally by type (warehouse, trucking, freight, or shipping)	Employers, employees, and the average square footage per employee
Wholesale	Nationally by type (sales, manufacturing, brokers, or truck/trailer operators)	Employers and employees
Construction	By state and type (private, federal, state, or local)	Employees, seasonal workers, and average wages
Financial services	By state, county, type (private, federal, state, or local), and subtype (banks, field offices, or service centers)	Employers, employees, and average wages

Table 11.3 (cont.)

Sector	Data distribution	Further detail
Real estate/retail sales	By state and type (agents, property managers, landscaping, sales, accounting, etc.)	Employees and average wages
Transportation	By state, type (water, air, rail, or ground), and subtype (pilot, ship captain, taxi, school bus, truck driver, maintenance, or clerks)	Employees and seasonal employees
Postal/courier	By state, type (US Postal Service, UPS, FedEx, etc.), and subtype (sorting, delivery, customer service, etc.)	Locations and employees
Nonresidential health care	By state, type (dialysis, chemotherapy, critical access hospitals, clinics, pharmacies, etc.), location, and stations/beds per location	Staff and average patient volume

Additionally, we discovered that some tests are easier for certain populations to use than others, such as sputum versus nasal swabs or devices that require smartphone apps to interpret results versus those with a visual result display. These types of test characteristics had significant implications for vulnerable populations, such as children, the elderly, those with limited technology or English skills, and people with disabilities.

We found that companies that designed tests to have a broad appeal across many different use cases and populations experienced the most commercial success. Companies that did not consider all potential use cases and populations when designing their products and devices were mostly successful in niche markets and among niche customers.

3. **Purchasers did not just need tests; they needed comprehensive testing solutions.** Most purchasers needed assistance with implementation and logistical support, such as staffing, workflows, personal protective equipment (PPE), software, and protocols. This issue became one of the biggest barriers to testing in schools in the fall of 2020. Schools, employers, congregate living facilities, and others needed a complete testing program at an affordable price per test to utilize the millions of test kits purchased and distributed by the federal government. Self-administered tests in particular needed technology and software to report, and track, test results in nonclinical settings. As noted by a global community relief organization: "Organizations that need testing don't know how to implement it. I can have the tests, but I don't know how to go about using them."

4. **Some industries were early adopters of testing while others lagged behind.** Various factors influenced whether, and how likely, organizations were willing or able to implement testing programs. The film industry and professional sports, for example, were early adopters due to the nature of in-person work, the financial resources

Table 11.4 External stakeholders

Government

Advanced Research Projects Agency for Health (ARPA-H)

City of Albuquerque

Manufacturing Extension Partnership (National Institute of Standards and Technology)

State of Ohio

State testing coordinators

Customers/employers

ALung

AccuTec Blades

Altisource

American Textiles

Ameritech

Becton Dickinson

Bilec Medical

Cadence

Capgemini

Coca Cola

Eat n' Park

Eaton

Ensign Plastics

Express Med

GECU

Goodman

Google

Grotte Business Partners

Hello Alice

Home Depot

JP Morgan

Lifeline Ambulance

Major League Baseball

Microsoft

Mighty Hook

Morgan Stanley

National Basketball Association

National Football League

Pelican

Rekon Productions

Sabic

SQUAN

Startbrite

Distributors/suppliers/ retailers

Abil

Adnas

Albine

All Clear Health

Amazon

Avestria

Azova

Balance Biotech

Biotia

C2 Sense

Carbon Health

Cardinal Health

CLX Health

Color Health

Cosmos Health

CVS Health

Early Testing Solutions

eMed

Everlywell

Global Direct Medical

Grapefruit

Hamilton Health Box

Helix

Henry Schein

Integrum Science

Keele Medical

Lighthouse Lab Services

Mologic

NUMI Health

Perkin Elmer

Pravici

Primary.Health

Project N95

Recuro Health (Udo Test)

SHIELD-UofI

Test Zone Dx

Thermo Fisher Scientific

UnitedHealthcare

Vault Health

WREN Labs

Walgreens

Foundations/nonprofit organizations/research

Air Force Research Labs

Ardelis

Arizona State University

Bill and Melinda Gates Foundation

C19 Response Advisors

CORE Response

COVIDCheck Colorado

Emergent

Health Advances

Indian Health Service

Johns Hopkins Center for Health Security

LydaHill Foundation

Medtech Crossroads

MIT

Rockefeller Foundation (K–12)

National Testing Action Program (NTAP)

Tribal Nations FEMA representative

Ysleta/Tigua Health Services

Industry groups

Arizona Technology Council

Association of Chamber of Commerce Executives

Angel Capital Association

Back2Cruise

Borderplex Alliance

Business Group on Health

Greater Houston Partnership

Health Industry Distributors Association

Idaho Economic Development Association

Impact Washington

Lubbock Economic Development Alliance

Medical Device Manufacturers Association

Table 11.4 (Cont.)

	Investors/financial industry	Miscellaneous
Stryker Medical		Large regional YMCA
The Cronos Group	Brevet Capital Management	Urban restaurant owner with five locations
TransUnion	Flare Capital	
Ureeka	Genoa Capital	Martial arts gym
Midwest manufacturing plant	Google Ventures	Public university (20 000+ students)
Fortune 100 global manufacturer with domestic/international locations (2 000+ employees)	Hollywell Partners	
	RA Capital	Small, private school (day care to eighth grade)
	WaterStreet	
Fortune 500 global manufacturer with domestic/international locations (< 300 employees)		

Note that this list is not comprehensive.

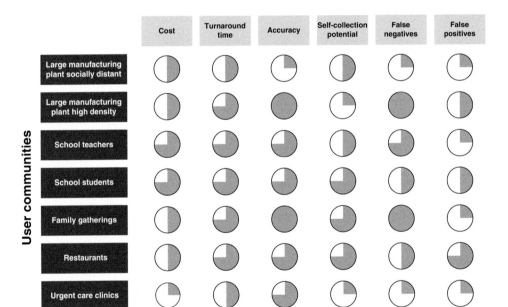

Figure 11.2 Importance of testing components from the perspectives of different users.

available, and the financial risks of being shut down in these industries. By contrast, employers in general, prisons, and nursing homes struggled to launch testing programs because of limited resources, safety concerns, and a lack of guidance on how to establish and manage testing programs.

Table 11.5 Purchaser perceptions of barriers to testing

Perceived barriers	True barriers (major)	True barriers (minor)
Reduced access to tests or delayed turnaround times: "At the beginning, you couldn't even get tests. When you could, it took 7 −14 days to get results. So, what's the point?" (vice president, facilities management)	Testing costs in the context of other costs: "We see no reason to bring back our staff to the office yet. Returning to office would mean additional expenses with PPE, sanitization, and testing." (vice president, human resources)	Access to test kits: "Practically speaking, I'm not sure we'd have access to enough test kits at a low enough cost to allow broad testing." (senior vice president, human resources)
Effectiveness of testing: "This just adds a false sense of security that everyone has been tested, and so it's safe." (vice president, human resources)	Operational challenges: "Proper care and isolation areas would need to be set up to ensure that individuals would not be unnecessarily exposed to COVID-positive employees." (program manager)	Cost and breadth of testing: "We have thousands of employees across 48 states. Cost would be a major factor in deciding whom to test and how frequently." (senior vice president, human resources)

5. **High costs and limited capacity in the early stages prevented greater uptake.** Initial community, school, and workplace testing programs were expensive and required medical personnel to administer and interpret POC tests, laboratories to process laboratory-based polymerase chain reaction (PCR) tests, and support staff to manage testing operations. Media reports of long lines and high turnaround times at public health testing sites further discouraged would-be purchasers, even as these challenges subsided. Many organizations that sought out testing early on received multiple bids and decided testing was too expensive or resource intensive. Many adopted other mitigation strategies or extended work-from-home policies and did not seek out testing in later phases of the pandemic due to these continued perceptions, even as testing became faster, cheaper, and easier to manage.

6. **A shifting consensus and public understanding of test reliability impacted market demand.** The understanding of the accuracy and sensitivity of various test types was evolving in real time, and this created both barriers and opportunities for wider adoption. The rapid antigen assay is the most prominent example. In August 2020, the White House announced a deal to purchase 150 million POC rapid antigen tests[1] with the intention being for states to distribute them to schools and long-term care facilities. As mentioned earlier, one barrier was that schools needed a full-package solution, not just test kits. The other initial major barrier was the confusion as to whether rapid antigen test results could be trusted in asymptomatic individuals. Clinical and nonclinical decision-makers alike knew that PCR was the "gold standard." Many public health experts were concerned about the potential for presymptomatic or asymptomatic individuals to unknowingly spread COVID-19 to others if schools relied on negative

rapid antigen tests to resume in-person learning. Concerns over false negatives were even greater when it came to high-risk settings and vulnerable populations, such as nursing homes. As a result, millions of test kits sat in state warehouses, with their expiration dates fast approaching.

In time, pilot projects and prepublication academic studies demonstrated important advantages of rapid antigen testing programs that alleviated most experts' concerns. These included low prices and moderate accuracy/sensitivity in high viral loads, namely when people are most contagious. Unlike PCR, rapid antigen tests do not continue to display a positive result for weeks or months after people are no longer contagious, which could unnecessarily delay students or employees from returning to school/work. By early 2021, the scientific community was more united in its messaging that the benefits of rapid antigen outweighed the risks, and purchaser demand soared.

Similar tipping points occurred with other diagnostic products, such as home tests; public health experts were initially hesitant to endorse home tests due to concerns over accuracy, usefulness, and the ability of laypersons to properly self-administer. These concerns, while potentially warranted, impacted the timing and long-term commercial success of many diagnostic products.

7. **Companies did not understand the appropriateness of testing as a primary, or complementary, mitigation strategy.** Most stakeholders understood the necessity of access to frequent testing. However, they did not necessarily understand their role in testing or the appropriateness of testing in certain environments where other mitigation measures were already in place (masking, social distancing, hand washing, etc.). Because of this confusion, we found that many organizations adopted an all-or-nothing approach. Some employers expressed concerns that, if they established routine testing programs at work, their employees would be less careful or engage in riskier behavior outside work. Stakeholders could have benefited from clearer guidance on the risk of transmission in each setting, the effectiveness of testing in the context of other mitigation measures, and tailored approaches based on various circumstances and goals. As a blades manufacturer noted: "What is the impetus to change – and incur the cost of testing – if we have no issues running now?"

8. **Purchasers did not understand the value of testing to ensure operational continuity.** We heard similar sentiments from many different organizations of all sizes, namely that unless testing could guarantee safety, they preferred to maintain work-from-home policies. In sectors where working from home was not an option, a better understanding was needed of the cost and benefits of testing compared, or in conjunction, with other, less expensive measures such as masking and social distancing.

Schools similarly could have benefited from cost–benefit analyses that examined not only testing and other mitigation measures, but also the broader context of long periods of time away from the classroom. While the speed with which schools shifted to distance learning was impressive, there was insufficient information about the value and effectiveness of in-person learning to justify the resources and logistics needed to provide on-site testing and return to classrooms full-time. For example, we did not know then the full extent and long-term impacts that distance learning would have on children and their caregivers in terms of learning loss, child abuse/neglect, family economic hardship, parental mental health, and substance use issues. In the future, school-based testing and associated costs should be placed in the context of the long-term socioeconomic costs of *not* testing.

Competitive Landscape and Pricing: At-Home Testing

While the Commercialization Team did not share any proprietary or confidential information with portfolio companies, we gathered publicly available data on non-RADx test manufacturers and suppliers, test types and characteristics, laboratory capacity, known partnerships, and government contract awards. We researched testing fees charged by laboratories, providers, and full-service testing companies; billing codes and reimbursement rates of health insurance carriers and government payers; Securities and Exchange Commission filings and publicly available sales forecasting reports; and advertised wholesale and retail prices for test kits. Finally, the Commercialization Team collaborated with other institutions and foundations in August 2020 to survey 3 870 consumers, 78 payers, and 250 employers about their attitudes toward, and willingness to pay for, at-home tests. We asked about trade-offs that consumers and purchasers were willing to forgo at various

Table 11.6 Market attitudes toward at-home testing

Population	Key insights
Consumers	• 83% expressed interest in rapid at-home testing
	• Results in < 24 hours was important
	• 69% found rapid at-home tests appealing when combined with an app
	• When presented with a range of testing options, "at home" was the most frequently selected response for preferred location
	• 66% were extremely interested in testing if it was free (to the consumer) compared with 39% interested if consumers needed to cover part of the cost
	• There were concerns about the accuracy of at-home tests
	• With testing that had higher than 80% sensitivity, there were concerns over out-of-pocket costs outweighing the benefits of accuracy
Payers	• 65% would be extremely likely to cover app-based at-home testing
	• 64% would reimburse policyholders $25–75 for at-home tests (i.e. around 50% of laboratory test prices at the time)
	• 26% would reimburse up to $25–35
	• 21% would reimburse up to $35–50
	• 17% would reimburse up to $50–75
	• Payers were primarily concerned about accuracy, reliability, and the potential for fraud, waste, and abuse
Employers	• 66% would pay $5–35 per test
	• 15% would pay $5–15 per test
	• 30% would pay $15–25 per test
	• 21% would pay $25–35 per test
	• On average, employers would be willing to pay $2.61 per employee per day
	• Employers with more employees were willing to pay more for testing (e.g. employers with 150+ employees would pay up to $3.76 per employee per day)
	• Employers were primarily concerned about accuracy and availability

price points, their level of interest in app-based devices, and other options for home-based diagnostics. We disseminated the pricing and survey information to portfolio companies through email newsletters and regular calls to inform their go-to-market strategies.

Core Function 3: Education and Business Support

The Commercialization Team provided education and training sessions for portfolio companies, covering topics identified as potential knowledge gaps in the internal capabilities assessments. We held a series of webinars, conducted 1:1 coaching sessions, and distributed materials via email to portfolio companies. These covered topics such as:

- frequent updates on user needs and the competitive landscape
- market research presentations and findings
- investment readiness – education on how to develop pitch decks, position the company for investment, and develop the company brand
- go-to-market strategy – identifying ideal use cases, the customer base, and product differentiators/value proposition; market forecasting and sales modeling; establishing and managing distribution; and partnering with technology platforms/testing providers
- fundamentals of government contracting – how to search for procurement notices, the minimum qualifications that most agencies require, types of contracts, subcontracting opportunities, business classifications as differentiators, and common win strategies
- marketing, sales – understanding the customer journey, appropriate pricing/competitor analysis, testing programs versus test products, logos/websites, presentations/videos, sales channels (business-to-business, business-to-consumer, public procurement, health care, etc.)
- corporate development – licensing and co-developing, strategic investments, and partnerships
- coaching – revising pitch decks, practicing presentations, refining value proposition and target customer segments, engaging financial versus strategic investors, scaling up and launching plans, and competitive positioning

In conjunction with the vendor support provided by the Deployment Core, the Commercialization Team provided tailored business support services to help incubators establish day-to-day business operations or to help mid-size companies expand. These services included financial modeling, talent acquisition, contract template development, and operations/logistics. Some portfolio companies took advantage of these offerings and some did not, while some engaged initially but then failed to follow through. Based on these experiences, future RADx-style initiatives should consider including clear developmental and operational milestones, tied to funding tranches, and establishing the criteria and a process for off-boarding companies that stagnate.

Core Function 4: Market Intelligence and Business Development

One of the Commercialization Team's most valuable functions was our real-time market intelligence and business development support. This included fundraising opportunities, purchaser–portfolio matchmaking, email newsletters with requests for proposal (RFP) opportunities, and email newsletters sharing news articles, market insight reports, and state and national policy updates. Many portfolio companies, especially incubators had little experience with business development and did not have the time or staff resources to continually monitor databases that post government contracting opportunities. Our team subscribed to one such database and identified state and federal RFPs for COVID-19 testing services. This information helped companies with small teams and limited resources stay up to date on market trends.

To further support portfolio companies' business development activities, we developed an unbiased matchmaking process to connect portfolio companies with potential customers, strategic partners, technology vendors, testing companies, and distributors. To match companies with third parties, we created interest forms that asked about preferred test characteristics, intended use cases, and other needs. We then sent these, blinded, to portfolio companies that met some or all of the criteria. If portfolio companies expressed an interest in connecting, the Commercialization Team facilitated introductions.

To support fundraising activities, the Commercialization Team convened two virtual investor forums, in January and May 2021. The first forum included 39 portfolio companies and 62 corporate (strategic partners), venture capital, and angel investors interested in COVID-19 diagnostics. We provided template slide decks and sample materials to portfolio companies that had never pitched to investors before. The companies prepared videos, one-pagers, and pitch decks. Some companies took advantage of the offer to conduct 1:1 coaching sessions to prepare for the event while others did not. A total of 325 meetings occurred during the January 2021 event, with 90% reporting that they planned to or had already scheduled follow-up meetings and 99% reporting they would participate again. Based on that success, we convened a second investor forum in May that included 44 portfolio companies and 46 investors, with a total of 170 participants breaking out into 150 follow-up meetings.

Case Studies

Company A, a PCR test maker, received a $6 million investment as a direct result of the introductions made during the investor forums.

Company B, maker of rapid antigen tests, had hired an executive who did not have experience pitching to investors. The Commercialization Team reviewed company B's pitch deck, provided feedback, and coached the executive on pitch presentations, including several practice sessions leading up to the investor forum. After a successful presentation, the executive became company B's designated representative for all presentations to investors.

One area that should be expanded upon in future pandemic-related efforts is connecting diagnostic companies with technology vendors and software developers earlier in the development process. Non-health-care purchasers needed comprehensive solutions that included being able to register users in a system other than a traditional electronic medical record, log test results, and report required information to public health agencies. As over-the-counter, fully self-administered tests began to dominate the market, the FDA issued a new requirement for diagnostic makers to provide a digital option for consumer reporting. Several RADx Tech companies developed web-based or native mobile applications while others partnered with technology vendors. The Commercialization Team hosted virtual "demo days" and provided opportunities for portfolio companies to connect with digital solution providers, but these should have happened earlier.

Core Function 5: Market Education

We used our established communication channels to educate stakeholders about the value of testing, new testing options through RADx that would be coming to market, how to choose the right test and right volume of tests for various use cases, and approaches to implementing testing programs. The RADx Commercialization Team hosted a series of webinars with would-be purchasers, including chambers of commerce executives, industry trade groups, businesses, schools/universities, academic and nonprofit organizations, and entities involved in implementing COVID-19 testing programs. Some of the specific topics covered included:

- test and assay types (antigen, PCR, lateral flow, etc.) and basic terminology that is familiar to clinicians but often confusing for purchasers (such as accuracy, sensitivity, and reliability) and how these terms relate to other trade-offs, such as desirable test characteristics and price
- test characteristics, including swab type (nasal or sputum), the devices and technology needed to run tests (visual reads or app-based results), price and price considerations (test kits plus other potential costs such as medical staffing and/or laboratory fees), and turnaround times
- the basics of test classifications (Clinical Laboratory Improvement Amendments (CLIA) versus CLIA-waived or over-the-counter with a prescription versus over-the-counter without a prescription) and how they relate to testing operations, such as which tests need to be administered by medical staff, which need to be administered by laypersons who have been trained and authorized to perform tests (e.g. teachers/school administrators under statewide CLIA waivers for schools), and which can be administered by non-trained laypersons (individuals)
- potential use cases for different types of tests, such as manufacturing, classrooms, office-based employment sectors, retail/hospitality environments, and health-care settings
- best practices for designing and implementing testing programs, including staffing, supplies, logistics, and operational considerations

In addition to webinars, RADx Tech, together with Massachusetts General Hospital and MIT, developed the website https://whentotest.org/, including the Workplace Testing Planner, to assist employers in estimating the number of tests they would need and how much workplace testing might cost. Launched in January 2021, the tool allows users to enter specifics about their job site, including the number of staff to be tested per day and the frequency of testing; it then populates detailed reports regarding estimated cost, speed, and the accuracy of various testing options. It also provides the option to overlay additional mitigation measures recommended by the Centers for Disease Control and Prevention (CDC) – such as masking, contact tracing, and social distancing – to provide a broader cost–benefit analysis (see Chapter 12 for more details).

RADx Tech launched a companion tool for consumers in November 2021. The When to Test Calculator for Individuals employs computer modeling to help people determine if they are at risk of contracting or transmitting COVID-19 based on variables such as vaccination status, transmission levels in their geographic community, and personal behaviors such as masking and social distancing. The website also links to testing options, such as how to order free home test kits through the mail and in-person testing locations by zip code.

In addition to these websites, the Commercialization Team published a playbook in March 2021 covering topics such as testing strategies, collection methods, communications to employees, personnel, physical spaces (layouts and workflows), sample transportation (for off-site and/or laboratory-based testing), testing program design and operation, and follow-up considerations such as isolation, contact tracing, and return-to-work policies.

Core Function 6: Regulatory and Policy Analysis

Throughout the RADx process, the Commercialization Team regularly identified and cataloged regulatory and policy issues that were negatively or positively impacting the commercial success of portfolio products. The ones that presented the greatest barriers to market entry and to widespread market adoption of new COVID-19 diagnostic technologies are presented in the following subsections.

CLIA Waivers for POC Testing

One of the most significant barriers to the early and widespread adoption of testing programs in employment and education sectors was the fact that rapid POC diagnostics can be administered only in certain clinical settings. POC tests require every test site to have either a CLIA certificate or a CLIA certificate of waiver (CLIA waiver). To receive CLIA certification, a laboratory must have a designated laboratory director with appropriate licensure and specially trained staff to administer tests and follow proper safety, privacy, documentation, and clinical protocols.

The CLIA program is a federal program regulated by the Centers for Medicare and Medicaid Services (CMS), but state agencies are responsible for laboratory oversight, applications, and renewals. States may also have their own licensure laws or additional regulations. As a result, in the initial stages of the pandemic, schools, workplaces, and community organizations had to contract with laboratories, medical staffing agencies, mobile clinics, or other CLIA and CLIA-waived entities to be able to run testing programs. These third-party contracts greatly increased the cost of testing and were scarce in many regions.

To address the CLIA waiver issue and support organizations, states took different approaches, with some states adopting policies that made it easy to set up testing programs and other states taking more restrictive approaches due to concerns over the ability of laypersons to understand and follow CLIA standards and proper testing protocols.

Most states issued blanket prescriptions, or "standing orders," authorizing COVID-19 tests without a physician having to individually assess each patient. These were usually signed by the state department of health's chief medical officer. Many states issued a statewide CLIA waiver and allowed entities such as schools, homeless shelters, and community-based organizations to apply to use the state's CLIA waiver for their testing programs. Not all states obtained and issued statewide CLIA waivers, however. Some required every school, homeless shelter, or community test site to apply for its own CLIA waiver.

Definitions of who was allowed to administer tests under a statewide CLIA varied, with some states allowing only school nurses and other medical paraprofessionals to administer tests and other states allowing teachers, principals, community health workers, workplace health and safety officers, and human resources professionals to be trained and authorized to administer tests. State agencies received hundreds or thousands of applications, which overwhelmed administrative capacity and created backlogs. Some states required test administrators to complete hands-on live (virtual) training with practice test kits, while others required test administrators only to watch online training videos on how to properly administer POC tests before approving an organization's application to use its CLIA. To our knowledge, no states allowed pharmacies to participate in statewide CLIA programs. They, too, had to go through the normal CLIA application process, which limited their ability to set up testing sites.

Texas stands out as one of the first states to tackle the CLIA issue head-on. In October 2020, the Texas Division of Emergency Management obtained a statewide CLIA waivers, issued a standing delegation order, provided online training to certify school nurses and nonmedical staff on how to correctly administer Abbott BinaxNOW tests (a POC rapid antigen test) and interpret results, and created a website and mobile app to support mandatory reporting requirements. PPE and test kits were distributed monthly. The Texas Department of Education cosponsored the program that ultimately covered more than 6 million students and staff at more than 10 000 school campuses across all 254 counties. The program expanded to include small businesses, restaurants, and other organizations that wanted to provide on-site rapid testing to support reopening plans and avoid closures.

Like Texas, California expanded its statewide CLIA program beyond K–12 education and allowed homeless shelters, day cares, after-school programs, agricultural sector employers, and non-profit and community-based organizations to participate.

This patchwork of policies created disparities, with some states having significantly more test sites and opportunities to access testing than others. To prepare for future pandemics, federal and state agencies should work together to develop protocols for allowing the use of POC tests in nonclinical settings. Rapid antigen lateral flow assays and some rapid PCRs, for example, have proven that they can be easily self-administered by laypersons, including school-age children, and correctly interpreted by laypersons in nonclinical settings. To construct a framework for widespread testing during a pandemic, regulators should therefore consider circumstances that could trigger the authorization to use POC tests in nonclinical settings, what type of training should be required to reduce safety and/or result interpretation risks, limits on the types of tests that can be performed and who can perform them, and other criteria.

Payment Policies

Many organizations failed, or were slow, to implement testing programs due to concerns about affordability and confusion around financial responsibility. Some full-service testing providers marketed their services as being "free" to the employer (or school district) with the intent to bill health insurance, but most insurance companies were not required to cover this type of testing. The USA's decentralized public health decision-making and multi-payer health-care system meant that *who* pays for tests and *when* varied from person to person, test site to test site, and state to state. As a result, not as many tests hit the market as quickly as they could have.

In March 2020, Congress passed and the president signed into law several pieces of legislation allocating billions of dollars to the COVID-19 response through the Coronavirus Preparedness and Response Supplemental Appropriations Act, the Families First Coronavirus Response Act, and the Coronavirus Aid, Relief, and Economic Security Act.

- Some provisions authorized the government to fund research for, and directly purchase, goods and services such as PPE, diagnostics, vaccines, and therapeutics
- Other provisions allocated funding for COVID-19 testing, including $1 billion to reimburse providers for claims for the uninsured and more than $200 million to the Indian Health Service, the Department of Veterans Affairs, and the Department of Defense's Defense Health Program (TRICARE)
- States also received billions of dollars to operate community and school-based test sites, with states individually having discretion on how to implement and fund these programs

The legislation mandated *most* private insurance plans, Medicare, and Medicaid to cover COVID-19 testing *for individual diagnostic purposes* without cost-sharing and provided 100% federal matching funds to state Medicaid agencies that chose to cover the costs of COVID-19 testing and services for people not otherwise eligible for Medicaid. Subsequent federal regulatory guidance clarified that health plans did *not* have to cover routine, asymptomatic testing, such as return-to-work or return-to-school testing. Some state health insurance regulators, however, issued their own bulletins notifying insurers that they *did* indeed have to cover surveillance testing.

These conflicting and confusing policies about which test sites were federally or state funded and which sites would bill insurance made it difficult for employers (and school districts) to know whether they or their insurance carriers would have to pay for on-site testing should they choose to offer it. To complicate matters further, students who attend the same school and employees who work at the same company are not necessarily covered by the same insurance carrier or insurance policies subject to the same state or federal regulations. One employee, for example, could be covered by an employer plan subject to state regulation and another employee could be covered by a spouse's plan subject to federal regulation.

The impact of public policy around who pays for testing and when meant that many organizations could not afford to run their own testing programs. In the early months of the pandemic, tests were scarce and testing companies were charging exorbitant fees. Even as self-administered and pooled testing options became more common, prices were still mostly unaffordable at the frequency required to maintain in-person operations. Moreover, each organization had to solicit bids and negotiate prices on its own. One way in which policymakers could have increased access to tests and supported widespread adoption of testing would have been to expand federally funded purchase orders and fee schedules. For example, in August 2020, the federal government negotiated $5 per test for Abbott BinaxNOW rapid antigen tests and distributed 150 million tests to states with the intention for states to give the tests to schools and nursing homes. The federal government could have continued to procure tests on behalf of all purchasers at this price and expanded the types of organizations that were eligible to receive them through the federal-to-state distribution arrangement to stabilize market volatility, but this did not happen.

In January 2022, the Biden Administration launched a similar initiative whereby the federal government purchased over-the-counter tests in bulk and shipped them directly to US households through the US Postal Service and made them available for pick-up at major retail pharmacy chains such as CVS, Rite Aid, and Walgreens. Many different brands serviced these contracts. The Biden Administration also issued an executive order, and subsequent regulatory guidance, requiring health insurers to cover over-the-counter tests up to $12 per test. These types of high-volume contracts and federally negotiated prices helped test makers project their sales and operations and reduced the burden on private purchasers to fight for contracts at significant markups.

Taking all of these factors together, policymakers should consider funding mechanisms and policy frameworks that would facilitate greater adoption and faster implementation of testing programs during future pandemics. These could include:

- federal or state purchase agreements (with multiple diagnostic makers) to reduce price volatility and make it easier for test makers to scale up manufacturing and operations
- centralized (federal or state) test kit distribution to increase access and reduce supply chain volatility – the framework could be expanded beyond the US Postal Service to include major couriers such as UPS, FedEx, and Amazon
- uniform payment and reimbursement policies to eliminate confusion over financial responsibility, such as requiring providers and payers to follow CMS fee schedules or paying for all testing through a single federal funding stream

Case studies from other countries may provide insights into streamlined funding mechanisms and distribution channels. In some European countries, for example, there was much broader access to fully government-funded community test sites (which reduced the need to establish work- or school-based testing programs) and test kits could be purchased from pharmacies at significantly lower prices than in the United States (or for free).

Privacy/Liability Issues

Like with the confusion over financial responsibility, we heard from many stakeholders that they hesitated to set up testing programs due to concerns over liability and privacy. It was not clear, for example, whether some employers (such as manufacturers and essential service providers) were *required* to provide testing as a means of compliance with state or federal occupational safety and health administration standards or whether they had the authority to *compel* workers to undergo testing and share test results with employers. Some guidance stated that employers could require employees to show proof of negative test results, but did not address frequency or time frames for testing nor did they address employers' responsibility to provide, or pay for, on-site testing as opposed to directing employees to seek community or off-site testing before coming to work.

Again, federal guidance was complicated by state and local agencies that issued their own bulletins. Many large employers have locations all over the country within different jurisdictions. This was one reason that office-based employers gave for repeatedly extending their work-from-home policies. In schools, testing was voluntary and required parental consent, which limited the effectiveness of testing programs and increased the total cost per test. Additionally, neither employers nor schools had clear guidance on their responsibility to conduct contact tracing or how to do it in a way that complied with privacy laws.

Stakeholders could have benefited from clearer guidance and liability protections. For example, schools and employers expressed significant concerns over compliance with the Health Insurance Portability and Accountability Act (HIPAA) of 1996, even though they are not HIPAA-covered entities. Employers and schools have their own privacy and confidentiality laws, and any third-party testing companies they hired would have had to be HIPAA-compliant. Privacy issues also arose around contact tracing. Local public health agencies were overwhelmed, and schools were asked (or required) to conduct contact tracing themselves. On-site testing creates additional privacy concerns because children who test positive need to leave campus as soon as possible, yet pulling them out of class discloses personal health information (their COVID-19 status) to other children. Some schools conducted testing before or after school to reduce this concern, but anecdotal evidence suggests fewer children participated when testing took place outside school hours.

It was also unclear what the minimum standards were for schools and workplaces to release them from liability, such as masking, ventilation, and disinfection protocols. Meatpacking plants and assembly lines where workers must be in proximity to one another, for example, could have benefited from clear minimum standards, which may have differed from offices with cubicle partitions, individual offices, and other environments with more spacing.

Policymakers and public health officials should anticipate concerns over privacy and liability before the next pandemic. Policies and guidance should consider:

- the circumstances under which on-site testing is required and providing guidance on the financial responsibility for testing
- requiring mandatory proof of negative test results, within a given time frame or at a specified frequency, for in-person attendance at work/school, concerts, large gatherings, travel, etc., with medical exemptions
- the responsibility to provide reasonable accommodation, as well as standards for acceptable forms of reasonable accommodation (distance learning/smaller class sizes, remote work), for those with medical exemptions
- the minimum safety precautions that must be in place to provide release of liability for positive cases
- providing clear guidance for non-compliance

Testing Guidance and Messaging

The demand for test kits varied significantly by region, with regions that encouraged stricter mask wearing and other mitigation strategies having higher test kit demand than regions with more relaxed mask wearing and mitigation approaches. As explained earlier, some entities may have been more likely to implement testing programs if the risks and benefits had been more clearly communicated and/or if testing protocols (types, frequencies, use cases, effectiveness, etc.) had been uniform.

Federal agencies were not aligned in their messaging, and state agencies exceeded or ignored federal guidance. Dozens of testing playbooks and best practices were issued by numerous governmental and nongovernmental organizations, but there was no uniform standard for each setting, population, or type of organization.

The Commercialization Team conducted an analysis in late 2020 of nearly 50 different playbooks on COVID-19 mitigation strategies. We entered the recommendations in each playbook into a database and analyzed them for consistencies/discrepancies in what they advised. Many more playbooks, particularly for educational settings, were published in 2021. However, of the ones we reviewed, we found that:

- infection control and prevention measures were the topics covered most thoroughly
- guidance across documents was generally consistent, and was often based on or contained references to the CDC

- the playbook of the National Community Pharmacy Association was the only one that we reviewed that included reimbursement/financial assistance guidance
- only five playbooks included guidance on test selection
- only eight playbooks included testing implementation guidance

Many of the regulatory and policy issues listed here remain unsolved as of the writing of this chapter and will have a continued impact on the deployment of rapid, user-friendly diagnostics during future pandemics. Outside the time constraints of a public health emergency, policymakers should take the time to build frameworks, guidance, and regulations that could be triggered in a public health emergency.

Core Function 7: Digital Solutions and Emerging Diagnostic Workflow

The pre-pandemic public health infrastructure was designed to support a traditional healthcare delivery model in which testing for infectious diseases relies on:

- clinical staff to collect patient information and virus samples, administer and interpret POC tests or safely transport samples and transmit the necessary information to laboratories, and report results back to patients, with connection to follow-up care if needed
- laboratory staff to receive (accession stage), analyze/process (result stage), and report test results to public agencies and providers (some private laboratories have patient-facing web portals or phone numbers through which patients can access results, but public health laboratories often do not)

In this model, diagnostic manufacturers' technological requirements are determined by provider and laboratory workflows, such as scannable barcodes and software that can transmit information between electronic health records and laboratory information management systems, and from laboratory information management systems to public health agency reporting databases. POC tests often have reader machines with specially designed interfaces and software capabilities. Once diagnostic supplies are purchased, manufacturers do not play any further role in test administration and processing.

Prior to the pandemic, home-based diagnostics were mostly limited to noninfectious diseases. For example, home pregnancy test results are easy to interpret and do not have to be shared with providers or public health agencies. They do not require any special software or technological components, although some manufacturers include QR codes or have created apps to provide instructional videos, results confirmation, or information on lot numbers and expiration dates.

The pandemic expanded the boundaries of our health-care system, necessitating products and infrastructure to be used by nonclinical staff and laypersons. Suddenly, communities needed user-friendly methods for collecting personally identifiable information, administering tests, interpreting results, and sharing results with public health agencies, employers, schools, concert/sports venues, and travel officials such as airline or cruise agents. Testing programs needed streamlined and secure software that was cheap and easy to use and could fulfill mandatory reporting requirements.

The RADx Commercialization Team communicated stakeholders' needs and challenges to portfolio companies and shared digital solutions and best practices that appeared to be working well in the field. We connected RADx companies with software developers and

Table 11.7 Changing diagnostic landscape

Traditional (pre-pandemic) diagnostic workflow	Emerging, rapid test workflow (on-site testing)
The patient seeks out testing in a health-care setting (doctor's office, urgent care, or clinic)	The patient (or a helper) registers themselves and enters information on a secure online portal (ideally before arriving at the testing site)
	This could include parental/employee consent forms
The provider collects patient information in an electronic health record, collects the sample from the patient, and submits a laboratory order	The patient (or helper) self-swabs and inserts the sample into the device
The test is sent to a laboratory where the laboratory receives, processes, and reports test results	The result is displayed via a visual read or an app
The laboratory shares the test results with the provider, who informs the patient For reportable communicable diseases, the laboratory shares the results with required public health agencies	The results need to be reported to public agencies, as well as to an employer, school district, etc.
The patient receives the test results by phone or through a patient portal	Employers/schools need to track all results over time
If indicated, the provider gives the patient treatment recommendations, which could include a prescription The public health agency calls the patient to conduct contact tracing	Patients need a way to show or submit the test result to third parties (a security guard, employer, airline, or school)

existing digital platforms, but this work should have been done much earlier in the process. Future diagnostics should evaluate technology needs early and often.

Prior to the pandemic, public health databases for receiving information related to reportable communicable diseases typically only received test results from CLIA and CLIA-waived entities, such as laboratories, clinics, and hospitals. Different states receive results in different formats (Health Level Seven [HL7] messages, .csv files, etc.), and their systems are often outdated and/or cumbersome to navigate. States may also collect different information, and data entry fields and categories may be different from what the CDC collects. These systems were not designed to be public-facing and easily accessible by employers, schools, or individuals, which created significant testing barriers. Organizations cannot run test sites if they have no way to report results.

During the pandemic, some states created pathways for nonclinical entities to be able to report test results by uploading Excel files or entering results via websites and mobile apps. In other states, positive home-based test results could be reported only if the person sought out a confirmatory, laboratory-based PCR test. This skews positivity rates because negative home test results go unreported. All stakeholders could have benefited from standardized data capture and exchange. A national reporting system that diagnostic makers could have integrated into their technology would have accelerated the commercialization process because it would have allowed for off-the-shelf, all-in-one solutions.

RADx-Initiated Reporting Solutions

In January 2022, RADx launched Mobile and At-home Reporting through Standards (MARS), a partnership between the National Institute of Biomedical Imaging and Bioengineering and the Office of the National Coordinator for Health Information Technology, to solve the COVID-19 self-test reporting drop-off. The goals were to:

1. design a system for encoding results and associated data in a health-care industry-standard format
2. identify one (or a small few) destination(s) where these results can be sent and subsequently retransmitted to appropriate state, federal, and related health systems
3. establish best practices for future reporting of remote diagnostics

In working with national and international health data organizations, MARS has developed, and as of December 2022 is still accepting public comments on, an HL7 v2 specification so that all interfaces are collecting the same type of information from users and transmitting it in a standardized way to a central reporting hub. MARS removes the burden of various jurisdictions (county and state public health agencies) having to collect at-home test results and report the data to the CDC.

Through RADx MARS, the NIH is also funding mobile app development, the adoption and implementation of the new reporting standards, and the development of user interfaces that are more user-friendly and meet equitability/accessibility requirements. Reporting systems, such as software companies, test manufacturers, and others facilitating over-the-counter reporting can send test results to one of two hubs:

1. the Association of Public Health Laboratories (APHL) AIMS+ platform – an informatics messaging services platform
2. ReportStream – an open-source platform created by the CDC in late 2020 to facilitate reporting of rapid antigen COVID-19 test results

There is no cost to onboard and transmit test results to state and federal systems through either hub, but reporting systems must be able to send messages that conform to a standard HL7 v2 specification to participate. In November 2022, RADx Tech published a website (https://learn.makemytestcount.org/) that allows users to anonymously report individual test results of any brand of at-home COVID-19 test. Further development of application programming interfaces (APIs) that integrate with existing student information management systems, human resources software, and other non-electronic health record platforms would make it easier for nonclinical entities such as schools and employers to submit batch test results.

Lessons Learned

In a crisis, the impact of diagnostic research and development is limited to the number of tests that make it into the hands of those who need to be tested. Detailed customer discovery and market research need to be conducted early and continually updated. Clinical teams should be in frequent communication with the commercial teams so that they can adapt and respond to the needs of and feedback from external stakeholders in real time before product finalization. As the science and understanding of the virus continuously evolves, so too do market dynamics, political and regulatory reactions, and technology needs. RADx proved incredibly nimble, but several environmental factors still affected the commercial success of RADx portfolio companies. The following recommendations summarize the tactics worth replicating and the challenges that must be anticipated, as described in this chapter:

- Establish communication channels between clinical and commercial teams to provide real-world experiences and market feedback
- Establish communication channels with the FDA, the CDC, and others to provide context for test classification review decisions, playbook development, etc.
- Conduct quantitative and qualitative market research analyses through surveys of a wide range of sectors that can be shared with diagnostic developers
- Convene roundtables and host webinars with two-way feedback to gather information as well as educate market players
- Provide internal and external resources to support business operations; do not restrict funding to research and development
- Consider additional pathways to help companies raise working capital, such as connection to lenders, government purchase orders, and/or matching funds
- Hold companies accountable through required milestones tied to funding tranches; create an offboarding process for companies that stagnate
- Recreate federal purchasing and distribution programs that increase access to no-cost testing by expanding US Postal Service programs to FedEx, UPS, Amazon, etc., and by streamlining pharmacy/retailer distribution without having to bill insurance
- Pair diagnostics with digital solutions, through either native software or external partnerships, before they go to market
- Develop a national communicable disease reporting system by creating uniform data collection and data transfer standards, establishing a framework for emergency-related access and connectivity for batch results, and implementing APIs for quick integrations with other software and reporting systems
- Create pandemic-related policy and regulatory frameworks that address CLIA waiver protocols when mass testing is needed in non-CLIA-waived health-care settings (pharmacies and residential care facilities) and/or nonclinical settings (homes, workplaces, schools, and public spaces)

Reference

1 White House, Statement from the Press Secretary regarding the Administration's purchase of 150 million rapid COVID-19 tests (August 27, 2020). https://tinyurl.com/ynjd6ajm.

Chapter 12

Testing Strategies to Mitigate COVID-19 Disease Spread

Paul Tessier and Anette E. Hosoi

Introduction

Taking measures to slow and prevent the spread of COVID-19 infection was an essential strategy for safely returning to work and school during the pandemic. The expansion of COVID-19 diagnostic testing across the USA was – and continues to be – critical to that effort. Testing can help people determine if they are infected with severe acute respiratory syndrome coronavirus 2 (SARS-CoV-2; the virus that causes COVID-19), regardless of whether they have symptoms, and thus if they are at risk of spreading the infection to others.

In the early months of the pandemic, diagnostic tests were made available at clinics and pop-up testing sites. Wherever possible, regular testing was instituted in settings where groups of people congregated regularly, such as schools, assisted living facilities, and businesses. Testing in non-health-care environments, however, proved to be complex. While universities and large businesses may have had the resources to deploy testing, kindergarten to 12th grade (K–12) schools, manufacturers, and other small businesses were less likely to have the requisite knowledge or resources available. Implementing testing within an organization also raises a number of questions, such as: Who should be tested? How often should testing be done? What type of test should be used? How does a testing program fit with other mitigation strategies (e.g. mask wearing, contact tracing, limiting unmasked group activities, and vaccination)? How much will it all cost? What are the risks of not testing?

In addition, small and medium-sized organizations interested in establishing a testing program did not have access to affordable and easily purchased tests, and this was exacerbated by the fact that most test manufacturers did not have the infrastructure to sell to small and medium-sized organizations that were new to testing.

This chapter summarizes the efforts of and the lessons learned by the Rapid Acceleration of Diagnostics (RADx®) Tech team in:

- providing science-based outputs to assess and guide specific mitigation and testing strategies
- demonstrating how COVID-19 prevention and containment efforts can most effectively be combined with the latest testing strategies to minimize the spread of the virus in a semi-contained organization (e.g. schools and businesses)
- delivering personal recommendations based on how likely an individual is to get COVID-19 and spread it to other people
- creating a marketplace for individuals and organizations to purchase testing solutions at a fair price

Efforts to Support Testing Adoption

Widespread, frequent testing is essential to the larger public health picture, helping investigators characterize the prevalence, spread, and contagiousness of the virus and its variants. Theoretically, if the USA had been able to test broadly and rapidly for COVID-19 sooner, and that effort was combined with other mitigations, we might have avoided a nationwide lockdown and its concomitant impacts on supply chains, work productivity, mental health, and more.

In the early months of the pandemic, there was significant confusion and concern on the part of the public and public health authorities around the likelihood and prevalence of asymptomatic spread. It is now recognized that a significant fraction of SARS-CoV-2 infections are transmitted by people who are not showing any symptoms. Identifying infected individuals while they are presymptomatic, as well as those who are asymptomatic, is critical to a successful testing strategy.

Testing strategies, including diagnostic testing (intended to identify current infection in individuals) and screening testing (intended to identify people with COVID-19 who are asymptomatic and do not have known, suspected, or reported exposure to SARS-CoV-2), can be used to achieve four primary goals:

1. minimize the initial spread and suppress the resurgence of outbreaks
2. lift confinement restrictions and enable individuals to return to normal activities such as school, work, and travel
3. gain intelligence on the evolution of the epidemic
4. enable treatment to start as soon as possible (the Test to Treat program, for example, provides same-visit testing and treatment for people who are at high risk of getting very sick from COVID-19)

At-home rapid tests, once available, became critical to slowing the spread of the virus. Awareness of one's own infection status encourages mitigation (e.g. self-isolation and wearing masks) to prevent spread. In other words, the ease with which people can know their COVID-19 status is directly correlated with how well prevention and treatment can be implemented. As of the writing of this chapter, RADx Tech has supported dozens of product teams with a cumulative production capacity of 4 billion tests under 50 US Food and Drug Administration (FDA) Emergency Use Authorizations (EUAs).

Considering that the public had never previously conducted self-testing at such a large scale, and to ensure that the unprecedented achievement of providing test kits to the country achieved the intended maximal impact, namely ending the pandemic, the RADx Tech team partnered with the Massachusetts Institute of Technology (MIT)'s Institute for Data, Systems, and Society (IDSS) and CIMIT to launch the website https://whentotest .org/ in early December 2020.[1] This site was dedicated to providing science-based outputs to assess and guide specific mitigation and COVID-19 testing strategies. The website includes two calculators (one for individuals and one for organizations), a comprehensive list of frequently asked questions targeted to each user group, and playbooks with detailed information for K–12 programs, testing implementation guidance, and laboratory pool testing.

The individual calculator ("COVID Risk Quiz") is a decision-support tool that delivers insights and recommendations based on how likely an individual is to get COVID-19 and spread it to other people. A user is guided through a short series of simple questions that cover the person's location, vaccination status, mask-wearing habits, and contacts and social gatherings. Based on these behaviors and the prevalence of disease in the person's location, the calculator suggests whether the person should consider COVID-19 testing and determines their risk of having or getting COVID-19 and their risk of spreading COVID-19. A link to the US Centers for Disease Control and Prevention (CDC) self-testing guidance assists people in getting an at-home COVID-19 test and provides instructions on how to use the test and interpret test results. Frequently asked questions in the individual calculator address COVID-19, mitigations, and testing. Topics include:

- the difference between polymerase chain reaction (PCR) and antigen tests
- the difference between isolation and quarantine
- how virus variants affect testing
- the impact of vaccines on an overall testing strategy
- how mask wearing affects test recommendations

The organization calculator ("Workplace Testing Planner") assists groups such as schools and businesses in developing a plan to minimize the spread of COVID-19 throughout their organizations. A user answers a series of simple questions that cover the organization's size, contact testing program, and location, in addition to employee testing participation, vaccination status, and rate of mask wearing. Based on these inputs, the calculator determines the recommended screening testing frequency and cost of testing for various types of testing technologies. The recommended frequency and cost of testing vary based on test performance, a factor that is built into the calculator. Users can readily explore different mitigation strategies – such as changing the company-wide mask-wearing policy – to find out how those changes impact recommended testing strategies and the accompanying costs. Different strategies can be compared in side-by-side tables.

Advanced users of the organization calculator can adjust underlying assumptions used in the calculations such as vaccine effectiveness, mask efficiency, basic reproductive number (R_0), and test performance parameters. Each setting has a tool tip to explain the function, and a video guide is available. Implementation details and additional test details – such as staffing requirements, equipment requirements (if needed), the number of people isolated or quarantined, and pooled test options – are also available.

As with the individual calculator, the organization calculator provides answers for company management to frequently asked questions such as:

- How do I know if I need to test at my organization at all?
- When can I stop testing?
- Where can I purchase the kind of test that the calculator recommends?
- What do we do when someone tests positive?
- What are the reporting and confidentiality requirements for COVID-19 test results?

In 2021, the When To Test initiative partnered with Project N95 to create a marketplace for individuals and organizations to purchase testing solutions at a fair price. Project N95 is a not-for-profit organization that was launched early in the pandemic to provide access to personal protective equipment for small organizations and individuals. Adding testing solutions to the platform was a natural fit to address the testing needs of these constituents. A shared goal of When To Test and Project N95 is to provide support for COVID-19 testing in non-health-care environments.

The RADx Tech team also launched a companion tool, My COVID Toolkit (which has since been integrated with When To Test), to educate the public on current facts, the optimal usage of test kits, and the importance of mitigation strategies, as well as to provide guidance on making smart choices. The website gives users the necessary information to make informed choices for their unique situation, whether that is going to work or school, doing everyday tasks such as grocery shopping, planning their social life, or attending special events. Simple safety measures are explained that can reduce an individual's risk of becoming infected and infecting others. The site also has information on available treatments, eligibility considerations for those treatments, and where and how to access treatment.

Test Types

The current diagnostic procedures for COVID-19 and its variants include two primary approaches: molecular tests and antigen tests.

Molecular tests detect genetic material from the virus, typically using a laboratory technique called real-time reverse transcription quantitative PCR. Not all molecular tests use PCR; however, this serves as the mainstay of COVID-19 diagnostic testing. Molecular tests amplify bits of viral ribonucleic acid (RNA) so that the viral infection can be detected. These tests also are referred to as nucleic acid amplification test (NAAT) assays. If SARS-CoV-2 is present in a person's nasal or saliva sample, even low levels of virus genomic material can be amplified into millions of copies during this assay. There are also point-of-care (POC) and over-the-counter (OTC) molecular tests. These tests typically use an isothermal amplification technique that is not as accurate as PCR.

Antigen tests detect proteins from the virus. Antigen tests are very specific for the COVID-19 virus but are not as sensitive as molecular tests. This means that a positive result is highly accurate, but a negative result does not rule out infection. They are also less expensive and generally faster than molecular tests. The consistent availability of rapid antigen tests for both POC and OTC use is necessary to contain the spread of infection and enable the reduction of activity restrictions. Rapid antigen tests must be performed frequently (e.g. two tests in sequence within a 24- to 48-hour period) to be effective.

In general, PCR tests pick up low viral loads, whereas antigen tests may not. That is why serial testing is needed with antigen tests. If someone is early in the infection cycle, they might have low viral load, which will likely increase as the infection continues and can be detected with a second antigen test. Both PCR tests and antigen tests can continue to give positive results even after someone is no longer considered infectious.

A third type of test – a so-called serologic test or antibody test – detects a prior infection in individuals through the presence of developed antibodies. Such tests are used to detect previous infections in people who had few or no symptoms and for surveillance and research purposes. Serologic tests provide intelligence on the evolution of the epidemic across the population.

With the continuous emergence of new variants of concern, which include mutations potentially affecting the nucleocapsid protein, the analytical performance of these assays should be frequently reevaluated. As described in Chapter 9, the RADx Tech initiative created a Variant Task Force (VTF) to assess the impact of emerging SARS-CoV-2 variants on in vitro diagnostic testing. The VTF is a cross-disciplinary and cross-organizational group of scientists and industry leaders with expertise in virology and diagnostic testing.

Working in tandem with clinical laboratories, the FDA, and the CDC, the VTF uses both *in silico* modeling and in vitro testing to determine the effect of SARS-CoV-2 mutations on diagnostic molecular and antigen tests.

In collaboration with ROSALIND (San Diego, California), the VTF developed a comprehensive platform – ROSALIND Diagnostic Monitoring (DxM) – that integrates bioinformatic modeling with clinical in vitro laboratory testing to assess the impact of SARS-CoV-2 mutations on both NAAT and antigen assays. (Refer to Chapter 9 for more information about ROSALIND.)

A Data-Driven Model to Mitigate Spread

Widespread testing is essential for understanding the extent of COVID-19, predicting peaks in contagion, anticipating where the next hot spots will emerge, and deploying resources to prepare for those surges. However, this is just the tip of the iceberg – the real potency of testing is not just in information, but in control.

The mathematical models behind the individual and organization testing recommendations provided by When To Test were developed to quantify the relationship between testing, risk, and control. These recommendations grew out of a partnership between the RADx Tech team and a volunteer, interdisciplinary team at IDSS assembled to analyze data associated with the COVID-19 pandemic in order to inform policymakers. The IDSS COVID-19 Collaboration, dubbed "Isolat," brought together faculty, postdoctoral researchers, and students from across IDSS, MIT, and around the globe.

Over the course of five months, Isolat met daily to discuss the findings of the various interconnected research projects. Different Isolat teams worked on forecasting waves or spikes in virus spread, modeling modes of transmission, assessing policies and economic effects, and exploring the impacts on more vulnerable communities to address equity in managing scarce resources. Team members also established a data lake that allowed researchers access to many relevant, up-to-date datasets.

Isolat brought insights to bear on many aspects of the pandemic, including the challenge of "hidden" carriers of the virus. At the onset of the pandemic, it quickly became evident that a significant fraction of the population was contagious but asymptomatic, while in others the disease was deadly; this combination is one of the most difficult scenarios to navigate. To understand the challenges associated with this particular mix of factors, consider the two extremes: Either most of the population experiences severe symptoms or most of the population is asymptomatic. In the first case, carriers can be rapidly identified through their symptoms and isolated to prevent spread. In the second, the virus spreads quickly through the population but does not have serious consequences (similar to the common cold). In the intermediate case, which corresponds with the COVID-19 scenario, asymptomatic people are difficult to identify and continue to interact with others, some of whom may die from the disease. Each of these interactions carries some probability that the virus will be transmitted and, if transmission occurs, consequences range from benign to deadly. Therefore, the most dangerous situation is one in which there are many hidden carriers and a significant proportion of the population has a severe reaction to the disease.

During a pandemic, strategies are required to deal with scenarios in which the agents spreading the disease may be unknown. To that end, Isolat created a model to quantify the power of testing in combination with other control strategies in semi-contained communities, such as schools and places of work.

The analysis is built on a simple counting exercise known in different disciplines as a control volume approach or queuing theory. The key idea is illustrated in Figure 12.1, which shows the movement of people into and out of different sub-populations: susceptible, infected, recovered, and isolated. There have been many excellent studies that consider different subdivisions from the ones we show here (e.g. many studies include a hospitalized subset); these finer distinctions are often necessary for logistics, planning, and allocating resources. However, for our simple estimate, we are primarily interested in the flow into and out of the "dangerous box" – the subpopulation of infected people who are not isolated but actively interacting with the community.

To control the spread of the virus, we need to limit the number of people in that "box." This can be done in two ways:

1. slowing the rate of people entering the box through mitigation strategies such as social distancing, improved hygiene, mask wearing, vaccination, and contact tracing
2. accelerating the rate at which we remove people from that population through testing, isolation, and quarantining

A great deal of our collective societal efforts, particularly in the USA, focused on practicing social distancing to reduce the mean number of people expected to become infected from one carrier. However, instead of relying predominantly on the first strategy, we can use this model to elevate the second strategy – testing and isolating people from the community while they are contagious – to develop a more balanced approach.

In typical model representations for the spread of diseases, people move among sub-populations (represented as moving from box to box in Figure 12.1). The rate at which people become infected is proportional to the reproduction number R_0 (pronounced "R-naught"), which represents the expected number of infections from one contagious individual in a naive population. When a person first becomes infected, they are not

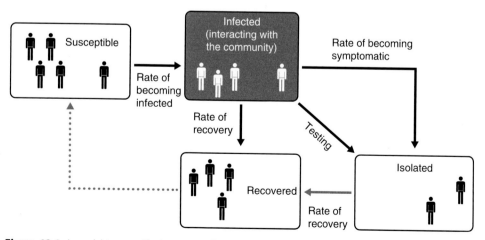

Figure 12.1 A model to quantify the power of testing in combination with other control strategies in semi-contained communities.

symptomatic and thus they move into the "Infected" box. From that box, each day presents four possibilities in our model:

1. with probability 1/D, the person recovers, where D represents the average recovery time in days – approximately 10 days for COVID-19
2. with probability S/D they become symptomatic, where S is the fraction of the infected population that develops symptoms (symptomatic people are immediately isolated)
3. with probability T_F they are tested; the test will reveal the infection and they are immediately isolated (this will be adjusted to account for test sensitivity)
4. they remain asymptomatic and undetected in the "Infected" box

This mean field approach suggests a simple strategy to estimate the value of testing in controlling the spread of the virus.[2] Essentially, we need to adjust the flow into and out of the "Infected" box such that the net number of people entering that box is less than or equal to the number exiting the box:

$$R_0/D \leq T_F + 1/D + S/D$$

So, what does testing buy us? Rearranging the equation yields the simple heuristic relationship:

$$R_0 \leq 1 + T_F D + S$$

This equation provides a rough estimate of the direct trade-off between social distancing and testing. In the absence of testing and isolation, we recover the standard criteria to control the spread of a disease, namely $R_0 \leq 1$. Increasing testing (increasing T_F) and/or isolating symptomatic individuals allows for less stringent social distancing requirements (a larger allowable effective reproduction number) without violating the inequality (i.e. keeping the spread of the virus contained).

Additional Strategies

As mentioned previously, controlling the spread of the virus can be accomplished through mitigation strategies such as social distancing, improved hygiene, mask wearing, vaccination, and contact tracing in addition to testing. These strategies play an important role in an overall mitigation plan and have a significant impact on testing requirements and therefore the cost of a testing program. In the model, these strategies appear as multipliers on R_0 that reduce the effective reproduction number.

COVID-19 is a highly contagious respiratory infection that is primarily spread when an infected person exhales droplets/particles containing the virus, which are subsequently inhaled by other people or land on their eyes, noses, or mouth. Thus, masks can be very effective at minimizing disease spread, with some mask types, such as the KN95 masks, being much more effective than others. To estimate the impact of mask wearing on the effective reproduction number, we turn to simple estimates for filtration.

In general, filters can be roughly classified by their filtration efficiency β, which represents the fraction of particles blocked by the filter (the "95" in KN95 masks means that the mask is rated to block 95% of particles larger than 0.3 microns, roughly the size of a typical viral particle).[3] Given that the models described earlier represent average spreading dynamics in a population, to estimate the impact of mask wearing on the effective reproduction number, we must know the approximate fraction of the population wearing masks, P. We can then use P to estimate what fraction of encounters are mitigated by one, two, or zero masks, for example, and use this estimate to modify the effective reproduction number:

$$(1-P\beta)^2 R_0 \leq 1 + T_F D + S$$

Note that if masks were perfect filters ($\beta = 1$) and 100% of the population wore masks ($P = 1$), we would not require any other mitigation strategies and the virus would be perfectly contained.

Another way to reduce the effective reproduction number (the left side of the equation) is through vaccination. Vaccines offer several benefits, including protection against severe illness and, in some cases, protection against transmission. Vaccine efficacy against severe illness has been remarkable throughout the pandemic. However, efficacy against transmission has varied as new variants arise, as our immune systems evolve, and as the vaccines improve. Consider a vaccine with efficacy ε against transmission, where ε represents the fraction of people who would have contracted the virus but do not on account of vaccination (e.g. if $R_0 = 4$, for every infected person we expect four more people to contract the virus). However, if everyone is vaccinated and $\varepsilon = 0.5$, then two of those four people are protected, and the effective reproductive number is 2. Once again, we can modify our heuristic relationship to account for vaccination, where f is the fraction of people who have been vaccinated:

$$(1-\varepsilon f)(1-P\beta)^2 R_0 \leq 1 + T_F D + S$$

Note that vaccines only modify the left side of the equation if they protect against *transmission*.

The final modification we will make to our model is to include the fact that tests are not perfect. There will be cases when the tested individual is carrying the virus, but the test fails to detect the carrier and returns a false negative. The probability of a false negative is reflected in the sensitivity, s_e, of the test. The sensitivity of PCR tests is close to 100%, whereas the sensitivity of antigen tests range can from 80% to 100%.[4] Including this consideration in the model, we arrive at our final expression:

$$(1-\varepsilon f)(1-P\beta)^2 R_0 \leq 1 + s_e T_F D + S$$

In the following section, "Examples of Different Mitigation Strategies," we will provide examples in which we use this expression to evaluate the testing needs of various organizations and the impact of other mitigations.

Clearly, vaccination is a powerful and important tool in reducing the spread of COVID-19. Vaccination reduces the risk of contracting and thus spreading the disease, although breakthrough infection is not uncommon. Thankfully, the risk of hospitalization and death is greatly reduced in breakthrough infections, but vaccination alone does not totally stem disease spread. The added strategies of contact tracing and the identification of hot spots and super spreaders can potentially further help to control spread.

While an optimal testing strategy would rely on perfect information about an individual's movements and behavior over time, these interactions can be approximated through methods such as contact tracing or through inferring their location from building entry. Individuals who are more likely to be infected owing to interactions with infected individuals or time spent in hot spots, for example, could be tested preferentially. Universities are one example of semi-contained environments that may have the capability to require those on campus to use their ID to enter buildings. The data of who enters where and when could then be used to estimate contacts between individuals. With this estimation, it is theoretically possible to identify locations or hot spots through which many people pass and which may amplify disease spread. It may also be possible to trace back the contacts of those who have tested positive, potentially filling in the gaps of traditional interview-based contact tracing. However, in practice, it has been found that the added overhead logistics associated with individual testing schedules, along with legitimate privacy concerns, are not worth the small gains in control. Throughout the pandemic, universities that instituted regular testing by and large adopted a constant regular testing cadence in their communities (rather than targeted individualized testing schedules). However, data from several studies show that congregating indoors with poor ventilation can cause higher levels of disease transmission. Identifying these hot spots and removing access to those spaces may be helpful in mitigating the spread.

Examples of Different Mitigation Strategies

In this section, we provide examples of how adjustments to mitigation strategies can affect the frequency and cost of testing required to prevent an outbreak, as demonstrated in the When To Test calculators.

Manufacturing Facility

This example is based on a manufacturing facility with 250 employees located in Hartford County in Connecticut on January 3, 2023.

Effect of Mask Wearing on Testing Requirements and Cost

Assume in this manufacturing facility:
- 80% of employees are willing to participate in a testing program
- there is an established contact tracing program
- 70% of employees are vaccinated

With 50% of employees properly and reliably wearing surgical masks, the organization would need to test employees three times a week with antigen tests, at a testing cost of about $5 000/week, to prevent a workplace outbreak. If proper and reliable mask wearing could be increased to 70%, testing would only need to be conducted every other week at a cost of $1 000/week.

Effect of Vaccination on Testing Requirements and Cost

Now assume in this manufacturing facility:
- 80% of employees are willing to participate in a testing program
- there is an established contact tracing program
- 70% of employees properly and reliably wear surgical masks

With 20% of employees vaccinated, the organization would need to test employees three times a week with antigen tests, at a cost of about $5 000/week, to prevent a workplace outbreak. If the vaccination rate could be increased to 65%, testing would only need to be done once a week at a cost of $2 000/week.

Effect of Contact Tracing on Testing Requirements and Cost

Finally, assume in this manufacturing facility:

- 100% of employees are willing to participate in a testing program
- 85% of employees properly and reliably wear *cloth* masks
- 75% of employees are vaccinated

Without a contact tracing program, the organization would need to test employees three times a week with antigen tests, at a cost of about $5 000/week, to prevent a workplace outbreak. If effective contract tracing was implemented, testing would only need to be done twice a week at a cost of about $3 000/week.

University

In this example, we consider a university during the spring semester of 2021. At this time, the sensitivity of common PCR tests was (conservatively) approximately 70% and the reported number of days that a person was contagious with COVID-19 ranged from 10 to 14.

Assuming the absence of social distancing measures on campus, the R_0 may be at the high end of the spectrum. If we consider $R_0 = 7$ with no masking and no vaccination, the university will need to test $(7 - 1) / (0.7 \times 12) = 71\%$ of the population daily. As this is unlikely to be a feasible long-term strategy, the university may decide to combine testing efforts with a sensible campus social distancing strategy, such as masking or vaccination requirements. However, these numbers also suggest that the university could handle quite severe fluctuations by temporarily ramping up testing frequencies until the surge subsides.

We can also approach this problem from the inverse perspective; if the university has resources to test everyone once per week, what additional mitigation strategies are required to keep the virus in check? If vaccines are not widely available (or do not protect against transmission), the university may consider masking as a second layer of defense. Using the expression derived above and isolating the masking parameters on the right-hand side, we find:

$$1-[(1 + s_e T_F D)/R0]^{1/2} = 1-\left[(1 + 0.7^*(1/7)^*12)/7\right]^{1/2} = 0.44 \leq P\beta$$

This can be achieved if > 46% of the population wears KN95 masks ($\beta = 0.95$) or if > 55% of the population wears surgical masks ($\beta = 0.8$). Unfortunately, the virus cannot be contained with this level of testing and cloth masks alone ($\beta = 0.3$).

Pooled Testing

Pooled testing is an available technique that can reduce testing costs. Also known as group testing, this approach is implemented by combining individual samples into a single pooled sample that is typically tested using reverse transcription PCR. If the pooled sample tests negative, all individuals in the pool are negative. If the pooled sample tests positive, each person in the pool must be individually tested to determine who is positive.

Pooling is most effective when the chance of positive detection of SARS-CoV-2 is low (the overall prevalence of COVID-19 within a community is less than 10%). As the prevalence increases, the optimal pool size goes down, as does the expected reduction in the total number of tests performed.

One pooled testing trade-off is the time to identify positive individuals, as a second test is typically required. The increased turnaround can result in a delay in isolating an asymptomatic person or in an individual starting treatment. There are techniques that can be used to automatically deconvolve the positive individuals from the original sample; however, these techniques are not in common use. During the COVID pandemic, few companies offered pooled testing and few organizations used pooled testing companies.

Slowing the Spread

In a pandemic with a highly infectious virus such as COVID-19, the timing of when people become infected can be an important determinant of societal impact. Spreading out the infections over time – which can be accomplished by using mitigations such as testing – can prevent the overburdening of our health-care system and result in better care. This gives public health agencies and the health-care infrastructure invaluable time to respond to the crisis. It also allows time for knowledge of how to treat patients and of available treatment options to develop. In addition, fewer workers are out sick, enabling essential services and business operations to continue.

While it is desirable to minimize the number of people who contract the disease during a pandemic, slowing the spread of the disease is important even if the total infected population (the area under the two curves in Figure 12.2) is equivalent.

Public Policy Impact on Testing

US government public policy had a tremendous impact on the approval, production, and availability of COVID-19 tests. At the start of the pandemic, there were no FDA-cleared tests for COVID-19 and the standard process for clearance would have taken significant investment and time. By January 2022, the US Government was procuring 1 billion tests to give to US citizens for free, and OTC tests were commonly in use.

The following is an overview of some of the key US government actions that affected testing.

- On February 4, 2020, the Secretary of Health and Human Services declared that there was a public health emergency, justifying the authorization of emergency use of in vitro diagnostics for detection and/or diagnosis of the novel coronavirus[5]
- On March 6, 2020, the FDA issued a guidance document describing a policy for laboratories to develop and validate tests before such tests had been issued an EUA to achieve more rapid testing capacity[6]
- On March 17, 2020, the FDA issued a guidance document describing a policy to help accelerate the availability of novel coronavirus (COVID-19) diagnostic tests developed by laboratories and commercial manufacturers during the public health emergency through an EUA.[7] That policy evolved and was revised on May 4, 2020 and one week later on May 11, 2020, then on November 15, 2021
- On March 27, 2020, the Coronavirus Aid, Relief, and Economic Security (CARES) Act was signed, which provided broad ranging remedial measures designed to curb the economic impact of the pandemic and included:[8]

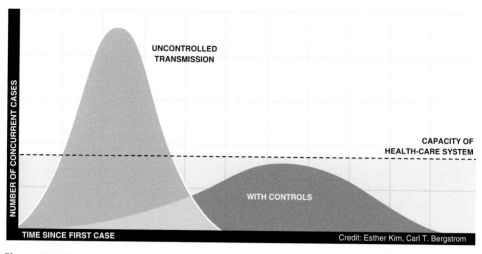

Figure 12.2 Flattening the curve relates to the control of a pandemic so the number of cases does not overwhelm a health system immediately. Modified image based on World Economic Forum figures. Source: www.weforum.org/agenda/2020/03/coronavirus-control-measures/.

- o modifying the FDA drug approval process, emergency paid sick leave programs, health insurance coverages for COVID-19 testing and vaccination, medical product supplies, and Medicare and Medicaid
- o providing $1.5 billion in investment from federal funding for the RADx program
- In April 2020, the RADx program was expanded to include RADx Advanced Technology Platforms (RADx-ATP) to increase testing capacity and throughput by identifying existing and late-stage testing platforms for COVID-19 that were far enough advanced to achieve rapid scale-up or expanded geographic placement in a short amount of time
- In June 2020, the RADx Tech II program was established to fill specific unmet national needs in two areas: (1) innovative, cost-effective, and accessible home and POC technologies that fill unmet national needs for screening, surveillance, diagnosis, and prognosis and (2) innovative methods and technologies that can be deployed in any setting (laboratory, POC, or home) that significantly advance SARS-CoV-2 variant testing capabilities
- In September 2020, the CDC reaffirmed its commitment to the significance of asymptomatic and presymptomatic transmission and reinforced the need to test asymptomatic persons
- In November 2020, the US government issued additional policy and regulatory revisions in response to the COVID-19 public health emergency instructing providers of COVID-19 diagnostic tests to make public their cash prices for those tests and establishing an enforcement scheme to enforce those requirements. The policy also required Medicaid programs to cover COVID-19 testing services[9]
- In January 2021, an executive order issued new guidance that removed barriers to COVID-19 diagnostic testing and vaccinations and strengthened the requirements for plans and issuers to cover diagnostic testing without cost sharing[10]

- In October 2021, the RADx program was again expanded to include the Independent Test Assessment Program (ITAP) to accelerate regulatory review and the availability of high-quality, accurate, and reliable OTC COVID-19 tests to the public, with the objective to quadruple the supply of at-home tests by the end of that year – up to 200 million at-home tests per month
- In November 2021, the Occupational Safety and Health Administration issued an emergency temporary standard stating that covered employers must develop, implement, and enforce a mandatory COVID-19 vaccination policy, with an exception for employers that instead adopt a policy requiring employees to either get vaccinated or elect to undergo regular COVID-19 testing and wear a face covering at work in lieu of vaccination[11]
- In January 2022, the US government required insurance companies and group health plans to cover the cost of at-home COVID-19 tests, thereby increasing access to free tests, and also announced the purchase of 1 billion tests to give to US citizens for free[12]

Conclusion

Many of the testing technologies and platforms developed for COVID-19 will allow the rapid development of tests for new pathogens that emerge, thus better preparing the nation to address a future pandemic. These products can also be applied to POC and OTC tests for diseases such as mpox, hepatitis, respiratory syncytial virus, influenza, HIV, and a variety of sexually transmitted infections. In addition, it has been shown that mass, at-home testing is a viable approach that is certain to continue in the future.

Lessons Learned

- Widespread, frequent testing is essential to characterize the prevalence, spread, and contagiousness of the virus and its variants. Widespread testing can also be useful in predicting peaks in contagion and anticipating where the next hot spots may emerge
- Screening (asymptomatic testing) for diseases in which a significant number of infected individuals are asymptomatic is important to identify and isolate infected but asymptomatic people who could spread the disease
- The implementation and effectiveness of complementary mitigations, such as mask wearing, isolation and quarantining, and vaccination, significantly impact testing requirements to control the spread of the virus
- Spreading out the infections over time – which can be accomplished by using mitigations such as testing – can prevent the health-care system from being overburdened and can buy time for the development of vaccines. In addition, in this way, the number of workers in a line of work that are out sick at any given time is less, allowing essential services and business operations to continue
- In addition to providing tests, it is necessary to provide education on testing and relevant mitigation strategies
- At-home testing raises the question of reporting results to characterize the prevalence, spread, and contagiousness of the virus
- Early testing with rapid results allows treatment to start as soon as possible, which can improve outcomes
- The public is accepting of, and capable of performing, self-testing

References

1. CIMIT, IDSS, and NIH RADx Initiative, When To Test (2020). https://whentotest.org/.

2. L. P. Kadanoff, More is the same; phase transitions and mean field theories. *J Stat Phys*, **137**, 5–6 (2009), 777–797.

3. W. Yim, D. Cheng, S. H. Patel, et al., KN95 and N95 respirators retain filtration efficiency despite a loss of dipole charge during decontamination. *ACS Appl Mater Interfaces*, **12**, 49 (2020), 54473–54480.

4. FDA, Template for developers of antigen tests (2021). www.fda.gov/media/137907/download.

5. US Department of Health and Human Services (HHS), Determination of public health emergency (2020). https://tinyurl.com/22252z7d.

6. FDA, Policy for diagnostics testing in laboratories certified to perform high complexity testing under the Clinical Laboratory Improvement Amendments prior to Emergency Use Authorization for coronavirus disease-2019 during the public health emergency; immediately in effect guidance for clinical laboratories and Food and Drug Administration staff; availability (2020). https://tinyurl.com/2s3efyse.

7. FDA, FDA issues temporary COVID-19 policy for receiving facilities and FSVP importers in meeting FSMA supplier verification onsite audit requirements (2020). https://tinyurl.com/mux3vbvr.

8. US Congress, H.R.748: Coronavirus Aid, Relief, and Economic Security Act or the CARES Act (2020). www.congress.gov/bill/116th-congress/house-bill/748.

9. US Department of Labor, Health and Human Services (HHS) and US Department of the Treasury, FAQs About Families First Coronavirus Response Act and Coronavirus Aid, Relief, And Economic Security Act Implementation Part 44 (2021). www.cms.gov/files/document/faqs-part-44.pdf.

10. J. R. Biden, Jr., National strategy for the COVID-19 response and pandemic preparedness (2021). https://tinyurl.com/ypeyuaju.

11. Occupational Safety and Health Administration (OSHA), Statement on the status of the OSHA COVID-19 vaccination and testing ETS (2022). www.osha.gov/coronavirus/ets2.

12. HHS Press Office, Biden-Harris Administration requires insurance companies and group health plans to cover the cost of at-home COVID-19 tests, increasing access to free tests (2022). https://tinyurl.com/47up6zz9.

A Pandemic Not Just of Infection but of Inequality: The Social Impact of COVID-19

Mara Aspinall and Liz Ruark

Introduction

It is hard to fully encompass or articulate the impact that the COVID-19 pandemic, caused by the severe acute respiratory syndrome coronavirus 2 (SARS-CoV-2) virus, has had on society in the USA and around the world. From the early days of denial through waves upon waves of cases and deaths to the sad recognition that the era of COVID-19 will likely never end, the last few years have been a tragedy of multiple dimensions.

Of course, the pandemic also shed light on the heroes among us, and many groups and organizations rose to the occasion. Work-from-home arrangements flourished, potentially changing the world of work forever. Digital innovations abounded. The reduction in traffic, and thus pollution, gave the planet a chance to breathe.

In this chapter, we focus on some of the most significant impacts of COVID-19 on US society, including many of the social ills it exposed, from income inequality and inequitable access to health care to the untenable burdens placed on public health workers. Our focus on the USA is not intended to minimize the fact that the disease has been confirmed in almost every country in the world or the fact that varied international responses to the virus – as well as demographic and economic differences among nations – have led to vastly divergent pandemic impacts. While we do not speak to the global experience here, many of the societal implications covered in this chapter are not unique to our nation and have been experienced around the world.

Direct Impacts of the Pandemic

The pandemic's disproportionate effects on the health and economic well-being of racial minorities, underserved communities, and low-income workers across the country have been heartbreaking. Data from the Centers for Disease Control and Prevention (CDC) show that, during the worst of the pandemic, Black, Hispanic/Latinx, American Indian, and Alaska Native people were hospitalized and/or died of the disease at rates more than 1.5 times higher than Caucasians, even when other socioeconomic differences were accounted for.[1] The death rates of Black and Hispanic/Latinx people during that phase were the highest of all, leaving their children with fewer caregivers.[2-4]

According to one study, adults aged 25 to 64 with a low socioeconomic position (SEP) were "five times as likely as high-SEP adults to die from COVID-19, and intermediate-SEP adults were twice as likely as high-SEP adults to die."[5]

Myriad reasons contribute to this disparity.[6] For example:

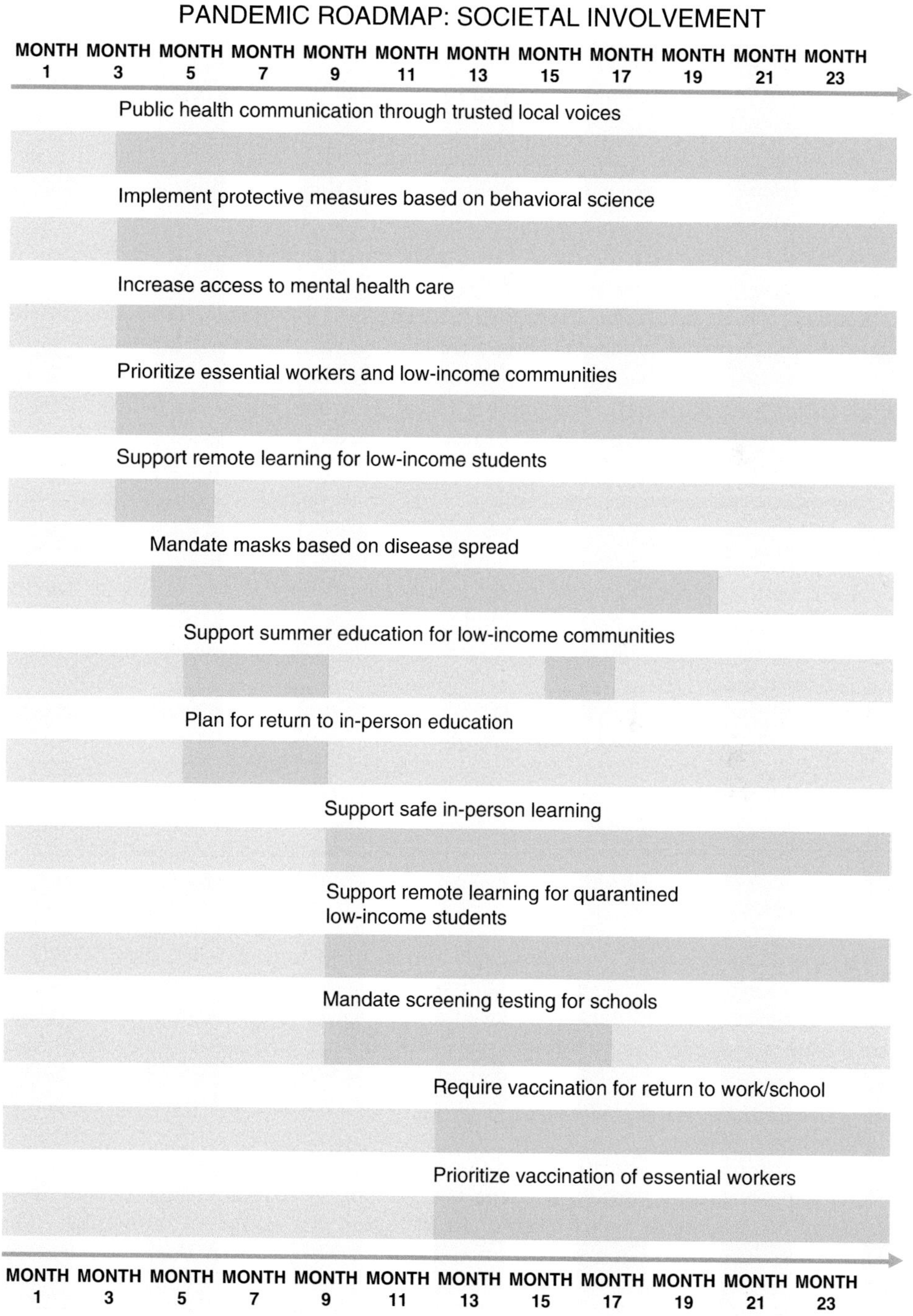

PANDEMIC ROADMAP: SOCIETAL INVOLVEMENT

MONTH 1	MONTH 3	MONTH 5	MONTH 7	MONTH 9	MONTH 11	MONTH 13	MONTH 15	MONTH 17	MONTH 19	MONTH 21	MONTH 23

Public health communication through trusted local voices

Implement protective measures based on behavioral science

Increase access to mental health care

Prioritize essential workers and low-income communities

Support remote learning for low-income students

Mandate masks based on disease spread

Support summer education for low-income communities

Plan for return to in-person education

Support safe in-person learning

Support remote learning for quarantined low-income students

Mandate screening testing for schools

Require vaccination for return to work/school

Prioritize vaccination of essential workers

MONTH 1	MONTH 3	MONTH 5	MONTH 7	MONTH 9	MONTH 11	MONTH 13	MONTH 15	MONTH 17	MONTH 19	MONTH 21	MONTH 23

Figure 13.1 This roadmap depicts the vital activities, their chronology, and an estimated time frame in months. In the case of the SARS-CoV-2 pandemic, month 1 was December 2019, the month in which the virus was isolated, sequenced, identified, and published.

- Communities of color are at increased risk of experiencing serious illness if they become infected with the virus, due to them having higher rates of certain underlying health conditions than white people
- Communities of color are more likely to be uninsured than white people and thus face increased challenges accessing COVID-19-related testing and treatment
- Communities of color, underserved communities, and low-wage workers face increased financial and health risks associated with COVID-19 due to economic and social circumstances

Unfortunately, because infection rates were higher among these groups, their incidence of long COVID, with all its concomitant effects, will likely be higher as well.

Another early marker of the disproportionate effects of the virus on these communities arrived during the very first months of the pandemic, when 22% of small businesses closed. The loss devastated Black-owned small-business owners in particular: 41% of their companies failed during this time. The number of Latinx-owned businesses fell by 32% and Asian-owned businesses dropped by 26%. Meanwhile, 17% of white-owned small businesses were shuttered.[7]

Low-income workers bore the brunt of COVID-19-related workplace closures and absences. As an example, in the initial surge of the omicron variant in the winter of 2021–2022, 6 in 10 adults with household incomes under \$40 000 had to miss work for COVID-19-related reasons, according to the Kaiser Family Foundation (KFF) COVID-19 Vaccine Monitor.[8] That meant a significant financial hit; nearly 50% of adults in that income bracket reported difficulty paying bills, compared with fewer than 15% of those with incomes of at least \$90 000 a year.

Why the dichotomy? In part it arose because of drastic differences in workplace flexibility. As the KFF reported in March 2022:

> One-third (32%) of workers in households with incomes below \$40,000 report getting paid time off if they [got] sick from COVID-19, compared to more than half (57%) of those earning \$40,000 or more. Similarly, 3 in 10 (28%) lower-income workers report having paid time off if they [needed] to quarantine following a COVID-19 exposure, compared to half of higher-income workers.[8]

These workers were also – unsurprisingly – more likely to go to work with COVID-19 symptoms, to avoid losing income. In addition, many lower wage employees were considered "essential workers" during the lockdowns of spring 2020, which meant that they were unable to sequester themselves at home during the pandemic's first surge. When they tested positive, their living conditions often meant that they were less likely to be able to effectively isolate themselves from other members of their households, which often included multiple generations.

Due in large part to a history of environmental racism, the communities in which people of color and low-income workers live tend to have more industrial companies and heavy manufacturers, leading to higher levels of air pollution, placing these communities at an even greater risk of poor outcomes from COVID-19. The fact that Black communities shoulder a disproportionate burden of the nation's pollution is not news; numerous studies have found that Black Americans are subjected to higher levels of air pollution than white Americans, regardless of their income level.[9] This problem was further exacerbated when regulations were suspended or relaxed and the Environmental Protection Agency postponed assessing penalties for environmental violations.

Just as income inequity and its consequences were compounded by the pandemic, so too were gender inequities, particularly for less-educated women. From February to May 2020, the Pew Research Center reported that roughly 11.5 million women lost their jobs, compared with 9 million men.[10] However, those job losses were concentrated primarily among women without a college degree – the employment of women who held at least a bachelor's degree grew by 3.9% between 2019 and 2021. By comparison, the number of women in the labor force without high-school diplomas decreased over that time by nearly 13% (compared with a decrease of approximately 5% among equivalently educated men).[11]

Indirect Impacts

The downstream consequences of COVID-19 were also worse for people of color and low-income workers. A classic example was access to routine health care. During the first year of the pandemic, Black and Hispanic/Latinx adults were significantly more likely to delay medical care or miss it altogether than white adults (13.3% and 16.2%, respectively, versus 8.7%, according to the Urban Institute's Health Reform Monitoring Survey).[12] During this time, adults with family incomes below 250% of the federal poverty level were more likely to avoid care both for themselves and for their children than adults with higher incomes (14.9% versus 8.2% for self-care; 12.3% versus 6.5% for children's care).[13] This disparity will outlast the pandemic for a variety of reasons, not least because of the impact on children of low-income families.

One hugely significant pandemic takeaway was the nation's rediscovery of the central place of public schools in our communities. In addition to education, these schools provide critical services that either are difficult to recreate successfully online (e.g. face-to-face socialization and physical education) or cannot be shifted to a virtual platform at all (e.g. free and reduced-cost meals). Approximately 35–40% of children's daily nutrition comes from meals they eat at school.[14] Without these provisions, children are at a further disadvantage.

Making the situation even worse, as reported by the news site The74Million in its series "COVID's K-Shaped Recession and the Looming Classroom Crisis," children in low-income families tended to remain in remote learning for much longer than those in more affluent areas.[15] According to one McKinsey study, in December 2020, schools with more than 50% Black students were 20 percentage points more likely to be in remote learning situations (69% of such schools were remote) than schools with 50% or more white students (49% of such schools).[16] While many districts took swift steps to ensure that students had access to computers and free internet, the reality remained that low-income students and students of color were less likely to have dedicated access to a computer or to a consistent internet connection – the minimal requirements for remote learning. As a result, on average, white students lost five to nine months of math learning, while students of color lost 12 to 16 months.[17–19] Over the course of the pandemic, many students of color disappeared from school altogether.[20]

A working paper from the Annenberg Institute for School Reform at Brown University documented the dismal result: Over the course of the pandemic's first two years, the performance gap between students at relatively high-poverty schools and those at relatively low-poverty schools grew by 15% in reading and 20% in math.[21] Data from the National Assessment of Educational Progress report covering reading and math assessments of nine-year-olds from 2020 to 2022 not only confirmed an increasing divergence between the top

READING

Percentile	2020 score	Change	2022 score
90th	267	↓ 2	265
75th	247	↓ 3	244
50th	224	↓ 4	219
25th	196	↓ 8	188
10th	164	↓ 10	155

MATHEMATICS

Percentile	2020 score	Change	2022 score
90th	286	↓ 3	283
75th	267	↓ 5	262
50th	245	↓ 8	238
25th	219	↓ 11	208
10th	191	↓ 12	178

Figure 13.2 National Assessment of Educational Progress report covering reading and math assessments of nine-year-olds from 2020 to 2022.

and bottom scores but showed that, overall, "Average scores for age-nine students in 2022 declined five points in reading and seven points in mathematics compared to 2020. This is the largest average score decline in reading since 1990, and the first ever score decline in mathematics."[22]

A Mental Health Pandemic

It should perhaps come as no surprise that the pandemic sparked or amplified serious mental health problems among people of all ages, including depression, anxiety, and post-traumatic stress. This distress led to a significant increase in deaths associated with alcohol, drugs, and suicide, which collectively took the lives of 186 763 US citizens in 2020. This represented a 20% one-year increase in the combined death rate and the highest number of substance-misuse deaths ever recorded for a single year, according to a report by Trust for America's Health and Well Being Trust.[23]

The loss of in-person school time, combined with other pandemic stressors, took a significant toll on children's mental health in particular. For nearly 150 000 children, those stressors included the death of a caregiver – a loss that was up to 4.5 times more likely to affect children of racial and ethnic minority groups, including indigenous people, than non-Hispanic white children.[4, 24] A 2021 *JAMA Pediatrics* meta-analysis of 29 studies, which together included 80 879 children and adolescents, found that the worldwide prevalence of depression and anxiety symptoms doubled over the course of the pandemic to that date.[25] That study and others have shown that girls, young people in the lesbian, gay, bisexual, transgender, and queer/questioning (LGBTQ) community, and children in racial and ethnic minority groups were the most likely to experience these issues.[26]

However, this challenge was not limited to any one group of young people. In a national study, 70% of public schools reported an increase in the percentage of their students seeking mental health services at school, and 76% reported an increase in staff voicing concerns about students exhibiting symptoms of depression, anxiety, and trauma.[27, 28] By late 2021, the situation had grown so dire that the American Academy of Pediatrics, the American Academy of Child and Adolescent Psychiatry, and the Children's Hospital Association together issued a joint declaration of a national emergency in child and adolescent mental health.[29]

Unfortunately, no demographic was spared the mental health impacts of the pandemic:

- Adults in households with job loss or lower incomes reported higher rates of symptoms of mental illness
- For people with chronic illness, the already high likelihood of having a concurrent mental health disorder was potentially exacerbated by their vulnerability to severe illness from COVID-19[30]
- A recent study also found that 18% of individuals who received a COVID-19 diagnosis were later diagnosed with a mental health disorder[31]
- Older adults were also more vulnerable to severe illness from COVID-19 and experienced increased levels of anxiety and depression during the pandemic[32]
- Women with children were more likely to report symptoms of anxiety and/or depressive disorder than men with children (49% versus 40%, respectively)
- Non-Hispanic Black adults and Hispanic or Latinx adults were more likely to report symptoms of anxiety and/or depressive disorder than non-Hispanic white adults

However, during this war against the virus, the toll may have been hardest on those who were on the front lines. For the fight against COVID-19, that meant health-care workers and public health workers. By May 2022, these groups had spent more than two years facing continuous crisis conditions, not to mention harassment (discussed later in "A Country Divided: Masks, Testing, and Vaccines"). At that point, the Surgeon General issued an Advisory – that is, a public statement "reserved for significant public health challenges that need the American people's immediate awareness" – on addressing health worker burnout.[33]

"Burnout" itself has a specific definition. As the Advisory explains, burnout is "an occupational syndrome characterized by a high degree of emotional exhaustion and depersonalization (i.e., cynicism), and a low sense of personal accomplishment at work." Health-care workers as a group had been experiencing burnout at high rates well before the pandemic began, due to a wide array of factors. COVID-19 made every one of those problems worse. As the Advisory explained, "Throughout the pandemic, health workers have reported high rates of stress, frustration, exhaustion, isolation, feeling undervalued, loss of sleep, anxiety, increased risk for substance use, and suicidal ideation."

Many of the causes behind these numbers were present before the pandemic – from structural racism and incredibly long working hours to mountains of paperwork and poorly coordinated care networks, and more. Other causes, such as overflowing hospitals and intensive care units and the devastating loss of patient after patient, bore the hallmark of an infectious disease out of control.

The Dangers of Misinformation

As the virus continued to spread and mutate, so too did misinformation about it. Unfortunately, COVID-19 misinformation is only the latest expression of new and enduring myths and conspiracies that are (re)framed to fit current contexts and that operate where psychological, social, economic, technological, and political dynamics interconnect. The political dynamics, in particular, resulted in a tide of cherry-picked data and sound bites that undermined health officials' warnings about the seriousness of this disease during the early months of the pandemic. Fueled by the current media ecosystem, which incentivizes the spread of misinformation, and further exacerbated by the viral effects of social media, medical misinformation is now pervasive, standing as one of the top threats to public health worldwide.

The internet has become a primary source for medical and health information during the digital age. With health misinformation existing alongside, overshadowing, or even discrediting factual sources across online platforms, internet users remain extremely vulnerable.

In clinical settings, providers have been forced to grapple with this challenge. Yet addressing misinformation in person with patients has been largely left out of medical education and training. To this end, Harvard Global Health Institute, the Technology and Social Change Project at the Harvard Shorenstein Center, First Draft, and others collaborated to create the MisinfoRx tool kit (https://misinforx.com/), which was designed for providers across the spectrum of care. Grounded in the science of misinformation, the tool kit provides strategies for addressing patient-held misinformation in clinical settings.[34]

A Country Divided: Masks, Testing, and Vaccines

Throughout the pandemic, and true to this current moment, positions for and against the virus mitigation measures of mask wearing, diagnostic testing, and vaccines bitterly divided families, communities, and the entire country. Positions on mask wearing cleaved along political lines from the very beginning. Research has shown that the most reliable indicator of when a mask mandate was issued in a state depended primarily on the political party of the state's governor: States with Republican governors issued mask mandates significantly later than other states.[35] At the county level, the likelihood of individuals wearing masks in public also tracked with their political affiliation.[36]

The debate was not merely contentious – it became outright violent at times. Irate citizens who felt that mask mandates infringed on their individual rights subjected public health workers and health-care providers to daily verbal abuse. School-board meetings across the country devolved into screaming matches, as anti-mask parents threatened school officials for following CDC guidelines regarding mask wearing in schools. In the end, what could have been an inexpensive, easy-to-use public health tool against all respiratory viruses was lost to partisanship.

While it was not the lightning rod that masking became, testing also became divisive. Early in the pandemic, the debate between those calling for ubiquitous testing and those saying we cannot or do not need to do it became a roadblock to widespread, urgent action.

And, of course, the final significant tool, and the one with initially the most potential to bring the virus to its knees, was vaccination. Unfortunately, vaccines also lost ground to misinformation and politicization. Exposure to online vaccine misinformation has been shown to reduce intent to receive a COVID-19 vaccine by up to 8.8%.[37] Anti-vaccine accounts across Facebook, Instagram, and Twitter held a following of 59.2 million users in December 2020, and their effects were marked: Exposure to the misinformation they purveyed was also shown to reduce the intent to receive a COVID-19 vaccine by up to 8.8%.[38] And politics took another bite: According to the KFF, by January 2022, political affiliation was responsible for a 13% difference in vaccination rates at the county level.[39]

As a significant number of US citizens became convinced that public health measures were putting their individual freedoms at risk, their willingness to follow public health officials' recommendations in general decreased. Officials instead became the target of vitriol. According to a Johns Hopkins Bloomberg School of Public Health study, 1 499 reports of harassment were filed by local health departments during the first 11 months of the pandemic. Of the departments surveyed, more than half (57%) had been harassed.[40]

By early 2022, a survey of nearly 45 000 state and local public health workers found that 20% described their mental health as either fair or poor; more than half reported symptoms of post-traumatic stress disorder.[41] Unsurprisingly, the Johns Hopkins Bloomberg School of Public Health study found that "across state and local health departments, 222 public health officials left their positions during [the pandemic's first 11 months]. Over one-third of those departures – 36 percent – involved officials who had experienced some form of harassment."[40]

Ongoing Impact of Disease: Long COVID

For most survivors, the direct health consequences of COVID-19 are relatively short-lived, typically lasting one to three weeks. It is now clear, however, that anywhere from 10% to more than 50% of people who recover from COVID-19 will suffer from post-acute sequelae of SARS-CoV-2 infection; in one 2023 study, 72% of participants were affected.[42, 43] Better known as long COVID, this syndrome is defined as COVID-19-related symptoms that may persist for four weeks or more after infection.[44] These symptoms may include physical and/or mental disabilities, such as "brain fog," a disorder of executive function.[45] While researchers debate the precise number of people suffering from long COVID, there is no argument about the two central issues: Long COVID is a real disease and no treatments for it have yet been proven to be effective.

Once again, social inequities are highly relevant here, as low-income and frontline workers do not have the privilege of working from home while they recover and gain strength. Many also do not have the privilege of receiving care at one of the few long COVID specialty centers in the USA.

The Silver Lining: Positive Consequences of the Pandemic

As evidenced by the statistics discussed in this chapter, the negative societal consequences of the COVID-19 pandemic have been overwhelming. However, during any world-changing event, no matter how traumatic, there are always bright spots.

First, for at least a little while, communities came together to help each other. Heartwarming stories abound and include neighbors helping neighbors, communities leaving meals at the doorsteps of those who could not or would not leave their homes, students celebrating their online teachers, and the public celebrating health-care professionals. It felt, during the first few months, like a worldwide shared adventure – probably because the average person did not understand how long the "adventure" was going to last.

However, some positive outcomes from the pandemic appear to be long-lasting, too. Physicians, nurses, and other health-care professionals have rallied to identify a standard of care for COVID-19 patients, sharing clinical protocols across countries and between nations. A new industry of research preprints has blossomed, allowing researchers and clinicians to read and act on data 3 to 12 months earlier than they would have been able to do if the articles had had to wait for peer review and formal publishing.

Innovation has flourished in the life sciences industry, with regard not only to vaccines but also to diagnostics, which showed impressive improvements in miniaturization and cost reduction. Polymerase chain reaction (PCR) testing, which had previously been limited to laboratory environments, can now be performed in the clinic or the home using a handheld instrument that costs less than $100. New molecular technologies such as loop-mediated isothermal amplification (LAMP) tests have also emerged as strong contributors to testing, even in the over-the-counter space.

Other unintended and positive consequences of the pandemic response include:

- the rise of remote work, especially in the knowledge economy
- an improved understanding of what works in remote education and what does not
- increased emphasis on at-home over-the-counter testing by the diagnostics industry and increased acceptance by the public
- a recognition of the broad utility of wastewater testing for disease surveillance
- the normalization of mask wearing in public when one is ill
- an increased focus on mental health, including the critical role that human interaction plays
- the realization that more viral diseases may have a "long tail" than was previously understood
- government and business willingness to increase funding for improved ventilation and air cleaning in buildings

What Might Have Helped?

So, could the negative societal repercussions of COVID-19 have been avoided or, at the very least, mitigated? Discussion about how our pandemic response could have been better (or worse) will last longer than the pandemic itself. While it is hard to identify a magic bullet that would have changed everything, there are two areas in which we as a nation clearly could have gotten things right even without the benefit of hindsight.

We Could Have Used What We Already Knew

Most fundamentally, preparedness plans either did not exist or were not used. Reportedly, the Trump Administration never acknowledged the Obama Administration's pandemic/epidemic plan.[46] In the private sector, while many companies had emergency preparedness plans, only 20% of them had any plans for a disease-based emergency, according to an Arizona State University survey of small and large businesses.[46]

Communication from those leading the nationwide pandemic response was poor or thwarted, with leaders either unwilling or unable to use known, effective strategies for communicating about the pandemic with the general public. Experts in science communication knew how to do this properly. In July 2020, the National Academies of Sciences, Engineering, and Medicine published a report that was essentially an instruction manual on the subject.[47] It detailed 10 key risk-communication strategies that public health decision-makers and communicators could have used:

1. Use clear, consistent, and transparent messaging
2. Avoid undue attention to the frequency of socially undesirable behaviors
3. Foster a sense of efficacy and avoid fatalism
4. Appeal to the collective good of one's community
5. Use messengers trusted by the target audience
6. Tailor the framing of the message to the audience
7. Link prevention behaviors to people's identities
8. Highlight social disapproval of a target audience member's failure to comply when it occurs
9. Highlight the growing prevalence of behavior change within the target audience when it occurs
10. Avoid repeating misinformation, even to debunk it

The report also detailed five key habit-promoting strategies for normalizing the use of protective measures and increasing the likelihood of behavior change:

1. Make the behavior easy to start and repeat
2. Make the behavior rewarding to repeat
3. Tie the behavior to an existing habit
4. Alert people to behaviors that conflict with existing habits and provide alternative behaviors
5. Provide specific descriptions of desired behaviors

The items on these lists were not guesses. They were evidence-based strategies that were known to work effectively. If properly employed, these methods would have helped the lay public understand the evolving health situation and encourage and normalize behaviors that would mitigate the spread of disease. These strategies might have also helped the nation to avoid one of its great pandemic failures: the widespread loss of trust in public health and medical experts – a trust that will take years to rebuild.

We Could Have Addressed Systemic Inequities in Our Response

The country's systemic inequities should have been accounted for at both the federal and the state levels as a central part of the pandemic response. That could have enabled both government and businesses to take proactive steps to avoid the consequences detailed in this chapter.

On a practical level, these steps could have included more programs to directly address the needs of low-income communities, as well as the needs of frontline workers who could not work from home. Such programs – funded by public health systems, private industry, or both – could have enabled frontline workers to test freely (especially early on, when testing was restricted). When workers tested positive, such programs could have provided housing in which to isolate these individuals and associated services to meet the needs of workers and their families during that time.

A major initiative to support both the quality of remote kindergarten to 12th grade education in underserved communities and the swift and safe return of those students and teachers to the in-person classroom might have mitigated the extensive learning loss that those communities suffered. The educational gaps that the pandemic exposed and exacerbated will impact society for too many years in the future. As we begin to look back at this pandemic, we need to look forward as well and plan to do better. We must rise above conscious and unconscious biases to save lives.

Lessons Learned

- Develop disease-based emergency plans and implement them at the start of a disease outbreak
- Implement clear, consistent, and frequent communication from those leading the nationwide/global pandemic effort
- Include more programs to directly address the needs of low-income communities, as well as the needs of frontline workers who cannot work from home
- Increase equitable access to full-time in-person learning by focusing on providing safety-optimized in-person learning options across grade levels
- Increase the emphasis on over-the-counter testing by the diagnostics industry and encourage increased acceptance by the public
- Increase government and business funding for improved ventilation and air cleaning in buildings

References

1. CDC, What is health equity? (2022). www.cdc.gov/healthequity/whatis/index.html (accessed January 30, 2023).

2. KFF, COVID-19 deaths by race/ethnicity (2022). https://tinyurl.com/bdh7mret (accessed January 30, 2023).

3. B. Dupré, C. S. Queen, S. Cahalan, et al., One million U.S. Covid deaths, *New York Times* (2022). https://tinyurl.com/35b4t22t (accessed January 30, 2023).

4. S. D. Hillis, A. Blenkinsop, A. Villaveces, et al., COVID-19–associated orphanhood and caregiver death in the United States. *Pediatrics*, **148**, 6 (2021), e2021053760.

5. E. B. Pathak, J. M. Menard, R. B. Garcia, and J. L. Salemi, Joint effects of socioeconomic position, race/ethnicity, and gender on COVID-19 mortality among working-age adults in the United States. *Int J Environ Res Public Health*, **19**, 9 (2022), 5479.

6. S. Artiga, R. Garfield, and K. Orgera, KFF: communities of color at higher risk for health and economic challenges due to COVID-19 (2020). https://tinyurl.com/2p8punv6 (accessed January 30, 2023).

7. C. K. Mills and J. Battisto, Double jeopardy: COVID-19's concentrated health and wealth effects in Black communities (2020). https://tinyurl.com/ycxp2m88 (accessed January 30, 2023).

8. A. Kirzinger, L. Hamel, G. Sparks, et al., KFF COVID-19 Vaccine Monitor: the pandemic's toll on workers and family finances during the omicron surge (2022). https://tinyurl.com/bdh8ks8u (accessed January 30, 2023).

9. L. Villarosa, Pollution is killing Black Americans. This community fought back, *New York Times* (2020). https://tinyurl.com/nnfdp7t6 (accessed January 30, 2023).

10. R. Kochhar, Hispanic women, immigrants, young adults, those with less education hit hardest by COVID-19 job losses,

Pew Research Center (2020). https://tinyurl.com/mv2fx5cz (accessed January 30, 2023).

11. R. Fry, Some gender disparities widened in the U.S. workforce during the pandemic, Pew Research Center (2022). https://tinyurl.com/4u824z5p (accessed January 30, 2023).

12. Urban Institute, Health Reform Monitoring Survey. https://tinyurl.com/ycx7upyv (accessed January 30, 2023).

13. M. Devitt, COVID-19 continues to cause some people to put off care, AAFP (2021). https://tinyurl.com/3e8yrew7 (accessed January 30, 2023).

14. UC Davis Health, Good food is good medicine. Are school lunches really important for your kid's health? (2019). https://tinyurl.com/mr223d5b (accessed January 30, 2023).

15. B. Hawkins, The 74. The fallout from the pandemic's K-shaped recession may be felt by students for years. How can schools head off this COVID classroom crisis? (2021). https://tinyurl.com/2p9bw3tx (accessed January 30, 2023).

16. E. Dorn, B. Hancock, J. Sarakatsannis, and E. Viruleg, COVID-19 and learning loss—disparities grow and students need help (2020). https://tinyurl.com/9ztjkxab (accessed January 30, 2023).

17. US Department of Education, Office for Civil Rights (OCR), Education in a pandemic: the disparate impacts of COVID-19 on America's students (2021). https://tinyurl.com/ycx8xrpk (accessed January 30, 2023).

18. F. Mitchell, COVID-19's disproportionate effects on children of color will challenge the next generation (2020). https://tinyurl.com/24byc5e2 (accessed January 30, 2023).

19. E. Oster, R. Jack, C. Halloran, et al., CDC: disparities in learning mode access among K–12 students during the COVID-19 pandemic, by race/ethnicity, geography, and grade level – United States, September 2020–April 2021. *MMWR Morb Mortal Wkly Rep*, **70**, 26 (2021), 953–958.

20. H. T. N. Korman, B. O'Keefe, and M. Repka, Missing in the margins 2020: estimating the scale of the COVID-19 attendance crisis (2020). https://tinyurl.com/yc86suzb (accessed January 30, 2023).

21. M. Kuhfeld, J. Soland, and K. Lewis. Test score patterns across three COVID-19-impacted school years (2022). www.edworkingpapers.com/ai22-521 (accessed January 30, 2023).

22. The Nations Report Card, Reading and mathematics scores decline during COVID-19 pandemic (2022). www.nationsreportcard.gov/highlights/ltt/2022/ (accessed January 30, 2023).

23. Trust for America's Health (TFAH), Well Being Trust (WBT), U.S. experienced highest ever combined rates of deaths due to alcohol, drugs, and suicide during the COVID-19 pandemic (2022). https://tinyurl.com/4n9zwc33 (accessed January 30, 2023).

24. A. Berman, Indigenous Alaskans died from COVID-19 at nearly three times the rate of white Alaskans, CDC report says, *Anchorage Daily News* (2022). https://tinyurl.com/zz35rxd3 (accessed January 30, 2023).

25. N. Racine, B. A. McArthur, J. E. Cooke, et al., Global prevalence of depressive and anxiety symptoms in children and adolescents during COVID-19: a meta-analysis. *JAMA Pediatr*, **175**, 11 (2021), 1142.

26. A. Paley. National Survey on LGBTQ Youth Mental Health 2021 (2021). www.thetrevorproject.org/survey-2021/?section=Introduction (accessed January 30, 2023).

27. T. Benton, W. F. M. Njoroge, and W. Y. K. Ng, Sounding the alarm for children's mental health during the COVID-19 pandemic. *JAMA Pediatr*, **176**, 4 (2022), e216295.

28. J. Washington, Stress up at school for students and teachers amid lasting pandemic, in Cleveland area and nationally (2022). https://tinyurl.com/5dyvjb72 (accessed January 30, 2023).

29. American Academy of Pediatrics, AAP-AACAP-CHA declaration of a national

emergency in child and adolescent mental health (2021). https://tinyurl.com/3y674fzx (accessed January 30, 2023).

30. B. G. Druss and E. R. Walker, Mental disorders and medical comorbidity. *Synth Proj Res Synth Rep*, 21 (2011), 1–26.

31. M. Taquet, S. Luciano, J. R. Geddes, and P. J. Harrison, Bidirectional associations between COVID-19 and psychiatric disorder: retrospective cohort studies of 62 354 COVID-19 cases in the USA. *Lancet Psychiatry*, **8**, 2 (2021), 130–140.

32. W. Koma, S. True, J. F. Biniek, et al., One in four older adults report anxiety or depression amid the COVID-19 pandemic (2020). https://tinyurl.com/4tp2thnm (accessed January 30, 2023).

33. V. H. Murthy, Addressing health worker burnout: the U.S. Surgeon General's Advisory on building a thriving health workforce (2022). https://tinyurl.com/mrw5a7e3 (accessed January 30, 2023).

34. A. Shajahan, I. Pasquetto, D. Winner, and L. Testa, The MisinfoRx gives health care providers the knowledge and training to tackle patient-held medical misinformation. https://misinforx.com/ (accessed January 30, 2023).

35. C. Adolph, K. Amano, B. Bang-Jensen, et al., Governor partisanship explains the adoption of statewide mask mandates in response to COVID-19. *State Polit Policy Q*, **22**, 1 (2022), 24–49.

36. L. H. Kahane, Politicizing the mask: political, economic and demographic factors affecting mask wearing behavior in the USA. *East Econ J*, **47**, 2 (2021), 163–183.

37. S. Loomba, A. de Figueiredo, S. J. Piatek, et al., Measuring the impact of COVID-19 vaccine misinformation on vaccination intent in the UK and USA. *Nat Hum Behav*, **5**, 3 (2021), 337–348.

38. Center for Countering Digital Hate (CCDH), The disinformation dozen (2021). https://counterhate.com/research/the-disinformation-dozen/ (accessed January 30, 2023).

39. KFF, KFF COVID-19 Vaccine Monitor. https://tinyurl.com/y2ydad84 (accessed January 30, 2023).

40. M. R. Fraser, Harassment of health officials: a significant threat to the public's health. *Am J Public Health*, **112**, 5 (2022), 728–730.

41. Public Health Workforce Interests and Needs Survey (PHWINS), The public health workforce in the COVID 19 era: younger, more diverse, with high levels of stress and intent to leave (2021). https://debeaumont.org/phwins/2021-findings/ (accessed January 30, 2023).

42. https://academic.oup.com/ofid/article/10/7/ofad233/7150886.

43. https://www.nature.com/articles/s41598-023-36995-4.

44. CDC, Long COVID or post-COVID conditions (2022). www.cdc.gov/coronavirus/2019-ncov/long-term-effects/ (accessed January 30, 2023).

45. E. Yong, One of long COVID's worst symptoms is also its most misunderstood, *The Atlantic* (2022). https://tinyurl.com/4fp67946 (accessed January 30, 2023).

46. ASU News, ASU releases first comprehensive survey on how companies are protecting their employees from COVID-19 (2020). https://tinyurl.com/mret76bf (accessed January 30, 2023).

47. D. Brossard, W. Wood, R. Cialdini, and R. M. Groves, Encouraging adoption of protective behaviors to mitigate the spread of COVID-19: strategies for behavior change (2020). www.nap.edu/catalog/25881 (accessed January 30, 2023).

Summary and Path Forward for Future Pandemics

Wade E. Bolton and Steven C. Schachter

Introduction

Facing emergencies always requires fast recognition of immediate crisis issues and prompt implementation of corrective actions. When the COVID-19 pandemic ensued and began to overwhelm our health-care systems, we found ourselves in a profound and far-reaching crisis that needed immediate attention.

The nation was ill-prepared and bereft of most means to diagnose the disease, leaving physicians and caregivers few tools to provide the medical direction for their patients that was desperately needed. Once the unknown disease was characterized and the virus was identified, the next most important step was to secure an accurate diagnostic test(s). Addressing this purpose, Rapid Acceleration of Diagnostics (RADx®) was created (as addressed in Chapter 4) to bring robust COVID-19 tests authorized by the US Food and Drug Administration (FDA) to the market as quickly as possible in sufficient quantities to address the national needs. RADx was established with the collaborative interaction of many experts, many of whom contributed to this book.

As our nation had experienced pandemics prior to COVID-19, RADx leadership began to search for guiding documents that would help define our path forward and provide us with a template that would quicken the pace of our response and provide documented and qualified processes. We hoped to benefit from lessons previously learned and take a previously well-validated "roadmap" and diligently march forward. It came to our profound surprise that there was no guiding document. There were no lessons learned. There were no roadmaps.

What we did have was years of experience in diagnostic assay development, product development, and management. With these tools and a group of scientists, engineers, product and marketing professionals, manufacturing experts, and many more, we tirelessly took charge and marched forward, developing the plans, processes, and tools in real-time with a sense of urgency. As we began to interact with other colleagues associated with therapeutics, prophylaxis, and other disciplines associated with our efforts, we found that many of them were experiencing the same conundrum: an urgent and profound task with few if any guiding documents.

More than three years after the emergence of severe acute respiratory syndrome coronavirus 2 (SARS-CoV-2), despite many challenges, we managed to achieve some great accomplishments, many of which are detailed in this book. However, during this time, we also identified alternative pathways and processes after experiencing some setbacks. The authors in this book, from different disciplines associated with the pandemic process, felt we needed to pass on the lessons we have learned and put together a more comprehensive roadmap that can be built upon in response to the next pandemic that emerges. Our

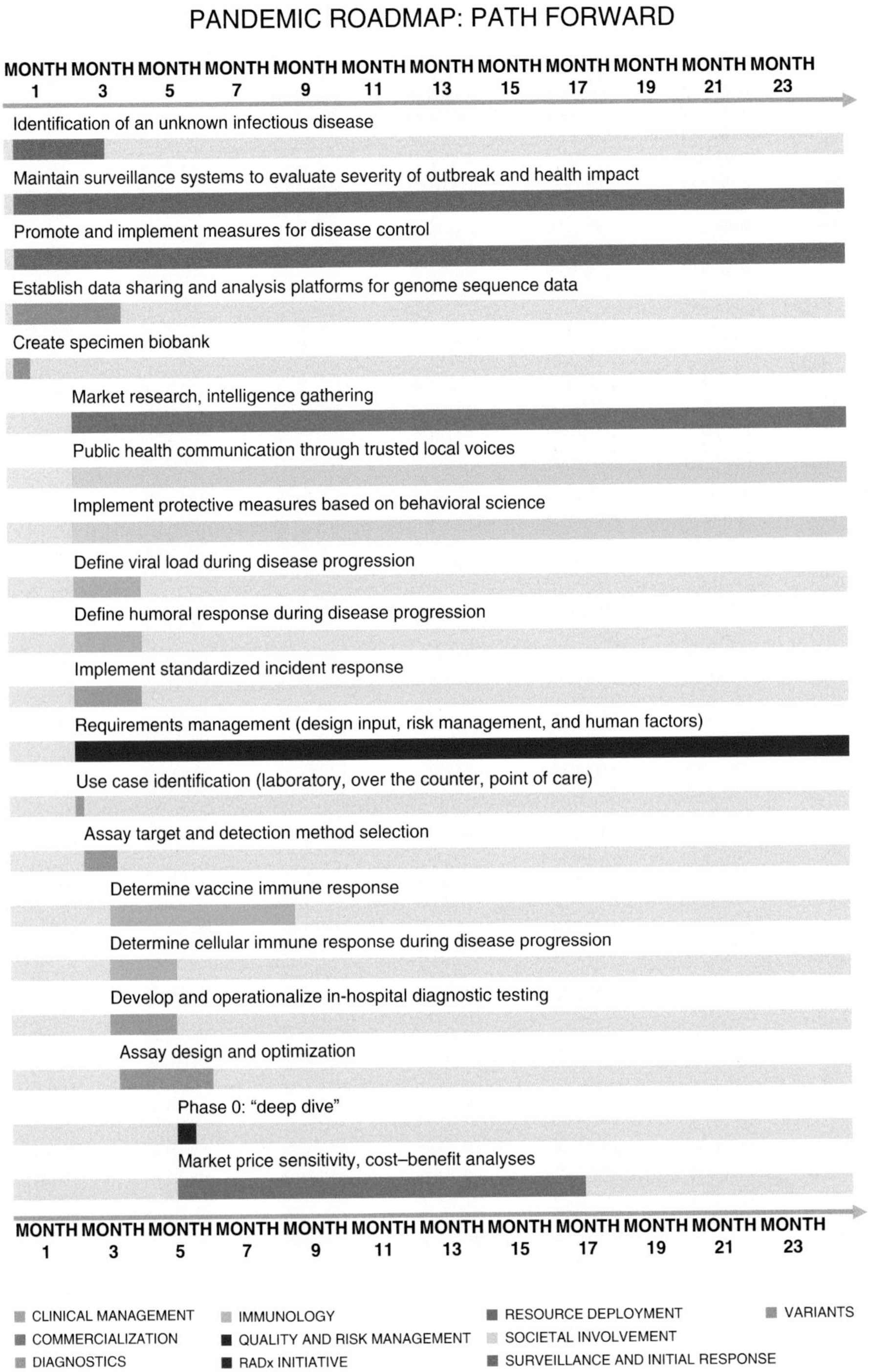

PANDEMIC ROADMAP: PATH FORWARD

MONTH MONTH MONTH MONTH MONTH MONTH MONTH MONTH MONTH MONTH MONTH MONTH
1   3   5   7   9   11   13   15   17   19   21   23

Identification of an unknown infectious disease

Maintain surveillance systems to evaluate severity of outbreak and health impact

Promote and implement measures for disease control

Establish data sharing and analysis platforms for genome sequence data

Create specimen biobank

Market research, intelligence gathering

Public health communication through trusted local voices

Implement protective measures based on behavioral science

Define viral load during disease progression

Define humoral response during disease progression

Implement standardized incident response

Requirements management (design input, risk management, and human factors)

Use case identification (laboratory, over the counter, point of care)

Assay target and detection method selection

Determine vaccine immune response

Determine cellular immune response during disease progression

Develop and operationalize in-hospital diagnostic testing

Assay design and optimization

Phase 0: "deep dive"

Market price sensitivity, cost–benefit analyses

MONTH MONTH MONTH MONTH MONTH MONTH MONTH MONTH MONTH MONTH MONTH MONTH
1   3   5   7   9   11   13   15   17   19   21   23

- CLINICAL MANAGEMENT
- COMMERCIALIZATION
- DIAGNOSTICS
- IMMUNOLOGY
- QUALITY AND RISK MANAGEMENT
- RADx INITIATIVE
- RESOURCE DEPLOYMENT
- SOCIETAL INVOLVEMENT
- SURVEILLANCE AND INITIAL RESPONSE
- VARIANTS

Figure 14.1 Important activities from each chapter compiled in chronological order. In the case of the SARS-CoV-2 pandemic, month 1 was December 2019, the month in which the virus was isolated, sequenced, identified, and published.

EUA, Emergency Use Authorization.

PANDEMIC ROADMAP: PATH FORWARD (CONT.)

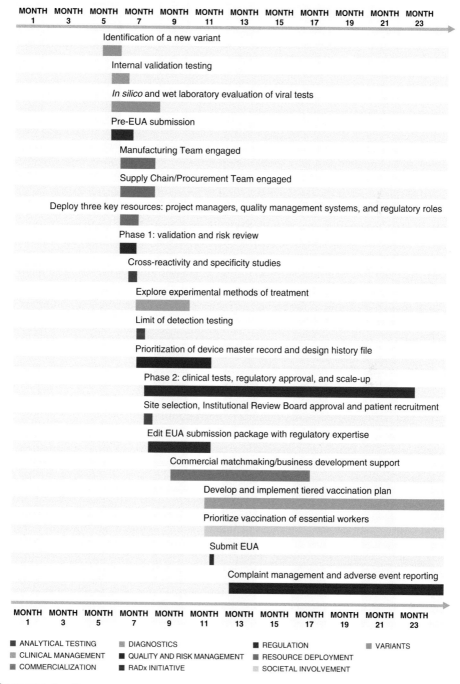

Figure 14.1 (cont.)

colleagues in the future will then have a suggested list of things to consider and things to avoid, plus a general path to follow that can be modified depending on the characteristics of the pathogen in question.

In this chapter, we will compile a comprehensive, chronological roadmap, summarize the lessons learned from individuals who were on the front line to battle COVID-19, and make recommendations on how to manage these efforts in an organized and timely manner.

Pandemic Roadmap Highlights

The professionals who are brought to the forefront in emergencies are often trained and experienced to a depth that enables them to address the challenge in front of them with the tools of their discipline(s). The problem is that many disciplines must be engaged promptly and must come together in a fully orchestrated manner. Handoffs from one discipline to another are often necessary as a pandemic emerges and begins to spread (many of which are discussed in this book). If the timing of the handoff is wrong, there can be significant delays as one discipline catches up to the other. It is much like a relay race, where the next runner must be in place to accept the baton from the previous runner. We have all seen cases of the timing in a relay race being off and indeed, in some cases, the baton is dropped and the team fails. In our case, lost time in scientific and informational handoffs could mean lost lives. That is unacceptable. The contributors to this book and our numerous colleagues felt it was our obligation to assemble a comprehensive roadmap that could be used as a guidance document to identify some of the pivotal activities necessary in a pandemic situation and how they relate to other disciplines.

In Figure 14.1, we have compiled the very high-level activities from the roadmaps in each chapter and have indicated when the associated activities began and their approximate length of time. This allows readers to see the time course of the assigned activities and their temporal interrelationships. The figure represents a simplification of an incredibly complex network of issues and processes in the COVID-19 pandemic, each stage of which required discovery and timing coordination. This is a representation of what we did in real time, and the activities outlined in this roadmap allowed the nation to respond in a historic manner. The result was FDA Emergency Use Authorization (EUAs) for multiple submissions and the introduction of billions of COVID-19 tests (laboratory-based, point-of-care [POC], and over-the-counter [OTC] tests) as illustrated in Figure 14.2.

As a new virus emerges, the first battlegrounds are in clinics and hospitals. Medical professionals begin surveillance and the initial clinical response, including identifying patients, undertaking contact tracing, and implementing containment measures such as personal protective equipment (PPE) and isolation practices. Early clinical intervention is based primarily on treating symptoms. These treatments evolve based on clinical results and scientific data as they become available. After identifying and sequencing the virus, medical staff can refine their treatment approaches to the specific virus with molecularly designed therapeutics.

The next area of focus is immunology. The goal is to investigate and understand the body's response to the new virus, especially the immune response. For example, how does the immune system respond to the virus? What are the limitations in the response and how can we correct them? Finally, how do we use the characterized immune response to better develop a vaccine or antibody-based therapies?

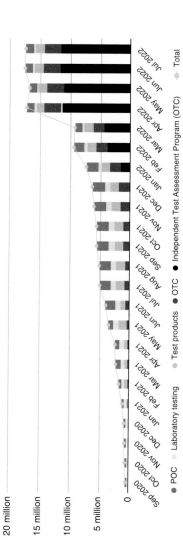

Figure 14.2 The number of tests produced per day. This represents items that were manufactured, including laboratory-based technologies, POC and home tests, and laboratory products. Descriptions of these technologies can be found on the RADx Tech/ATP Phase 2 awards page.[1]

Next, there is a parallel wave of areas of focus and activities to develop diagnostic tests, vaccines, and therapeutics. And, as strides begin to be made in the development of diagnostics (as well as vaccines and therapeutics), the societal impact of the tests needs to be considered in terms of distributing tests efficiently and equitably with minimal disruption to society.

Comprehensive Pandemic Response Roadmap

As indicated in its title, the main objective of this book is to provide a well-validated roadmap for our future colleagues when a new pandemic emerges. Certainly, it is impossible to capture everything in this book that needs to be executed when new pandemics occur, but we can provide guidance on expectations and timelines for the implementation of pandemic control and containment. To accomplish this task, we thought it best to capture as many components as possible and compile them in one place: the Pandemic Response Roadmap is available digitally at www.pandemicresponseroadmap.org. While we want to be clear to the reader that not all issues and items are considered, the path forward is written through the lens of a comprehensive response driven by diagnostic and screening tests with FDA EUAs designed for laboratory platforms, POC settings, and the home distributed OTC.

Lessons Learned

One may assume that the most valuable aspect of our efforts was to make suggestions to companies on what to do in a particular situation, and this was true in many cases, but we found that the most valuable advice for our companies was telling them what *not* to do. You see, individually, as we gain experience over years in our selected professions, we inevitably make mistakes, and these are valuable lessons. Mistakes can cause undue delays and significant cost increases and, if bad enough, can completely derail a project. However, when responding to a pandemic, any time delay translates to disease spread, increases in morbidity, and potentially preventable death – the stakes could not be higher. Therefore, we were in constant surveillance mode in these projects to identify potential pitfalls/mistakes before their occurrence so that the mistake could be avoided or mitigated, as otherwise the projects could be significantly delayed.

In every chapter of the book, our colleagues have identified those "aha" moments, that is, moments when we realized that the approach that we took was suboptimal. We like to call these lessons learned, and we want to be sure that, in the next pandemic, these will be considered prior to implementing a response. The lessons learned are discussed in context in their respective chapters, so we will not repeat all of them here. However, we felt it was important to capture those that were or could be particularly onerous, and these can be seen in Table 14.1.

Summary

The COVID-19 pandemic provided us the opportunity as a nation and as a global team to use all of the resources we had at our disposal to respond in a timely manner and with concerted effort. There were heroic efforts made by individuals who dedicated themselves unselfishly to this cause and worked untold hours. In these efforts, we had to be laser-focused. We could not allow ourselves to say, "we can't do this"; instead, we had to say, "this is how we can do this." We could not let ourselves be unraveled by an atmosphere of political

Table 14.1 Compilation of high-level lessons learned

Chapter area	Lessons learned
Surveillance and initial response (Chapter 1)	Recognize early any infectious ailments with unique clinical manifestations different from known diseases
	Immediately report all suspicious or confirmed infectious diseases to health authorities and international health forums
	Develop surveillance programs in different areas related to patient care, disease spread, control countermeasures, diagnostics, therapies, and vaccination programs. Secure appropriate data analysis, integration, interpretation, and broad distribution as required
	Develop robust programs of pandemic control in coordination with national and international health organizations (World Health Organization, US Centers for Disease Control and Prevention, Chinese Center for Disease Control and Prevention, UK National Health Service, and country health ministries)
Immunology (Chapter 2)	Determine and publish viral sequences as rapidly as possible such that diagnostic, therapeutic, and prophylactic targets can be proposed as early as possible
	Map viral load and antibody production of patients throughout the disease lifetime to assist as a tool to determine therapeutic efficacy
	If asymptomatic individuals are identified, determine viral load and viral transmissibility potential
	Identify multiple viral targets for diagnostic, therapeutic, and prophylactic development to ensure coverage if variants emerge
Clinical management (Chapter 3)	Streamline information using a standardizing incident response system to ensure that all resources are allocated to the site that is in the most need
	Explore experimental methods of treatment to provide all efforts of treatment for patients. While some experimental methods may fail, others may be successful, such as delayed intubation and the use of steroids
	Develop a geographic-based model and safe storage for reuse of PPE. This will extend supplies until replenishment
	Distribute vaccines through a tiered system, prioritizing distribution to essential health-care workers. For example, include staff in emergency departments and critical care units in the first tiers, shortly followed by immunocompromised patients and patients with multiple comorbidities

Table 14.1 (cont.)

Chapter area	Lessons learned
RADx process (Chapter 4)	Accelerate and expand the RADx Tech process to ensure the timely development and distribution of diagnostic tests
	Accelerate the development and distribution of POC and home-based diagnostic tests
	Expand engagement with public health authorities to enhance the public's acceptance of self-testing and reporting test results
	Collaborate with governmental authorities to inform national policies
Resource deployment (Chapter 5)	Establish a process to fuel consistency across a vast variety of RADx projects and reduce variability in failure
	Find alternatives to items with long lead times coming from offshore suppliers, as expediting such products is more difficult than dealing with US suppliers
	Implement accessibility efforts early on in test development to improve the level of access across the entire population. Intercepting a test in the middle of development poses challenges that could have been mitigated earlier in the development process
	Introduce resources gradually when supporting companies that are developing diagnostics. Assigning multiple resources to a small company could easily overwhelm it by doubling the company's size overnight
Quality and risk management (Chapter 6)	Implement a digital document repository/electronic quality management system (QMS) quickly to give all team members access to documentation and create a single source of information, even when team members cannot meet physically
	Re-prioritize QMS processes from what is typically done to first quickly establish the specifications for how to make the device and scale up manufacturing; the remainder of the QMS documents should be completed later, after EUA submission
	To ensure trust in the data generated from prototypes, create lightweight equipment and materials management processes and implement laboratory practices/training
	Utilize risk management tactically to find and mitigate risks early
Diagnostic assay development (Chapter 7)	Encourage developers to pivot toward lyophilized reagents, as many POC Clinical Laboratory Improvement

Table 14.1 (cont.)

Chapter area	Lessons learned
	Amendments (CLIA)-waived or OTC settings do not have the necessary equipment for cold chain reagents
	Include a sample inactivation buffer (eliminating the need for biohazard disposal). CLIA-waived POC tests, require biosafety and proper disposal
	Ensure CLIA-waived tests have fewer than three steps, as the complexity of a workflow can make the usefulness of a test obsolete in a POC or OTC setting
	Consider test design carefully, as complicated designs with high manufacturing costs, complex assembly, and many components can lead to a cost of goods that makes the test unattractive for POC or OTC settings
Verification and validation (Chapter 8)	Put a plan in place to sequence a higher percentage of positive samples from the beginning of the next pandemic and simultaneously study viral evolution
	Preserve the capacity to culture virus from remnant clinical samples, as we did in this pandemic
	Be aware of temperature extremes at outdoor mobile sites. Refrigeration is needed for all sample types and some devices may require ambient temperatures
Variants (Chapter 9)	Ensure data sharing and open sequence sharing for coordinated global monitoring of variants
	Vary target selection for both vaccines and diagnostics; do not concentrate efforts on a single portion of the genome
	Ensure a robust bioinformatics platform, such as the ROSALIND Diagnostic Monitoring system, is put in place, as this is fundamental to speeding up the selection of suitable variant samples for testing and assessing the risk of decreased test sensitivity with new variants
	Have a large, reliable number of samples from a large geographic area; this enabled the RADx Variant Task Force to identify, order, and test rare variants before they became prevalent in the population
Regulatory aspects (Chapter 10)	Consider that EUAs typically require smaller amounts of data than full authorizations, and some requirements may be addressed in ongoing studies as post-market commitments as part of the conditions of authorization
	Ensure fluid communication with health authorities to aid in the determination of appropriate use cases and use settings for proposed testing technologies. Direct and frequent communication between RADx and the FDA

Table 14.1 (cont.)

Chapter area	Lessons learned
	allowed for efficient information sharing as the virus evolved and pandemic needs shifted
	Develop tests earlier for the POC and OTC markets – this pandemic enabled widespread POC and home self-testing, something that previously had not been achieved. The RADx initiative created important right of references for test developers, including bridging the gap for pediatric self-swabbing and determining the effective testing frequency for serial home testing
	Consider developing a multiplex test quickly after the introduction of a singleplex test for new respiratory infections. In the wake of the COVID-19 pandemic, there is a strong continued desire to have multiplex tests for respiratory illness (COVID-19, influenza A, influenza B, respiratory syncytial virus, etc.) for differentiating respiratory illnesses in both POC and home settings
Commercialization and market assessment (Chapter 11)	Conduct quantitative and qualitative market research analyses through surveys of a wide range of sectors that can be shared with diagnostic developers
	Create pandemic-related policy and regulatory frameworks that address CLIA-waiver protocols for mass testing in non-CLIA-waived health-care settings (pharmacies, residential care facilities) and/or non-clinical settings (home, workplace, school, public spaces)
	Establish communication channels between clinical and commercial teams to provide real-world experiences and market feedback
	Recreate federal purchasing and distribution programs that increase access to no-cost testing by expanding US Postal Service programs to FedEx, UPS, Amazon, etc., and by streamlining pharmacy/retailer distribution without having to bill insurance
Testing strategy (Chapter 12)	Ensure widespread and frequent testing, which will help investigators to characterize the prevalence, spread, and contagiousness of the virus and its variants. Widespread testing can also be useful in predicting peaks in contagion and anticipating where the next hotspots may emerge
	Conduct screening (asymptomatic testing) for diseases in which a significant number of infected individuals are asymptomatic to identify and isolate infected but asymptomatic people who could spread the disease

Table 14.1 (cont.)

Chapter area	Lessons learned
	Implement complementary mitigations (such as mask wearing, isolation and quarantining, and vaccination) and ensure their and effectiveness, as this can significantly impact testing requirements to control the spread of the virus
	Spread out the infections over time by using mitigations such as testing, which can prevent the health-care system from being overburdened and buy time for the development of vaccines. This can also mean that the number of workers in a line of work that are out sick at any given time is less, allowing essential services and business operations to continue
Societal impact (Chapter 13)	Develop disease-based emergency plans and implement them at the start of a disease outbreak
	Ensure clear, consistent, and frequent communication from those leading the nationwide/global pandemic effort
	Consider an initiative to support the quality of remote kindergarten to 12th grade education, particularly in underserved communities
	Include more programs to directly address the needs of low-income communities, as well as the needs of frontline workers who cannot work from home

turpitude and sometimes personal or corporate confrontations. We also had to be available whenever needed. Most companies and individuals were not attuned to this level of demand, but they became quickly aligned. In one of our early RADx faculty meetings, a team lead relayed a question asked by one of our participating RADx companies about the RADx expectations of company work hours. One of the RADx executives responded: "If necessary, we will work and be available 24/7, including holidays, since SARS-CoV-2 doesn't take any days off and nor should we!" With this level of dedication, collegiality, and spirit, the race to make SARS-CoV-2 testing available throughout our nation began. Our collective hope is that the information documented in this book, especially the lessons learned and the pandemic response roadmap, will be of value for global response teams during future pandemics.

References

1. National Institute of Biomedical Imaging and Bioengineering (NIBIB), Authorized tests for COVID-19 and multiplex diagnostics. www.nibib.nih.gov/covid-19/radx-tech-program/authorized-tests (accessed July 12, 2023).

Index

Printed in the United States
by Baker & Taylor Publisher Services